MICROSPHERES AND DRUG THERAPY

PHARMACEUTICAL, IMMUNOLOGICAL AND MEDICAL ASPECTS

Microspheres and Drug Therapy

Pharmaceutical, Immunological and Medical Aspects

Editors

Stanley S. Davis
Lord Trent Professor of Pharmacy, Department of Pharmacy,
University of Nottingham, University Park, Nottingham, U.K.

Lisbeth Illum
Senior Lecturer, Royal Danish School of Pharmacy,
Universiteitsparken 2, Copenhagen, Denmark

J. Gordon McVie
Head of Clinical Research, Netherlands Cancer Institute,
Plesmanlaan 121, Amsterdam, The Netherlands

Eric Tomlinson
Professor of Pharmacy, Department of Pharmacy, University of
Amsterdam, Plantage Muidergracht 24, Amsterdam, The Netherlands

1984
Elsevier
Amsterdam · New York · Oxford

ISBN 0–444–80577–X

Published by:
Elsevier Science Publishers B.V.
PO Box 211
1000 AE Amsterdam
The Netherlands

Sole distributors for the USA and Canada:
Elsevier Science Publishing Company, Inc.
52 Vanderbilt Avenue
New York, NY 10017
USA

Library of Congress Cataloging in Publication Data
Main entry under title:

Microspheres and drug therapy.

Papers presented at a meeting held in Amsterdam in 1983.
1. Microspheres (Pharmacy)--Congresses. Chemother-apy--Congresses. I. Davis, Stanley S. [DNLM: 1. Drug Therapy--methods--congresses. 2. Microspheres--congresses. 3. Vehicles--congresses.   WB 330 M626 1983]
RS201.M53M53   1984   615'.1   84-10159
ISBN 0-444-80577-X

PRINTED IN THE NETHERLANDS

Foreword

Microspheres are small solid particles that range in size from a few tenths of a μm up to several hundred μm in diameter. They may be prepared in different ways, including various polymerization processes and encapsulation. Microspheres have various applications in biology and medicine as they are of growing importance as carriers for drugs, for cell sorting, and as membrane probes.

An essential requirement of modern drug therapy is the controlled delivery of the pharmacological agent to its site(s) of action in the body in the correct concentration-time profile. The combination of drugs and microspheres allows the possibility of more selective administration. Similarly, the combination of antibodies and/or magnetic particles with microspheres can be applied to both in vivo targeting and the sorting of cells in vitro.

The preparation and evaluation of microsphere systems is multifaceted and requires a significant input from the various scientific disciplines. This book brings together authors from the fields of cell biology, immunology, pathology, physiology, biochemistry, pharmacy, physical chemistry, materials science, medicine, surgery and radiology, in order to provide a comprehensive review of the current and future developments in this field. It has been produced following a meeting of a group of expert participants in Amsterdam in the autumn of 1983.

The multidisciplinary nature of the subject has resulted in the book being divided into four sections. The first section deals with the biological target, and the interaction of microspheres with it. Section 2 examines the pharmaceutical aspects of microspheres, including their preparation and characterization, and also considers the use of microsphere-drug conjugates as probes of drug (membrane) action. The following sections describe the in vivo and in vitro targeting of microspheres. Thus, section 3 discusses passive targeting with microspheres, and covers occlusion techniques, cellular uptake and local use of microspheres, containing drugs. Section 4 deals with active targeting, and specifically the use of antibodies and magnetic particles as homing devices for both in vivo targeting and in vitro cell recognition.

The challenge of advanced drug delivery research and development is that they are multidisciplinary in nature. We hope that the design and content of this book helps meet that challenge and stimulates others to respond to it in a similar manner.

S.S.D., L.I., J.G.M., E.T.
December, 1983

Sponsorship

The Editors are most grateful to **Pharmacia Infusion AB (Sweden),** who largely sponsored the production of this book. In addition, we are most pleased to be able to acknowledge the support of the following pharmaceutical companies, who helped to sponsor the Meeting in Amsterdam:

Abbott (U.S.A.)
Beechams (U.K.)
The Boots Company (U.K.)
Ciba-Geigy (U.K.)
Ciba-Geigy (Switzerland)
Dumex (Denmark)
Eli Lilly (The Netherlands)
Fisons (U.K.)
Fujisawa (Japan)
Glaxo (U.K.)
Hoechst (U.K.)
ICI (U.K.)
Lederle (Cyanamid Benelux) (Belgium)
Lundbeck (Denmark)
May & Baker (U.K.)
Merck, Sharp & Dohme (U.S.A.)
Merck, Sharp & Dohme (U.K.)
Novo (Denmark)
Organon (The Netherlands)
Pfizer (Central Research) (U.K.)
Rhône-Poulenc Santé (France)
Searle (U.S.A.)
Smith Kline & French Laboratories (U.S.A.)
E.R. Squibb and Sons (U.K.)
UpJohn (The Netherlands)
Warner-Lambert (U.S.A.)
Wellcome (U.K.)

Contents

Section 1: Biological and biophysical factors

Section 2: Pharmaceutical and pharmacodynamic aspects

Section 3: Passive targeting — Occlusion, cellular uptake and local injection

Section 4: Active targeting in vivo and in vitro — Homing with antibodies and magnetic particles

xii

Contributors

W. Ansorge, European Molecular Biology Laboratory, Postfach 10.2209, D-6900 Heidelberg, F.R.G.

J.M. Bartlett, School of Veterinary Medicine, Purdue University, West Lafayette, IN 47907, U.S.A.

M. Beal, School of Pharmacy and Pharmacology, University of Bath, Claverton Down, Bath, Avon BA2 7AY, U.K.

S. Benita, Laboratoire de Pharmacie Galénique, Faculté de Pharmacie de l'Université Paris-Sud, Rue J.B. Clement, 92290 Chatenay-Malabry, France.

J.-P. Benoît, Laboratoire de Pharmacie Galénique, Faculté de Pharmacie de l'Université Paris-Sud, Rue J.B. Clement, 92290 Chatenay-Malabry, France.

L. Bergqvist, Department of Radiation Physics, University of Lund, Lasarettet, S-221 85 Lund, Sweden.

M.-C. Bissery, Michigan Cancer Foundation, 110 East Warren Avenue, Detroit, MI 48201, U.S.A.

W.E. Blevins, School of Veterinary Medicine, Purdue University, West Lafayette, IN 47907, U.S.A.

J.W.B. Bradfield, Department of Pathology, University of Bristol, Medical School, University Walk, Bristol BS8 1TD, U.K.

G. Bruno, MEDEA Research, Via Piscane 34/a, 20129 Milan, Italy.

J.J. Burger, Department of Pharmacy, University of Amsterdam, Plantage Muidergracht 24, Amsterdam, The Netherlands.

I. Caruso, Osspedale L. Sacco, Milan, Italy.

M. Chang, Jet Propulsion Laboratory, California Institute of Technology, 4800 Oak Grove Drive, Pasadena, CA 91109, U.S.A.

P. Charles, Department of Nuclear Medicine, Municipal Hospital, DK-8000 Århus, Denmark.

P. Couvreur, Laboratoire de Pharmacie Galénique, Université Catholique de Louvain, 73 Avenue Emmanuel Mounier, B-1200 Brussels, Belgium.

J. Cummings, Department of Oncology, University of Glasgow, 1 Horselethill Road, Glasgow, U.K.

D.J.G. Davies, School of Pharmacy and Pharmacology, University of Bath, Claverton Down, Bath, Avon BA2 7AY, U.K.

S.S. Davis, Department of Pharmacy, University of Nottingham, Nottingham NG7 2UH, U.K.

A.M. De Leeuw, Institute for Experimental Gerontology, T.N.O., Lange Kleiweg 151, 2280 HV Rijswijk, The Netherlands.

P.P. DeLuca, School of Pharmacy, University of Kentucky, Lexington, KY 40536-0053, U.S.A.

P. Edman, Division of Pharmacy, Department of Drugs, National Board of Health and Welfare, Box 607, S-751 25 Uppsala, Sweden

G.S. Elliott, School of Veterinary Medicine, Purdue University, West Lafayette, IN 47907, U.S.A.

A.T. Florence, Department of Pharmacy, University of Strathclyde, 204 George Street, Glasgow Gl 1XW, U.K.

J.F. Forbes, Department of Surgery, University of Melbourne, Royal Melbourne Hospital, Parkville, Australia 3050

S. Frøkjaer, Novo Industri a/s, Novo Allé, DK-2880 Bagsvaerd, Denmark.

M. Fumagalli, Ospedale L. Sacco, Milan, Italy.

S. Funderud, The Norwegian Radium Hospital, Oslo, Norway.

M. Garufi, MEDEA Research, Via Piscane 34/a, 20129 Milan, Italy.

E.M. Gipps, Victorian College of Pharmacy, 381 Royal Parade, Parkville, Australia 3052.

E.P. Goldberg, College of Engineering, Department of Materials Science and Engineering, University of Florida, Gainesville, FL 32611, U.S.A.

J. Grünberg, European Molecular Biology Laboratory, Postfach 10.2209, D-6900 Heidelberg, F.R.G.

P. Guiot, Laboratoire de Chimie Pharmaceutique, Université Catholique de Louvain, 73 Avenue Emmanuel Mounier, B-1200 Brussels, Belgium.

J.R. Hale, Francis Bitter National Magnetic Laboratory, Massachusetts Institute of Technology, Cambridge, MA 02139, U.S.A.

M. Hashida, Faculty of Pharmaceutical Sciences, Kyoto University, Sakyo-ku, Kyoto 606, Japan.

D.P. Howard, The Lilly Research Laboratories, 307 East McCarty Street, Indianapolis, IN 46285, U.S.A.

K. Howell, European Molecular Biology Laboratory, Postfach 10.2209, D-6900 Heidelberg, F.R.G.

I.M. Hunneyball, Research Department, The Boots Company, Nottingham, U.K.

H. Hvid-Hansen, Department of Nuclear Medicine, Municipal Hospital, DK-8000 Århus, Denmark.

L. Illum, Royal Danish School of Pharmacy, Universitetsparken 2, 2100 Copenhagen Ø, Denmark.

S. Inoue, Department of Synthetic Chemistry, Faculty of Engineering, University of Tokyo, Tokyo 113, Japan.

R. Iwaoku, Department of Pharmacy, Kumamoto University Hospital, Kumamoto 860, Japan.

H. Iwata, Department of Materials Science, University of Florida, Gainesville, FL 32611, U.S.A.

W. Janas, School of Veterinary Medicine, Purdue University, West Lafayette, IN 47907, U.S.A.

P.D.E. Jones, Department of Pharmacy, University of Nottingham, Nottingham NG7 2UH, U.K.

P.-E. Jönsson, Department of Surgery, University of Lund, Lasarettet, S-221 85 Lund, Sweden.

K. Juni, Department of Pharmacy, Kumamoto University Hospital, Kumamoto 860, Japan.

H.M.H. Kamel, Department of Pathology, Royal Infirmary, Glasgow, U.K.

M. Kanke, College of Pharmacy, University of Kentucky, Lexington, KY 40536-0053, U.S.A.

T. Kato, Department of Urology, Akita University School of Medicine, 1-1-1 Hondo, Akita 010, Japan.

J.T. Kemshead, Imperial Cancer Research Fund Laboratory, Guildford Street, London WC1N 1EH, U.K.

T. Kojima, Department of Pharmacy, Kumamoto University Hospital, Kumamoto 860, Japan.

T. Kondo, Faculty of Pharmaceutical Sciences, Science University of Tokyo, 12 Ichigaya Fungawara-Machi, Shinjuku-ku, Tokyo 162, Japan.

J. Kreuter, Institute of Pharmacy, ETH, Clausiusstrasse 25, CH-8092 Zürich, Switzerland

R. Langer, Massachusetts Institute of Technology, Department of Nutrition and Food Science, Cambridge, MA 02139, U.S.A.

V. Lenaerts, Laboratoire de Pharmacie Galénique, Université Catholique de Louvain, 73 Avenue Emmanuel Mounier, B-1200 Brussels, Belgium.

D. Leyh, Laboratoire de Pharmacie Galénique, Université Catholique de Louvain, 73 Avenue Emmanuel Mounier, B-1200 Brussels, Belgium.

B. Lindberg, Department of Chemical Research, Pharmacia AB, Box 181, S-751 04 Uppsala, Sweden.

W. Longo, Department of Materials Science, University of Florida, Gainesville, FL 32611, U.S.A.

K. Lote, Department of Radiology, Haukeland Hospital, N-5016 Bergen, Norway.

S. Margel, Department of Plastics Research, Weizmann Institute of Science, Rehovot, Israel.

J. Marqversen, Department of Nuclear Medicine, Municipal Hospital, DK-8000 Århus, Denmark.

J.G. McVie, Netherlands Cancer Institute, Plesmanlaan 121, Amsterdam, The Netherlands.

B.J. Meakin, School of Pharmacy and Pharmacology, University of Bath, Claverton Down, Bath, Avon BA2 7AY, U.K.

L. Molteni, MEDEA Research, Via Piscane 34/a, 20129 Milan, Italy.

R.M. Morris, The Lilly Research Laboratories, 307 East McCarty Street, Indianapolis, IN 46285, U.S.A.

M. Nakano, Department of Pharmacy, Kumamoto University Medical School, 1-1-1 Honjo, Kumamoto 860, Japan.

R. Nemoto, Department of Urology, Institute of Clinical Medicine, The University of Tsukuba, Sakura-Mura, Niihari, Ibaraki 305, Japan.

W. Norde, Laboratory for Physical and Colloid Chemistry, Agricultural University of Wageningen, De Dreijen 6, 6703 BC Wageningen, The Netherlands.

K. Nustad, The Norwegian Radium Hospital, Oslo, Norway.

R.C. Oppenheim, Victorian College of Pharmacy, 381 Royal Parade, Parkville, Victoria, Australia 3052.

G.A. Poore, The Lilly Research Laboratories, 307 East McCarty Street, Indianapolis, IN 46285, U.S.A.

F. Puisieux, Laboratoire de Pharmacie Galénique, Centre d'études Pharmaceutiques, Université Paris-Sud, Rue J.B. Clement, 92290 Chatenay-Malabry, France.

J.H. Ratcliffe, Department of Pharmacy, University of Nottingham, Nottingham NG7 2UH, U.K.

A. Rembaum, Chemistry and Biotechnology Research Section, Jet Propulsion Laboratory, California Institute of Technology, 4800 Oak Grove Drive, Pasadena, CA 91109, U.S.A.

G. Richards, Jet Propulsion Laboratory, California Institute of Technology, 4800 Oak Grove Drive, Pasadena, CA 91109, U.S.A.

N.E. Richardson, School of Pharmacy and Pharmacology, University of Bath, Claverton Down, Bath, Avon BA2 7AY, U.K.

R.C. Richardson, School of Veterinary Medicine, Purdue University, West Lafayette, IN 47907, U.S.A.

J.C. Riis Jørgensen, Department of Nuclear Medicine, Municipal Hospital, DK-8000 Århus, Denmark.

K.E. Rogers, Department of Biochemistry, Comprehensive Cancer Center, University of Southern California, School of Medicine, Los Angeles, CA 90033, U.S.A.

M. Roland, Laboratoire de Pharmacie Galénique, Université Catholique de Louvain, 73 Avenue Emmanuel Mounier, B-1200 Brussels, Belgium.

K.L. Ross, Department of Biochemistry, Comprehensive Cancer Center, University of Southern California, School of Medicine, Los Angeles, CA 90033, U.S.A.

G.P. Royer, Standard Oil Company (Ind), Naperville, IL 60566, U.S.A.

L.G. Salford, Department of Neurosurgery, University of Lund, S-220 07 Lund, Sweden.

T. Sato, College of Pharmacy, University of Kentucky, Lexington, KY 40536-0053, U.S.A.

E.M.A. Schoonderwoerd, Department of Pharmacy, University of Amsterdam, Plantage Muidergracht 24, Amsterdam, The Netherlands.

R. Schmid, SINTEF, Division of Applied Chemistry, N-7034 Trondheim-NTH, Norway.

U. Schröder, Department of Tumour Immunology, The Wallenberg Laboratory, University of Lund, P.O. 7031, S-220 07 Lund, Sweden.

J.A. Sefranka, The Lilly Research Laboratories, 307 East McCarty Street, Indianapolis, IN 46285, U.S.A.

A.E. Senyei, Molecular Biosystems Inc., 11180 Roselle Street, Suite A, San Diego, CA 92121, U.S.A.

H. Sezaki, Faculty of Pharmaceutical Sciences, Kyoto University, Sakyo-ku, Kyoto 606, Japan.

R.L. Silver, Michael Reese Hospital and Medical Center, Chicago, IL, U.S.A.

I. Sjöholm, Department of Drugs, National Board of Health and Welfare, Box 607, S-751 25 Uppsala, Sweden.

A. Smith, Research Department, The Boots Company, Nottingham, U.K.

T.D. Sokoloski, College of Pharmacy, Ohio State University, 500 West 12th Avenue, Columbus, OH 43210, U.S.A.

P.P. Speiser, Pharmacy Institute, ETH, Clausiusstrasse 25, CH-8092 Zürich, Switzerland.

A. Ståhl, Department of Tumour Immunology, University of Lund, S-220 07 Lund, Sweden.

G. Steele, Department of Pharmacy, University of Strathclyde, 204 George Street, Glasgow G1 1XW, U.K.

S.-E. Strand, Radiation Physics Department, University of Lund, Lasarettet, S-221 85 Lund, Sweden.

J.F.B. Stuart, Department of Pharmacy, University of Strathclyde, Glasgow, U.K.

F. Tågehøj Jensen, Department of Nuclear Medicine, Municipal Hospital, DK-8000 Århus, Denmark.

H. Teder, Department of Surgery, General Hospital, S-214 01 Malmö, Sweden.

C. Thies, Biological Transport Laboratory, Box 1198, Washington University, St Louis, MO 63130, U.S.A.

Z.A. Tökès, Department of Biochemistry, Comprehensive Cancer Center, University of Southern California, School of Medicine, Cancer Center, Los Angeles, CA 90033, U.S.A.

E. Tomlinson, Advanced Drug Delivery Research, Ciba-Geigy Pharmaceuticals Division, Horsham, West Sussex, U.K.

T.R. Tritton, Department of Pharmacology, School of Medicine, Yale University, 333 Cedar Street, P.O. Box 3333, New Haven, CT 06510, U.S.A.

R.F. Tuma, Department of Physiology, Temple University, Health Sciences Center, School of Medicine, Philadelphia, PA 19140, U.S.A.

J. Ugelstad, Laboratory of Industrial Chemistry, Norwegian Institute of Technology, The University of Trondheim, N-7034 Trondheim-NTH, Norway.

F. Valeriote, Department of Experimental Therapeutics, Michigan Cancer Foundation, 110 East Warren Avenue, Detroit, MI 48201, U.S.A.

N. Wakiyama, Sankyo Company, Tokyo 140, Japan.

B. Warburton, The School of Pharmacy, University of London, 29/39 Brunswick Square, London, U.K.

T.L. Whateley, Department of Pharmacy, University of Strathclyde, 204 George Street, Glasgow G1 1XW, U.K.

M. Wheatley, Department of Nutrition and Food Science, Massachusetts Institute of Technology, Cambridge, MA 02139, U.S.A.

R.H. Whitehead, Tumour Biology Unit, Ludwig Institute for Cancer Research, Parkville, Australia 3050.

K.J. Widder, Molecular Biosystems Inc., 11180 Roselle Street, Suite A, San Diego, CA 92121, U.S.A.

N. Willmott, Department of Pharmaceutics, University of Strathclyde, 204 George Street, Glasgow G1 1XW, U.K.

C.G. Wilson, Department of Physiology and Pharmacology, Queens Medical School, Clifton Boulevard, Nottingham, U.K.

L.B. Wingard, Jr., Department of Pharmacology, University of Pittsburgh School of Medicine, Pittsburgh, PA 15261, U.S.A.

E. Wisse, Department of Cell Biology and Histology, Free University of Brussels, Laarbeeklaan 103, 1090 Brussel-Jette, Belgium.

Y. Yoshida, Department of Synthetic Chemistry, Faculty of Engineering, University of Tokyo, Tokyo 113, Japan.

Section 1

Biological and biophysical factors

Microspheres and Drug Therapy. Pharmaceutical, Immunological and Medical Aspects
edited by S.S. Davis, L. Illum, J.G. McVie and E. Tomlinson
© *1984, Elsevier Science Publishers B.V.*
1

Structural elements determining transport and exchange processes in the liver

E. Wisse and A.M. De Leeuw

1. Introduction

Structural entities such as the liver lobule, vascular elements such as the portal vein, hepatic arteries, sinusoids, and central veins, the different cell types with their peculiar histological relationships and the various endocytotic and intracellular transport mechanisms all play an important role in our attempts to understand the function of the liver as a major and central organ in the processing of various vital metabolites. A variety of delicate structures are involved in the exchange processes between the blood and the hepatic cells which take up, metabolize, store, synthesize and excrete a number of endogenous products. The liver also plays an important role in the interaction with a number of injected compounds, particles and artificial vesicles, such as liposomes or microspheres. It is the aim of this chapter to review data concerning the structure and function of the liver tissue as far as they are relevant to transport, exchange and endocytotic processes.

As far as our own data are concerned, these are mainly based on perfusion-fixed rat livers (Wisse, 1970, 1972, 1974, 1977; Wisse and Knook, 1979; Wisse et al., 1974, 1976, 1980, 1982, 1983) prepared for transmission (Wisse, 1970, 1972, 1974) or scanning electron microscopy (Wisse et al., 1982, 1983). From these studies, it might be concluded that perfusion fixation is a prerequisite for the preservation of structural details and histological relationships in sinusoids, sinusoidal cells and the space of Disse. For this purpose, different methods for applying a perfusion type of fixation using needle (De Wilde et al., 1982; Muto et al., 1977) or surgical biopsies (Muto et al., 1977; Vonnahme, 1980; Wisse et al., 1974) of rat or human liver have been described. In addition, a number of functional data has been collected in studies making use of different types of isolated and purified sinusoidal cells (Knook and Sleyster, 1976; Knook et al., 1977), on cultures of these cells (De Leeuw et al., 1982, 1983) in which their endocytotic capabilities (Praaning-Van Dalen, 1983; Praaning-Van Dalen and Knook, 1982; Praaning-Van Dalen et al., 1981) or digestive capacity were studied (De Leeuw et al., 1983). In this chapter, we will discuss the liver lobule, the sinusoids, the sinusoidal cells, the process of endocytosis, the space of Disse, the parenchymal cells, and our conclusions.

2. The liver lobule

Different terms and models have been used to describe and explain why a certain amount of liver parenchymal tissue, as a functional unit, seems to be capable of performing the many different functions known to take place in the liver. In this chapter, we will restrict ourselves to the term liver lobule (Malpighi, 1666), defined as a unit of parenchymal tissue peripherally characterized by branches of the portal vein and hepatic artery and centrolobularly by a branch of the hepatic vein, i.e., the central vein (Fig. 1). In our opinion, this terminology is compatible with the fact that the blood enters the lobule via the portal tract through sinusoidal inlets and, after interaction with the tissue during passage through the sinusoids, leaves the lobule again through outlet sinusoids connected to the central veins. The proposed model of the liver acinus together with the distinction of zones I, II and III in the parenchymal tissue (Rappaport, 1973) is handicapped by semantic interdisciplinary disputes and the fact that a clear distinction between three zones in the tissue is not possible on the basis of any structural or functional phenomenon. Nevertheless, the existence of an important multifarious gradient oriented from portal to central regions and expressed in terms of function and structure has been generally accepted.

Important contributions to the knowledge of the structure and function of the liver lobule have been made by in vivo light microscopical studies (Koo et al., 1975; McCuskey, 1966; Platteborse, 1971; Rappaport, 1973; Reilly et al., 1981), by the vascular corrosion cast technique (Hase and Brim, 1965; Kardon and Kessel, 1980; Nopanitaya et al., 1978, Ohtani et al., 1983) and by laborious three-disemsional reconstruction using histological sections (Matsumoto et al., 1979).

In vivo light microscopy of the transilluminated liver is a powerful technique for visualizing cells and their interactions in a living state. At lower magnifications, the liver lobule can be observed as a microcirculatory complex. Three zones in branches of the portal vein can be discerned: a conducting, distributing and terminal part, the latter being in the order of about 60 μm in length (Rappaport, 1973) and 15–20 μm in diameter (Rappaport, 1973; Reilly et al., 1983). Sparse and rectangular side branches (Itoshima et al., 1974; Matsumoto et al., 1979; Wisse et al., 1983) distribute the blood into the periportal tissue until the tapering end portion of the terminal portal vein is reached. The larger ramifications of the portal vein, however, also seem to contribute blood to the surrounding tissue, since the tissue surrounding such branches seems to bear the characteristics of true periportal tissue (Hase and Brim, 1965; Matsumoto et al., 1979; Ohtani et al., 1983). Within the portal tract, the artery is not always easily seen (McCuskey, 1966; Ohtani et al., 1983); its diameter measures from 4 to 10 μm and occasional branches connect to sinusoids, as the so-called arteriosinusoid twigs (AST; McCuskey, 1966). Both arterial and portal injections of a blue dye (Platteborse, 1971) show a similar wave-like distribution pattern through the liver lobule towards the central vein, indicating the mixing of arterial and portal blood before reaching the parenchymal tissue, probably by arterioportal anastomosis. The normal transit time of indicator solutions through the liver lobule seems to

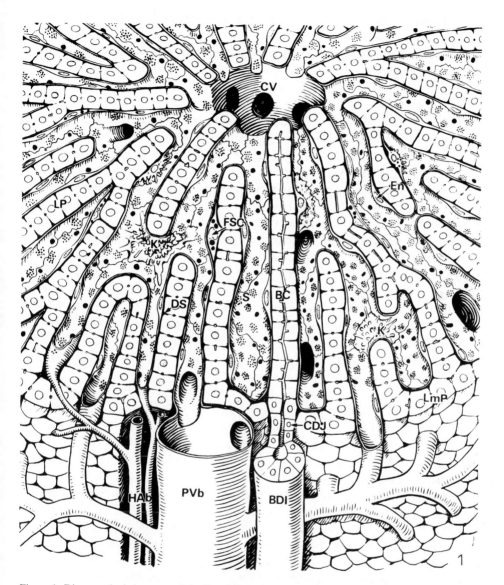

Figure 1. Diagram depicting part of the liver lobule. At the periphery of the lobule, the hepatic artery (HAb), the portal vein (PVb) and the bile duct (BDI) are connected to sinusoids and bile capillaries (BC), the latter through a ductus of Hering (CDJ). The blood flows from the periphery to the central vein (CV) through sinusoids (S) lined by endothelial cells (En). Other cell types are fat-storing cells (FSC), Kupffer cells (K) and parenchymal cells (LP), at the periphery locally arranged in limiting plates (LmP). From Muto (1975), with permission.

be in the order of 5–10 seconds (Goresky, 1982; Platteborse, 1971). The in vivo microscopy technique also demonstrates great differences in flow rate within the sinusoids (Koo et al., 1975; McCuskey, 1966) depending not only on possible connections to arterioles and the orientation of the portal to central axis but also on the interaction of sinusoidal cells bulging into the sinusoidal lumen (McCuskey, 1966). Direct shunting connections between the portal and central veins do not exist. Vasoactive substances (McCuskey, 1966; Platteborse, 1971; Rappaport, 1973; Reilly et al., 1981) or extensive endocytosis by sinusoidal cells directly influence the sinusoidal blood flow.

Vascular casts have clearly and beautifully depicted the existence of a peribiliary plexus fed by arterioles. Vascular connections between these arterioles, the peribiliary plexus, the portal veins and the sinusoids seem to exist (Hase and Brim, 1965; Kardon and Kessel, 1980; McCuskey, 1966; Nopanitaya et al., 1978; Ohtani et al., 1983; Platteborse, 1971; Reilly et al., 1981).

Three-dimensional reconstructions of the human hepatic lobular tissue seem to indicate that there is an almost equal number of branches of portal and central veins of comparable diameter (Matsumoto et al., 1979). Central veins which have a mean diameter of 25.1 μm (Reilly et al., 1981) receive a large number of sinusoidal outlet connections (Itoshima et al., 1974; Wisse et al., 1983) and can be easily recognized on this basis in scanning electron microscope (SEM) preparations. Morphological differences between endothelial cells from portal and central veins have been described (Wisse et al., 1983) and a clear morphological and functional distinction can be made between these endothelial cells and the sinusoidal endothelial cells (Wisse, 1970, 1972). Transitions between sinusoidal endothelial cells and the ones of the larger veins are abrupt and mostly occur at the orifices of sinusoidal inlet and outlet connections (Wisse et al., 1983).

3. Sinusoids

The liver sinusoid is a unique capillary and an important link in the hepatic microcirculatory chain (Figs. 3, 5). The cells forming this capillary are endothelial cells and the underlying fat-storing cells, both in contact with the microvilli of the parenchymal cells, keeping open the space of Disse. This specific structure of the liver sinusoidal wall is not observed in any other capillary or tissue in the body.

Sinusoids can be oriented in three different ways within the liver lobule: direct sinusoids running from portal to central parts of the lobule, branching sinusoids and interconnecting sinusoids (Koo et al., 1975). Due to this difference in sinusoidal orientation, blood flow will vary widely in these sinusoids; differences in red blood cell (RBC) speed of 270 to 410 μm/sec have been determined by in vivo light microscopy (Koo et al., 1975)

The direct sinusoids can have a length of 250 μm (Rappaport, 1973), which can be regarded as the radius of the liver lobule. With regard to the diameter of sinusoids, a number of values determined by different methods are to be found in the literature (see Table 1). Apparently, the diameter of sinusoids can be influenced by either pressure (e.g., during perfusion fixation) or preparative methods (such as critical point drying for SEM, introducing a 20–30% shrinkage). In a recent comparison of plastic-embedded material and critical point-dried material of rat livers perfusion-fixed at constant low pressure (10 cm H_2O), the sinusoidal diameter was found to vary from 3 to 12 μm (Table 2).

We were able to demonstrate significant differences in diameter between periportal and centrolobular sinusoids (Wisse et al., 1982, 1983; Table 2). In addition, periportal sinusoids are more tortuous than the straighter centrolobular ones (Fig. 2), which has also been reported in studies using the vascular cast technique (Hase and Brim, 1965). The resulting periportal sinusoidal anastomosis (Matsumoto et al., 1979) seems to be effective in distributing the blood received from the relatively few portal inlets and in reducing the flow rate (Koo et al., 1975) and pressure (Rappaport, 1973) when the blood enters the tissue.

The volume fraction taken by the sinusoidal lumen has been estimated by morphometric methods to be 10.6%, not including the space of Disse (Blouin et al., 1977), 26.7–30.3% (Lemoine et al., 1982), 11.1–14.1% (Miller et al., 1979) or 13% (Weibel et al., 1969). The sinusoidal space was found to be half of the total vascular space of the liver (25%) by using the multiple indicator dilution technique (Goresky, 1982), giving a value close to some of the morphometric data. In these studies, an increase in sinusoidal volume fraction going from periportal towards centrolobular regions

TABLE 1

Sinusoidal diameter as given by various authors

Reference		Sinusoidal diameter (μm)	Method
Grisham et al.	(1975)	20–40	SEM
Nopanitaya et al.	(1976)	20–40	SEM
Rappaport	(1973)	15–30	in vivo
Muto	(1975)	7–10	SEM
Motta	(1977)	7–10	SEM
Koo et al.	(1975)	6.3–6.6	in vivo
Reilly et al.	(1981)	5.5	in vivo
Wisse et al.	(1980)	3.4	SEM
Wisse et al.	(1983)	4.0–5.7	SEM

TABLE 2

Sinusoidal diameters compared in plastic-embedded and critical point-dried material

	Periportal	Centrolobular
Plastic-embedded	6.42 ± 0.12 μm	7.62 μm
Range	4–11 μm	5–12 μm
Critical point-dried	4.09 ± 0.06 μm	5.67 μm
Range	3–8 μm	3–9 μm

Values are mean $\pm$ S.E. Plastic-embedded material was examined using light microscopy, Critical point-dried material using SEM.

was also given: 26.7–30.3% (Lemoine et al., 1982) and 11.1–14.1% (Miller et al., 1979). Here again, different preparative techniques and experimental approaches might explain the variation in results. For uptake processes, the sinusoidal surface to sinusoidal volume ratio seems to favour uptake in the periportal areas (Gumucio and Miller, 1982). One might, however, argue that another ratio, i.e., endothelial surface to parenchymal cell volume ratio, might also be an important factor. This ratio seems to be higher in centrolobular areas, since the perimeter of sinusoids increases (Wisse et al., 1983) and parenchymal cells do not change their diameter or volume (Hemet et al., 1983; Loud, 1968). In addition to topographical differences in sinusoidal diameter, time-dependent variations due to the application of a number of vasoactive substances (McCuskey, 1966; Rappaport, 1973; Reilly et al., 1981; Wisse et al., 1980) or venous outflow obstruction (Nopanitaya et al., 1976) have also been reported. It is unknown so far whether lobular gradients will become more pronounced or be neutralized or converted during such dynamic changes.

4. Do blood cells fit into sinusoids?

As a result of comparing diameters of sinusoids with diameters of blood cells, one must assume special interactions between the two. Fresh red blood cells (RBCs) have a diameter of 7.65 μm (Eskelinen and Saukko, 1983) in the resting, discocyte state. This diameter changes to 5.8 or 5.9 μm in SEM preparations (Eskelinen and Saukko, 1983; Wisse et al., 1983). One may conclude that sinusoids are too small, especially the small sinusoids in periportal areas (see Table 2), to allow the RBCs to pass without considerable changes in their shape. RBCs happen to be very flexible (Skalak and Brånemark, 1969) and might rapidly adapt their diameter within 0.06 second to different shapes, described as umbrella, paraboloid or even torpedo shapes (Skalak and Brånemark, 1969). As a result, a single cell blood flow (bolus flow) consisting of a row of single cells separated by small volumes of plasma will exist in most sinusoids (Goresky, 1982).

In the case of white blood cells (WBCs), even more serious interactions might be assumed. Human WBCs in a globular, resting state have been accurately measured (Schmid-Schönbein et al., 1980a): lymphocytes, 6.2 μm (range 4–8 μm); neutrophils, 7.03 μm (range 5–8 μm); eosinophils, 7.3 μm; and monocytes 7.5 μm. These values differ from those in air-dried smear preparations, which give higher values due to the flattening of the cells. Apart from the somewhat greater values of WBC diameter,

---

Figure 2. SEM survey picture of a part of the liver lobule of a perfusion-fixed rat liver. Left, a portal vein; right, a central vein. Periportal sinusoids are narrow and tortuous; centrolobular sinusoids are wider and straighter.

Figure 3. SEM photograph of a rat liver sinusoid. A fenestrated endothelial wall separates the sinusoidal lumen (L) from the space of Disse (SD) and parenchymal cells (P).

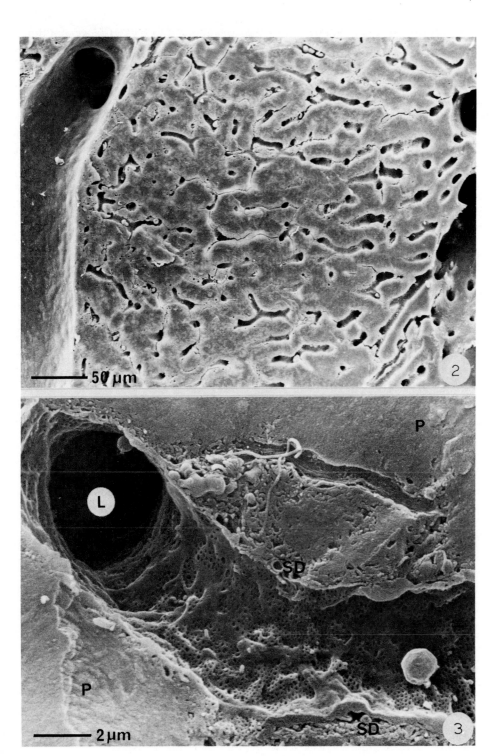

it is supposed that the volume and rigidity as compared to RBCs (Bagge and Bråne-mark, 1977) will result in regular WBC plugging (Bagge and Brånemark, 1977; Bagge et al., 1977a; Figs. 9, 10) at the portal inlets or at places where the perikaryons of sinusoidal cells bulge into the lumen (McCuskey, 1966; Fig. 9). This will result in interrupted flow (Bagge and Brånemark, 1977; Bagge et al., 1977a) and impressions of the endothelial wall and the underlying space of Disse (Fig. 11), which we proposed to call endothelial massage (Wisse et al., 1983). WBCs appear to adapt their shape more slowly (0.5–3 seconds and up to minutes) (Bagge and Brånemark, 1977; Bagge et al., 1977b) and in different, time-dependent phases as compared with RBCs and seem to be able to widen the lumen of small capillaries somewhat (Bagge and Brånemark, 1977). WBCs move more slowly in small vessels (Bagge and Brånemark, 1977; Schmid-Schönbein et al., 1980b) and are marginated by interactions with RBCs (Schmidt-Schönbein et al., 1980b). Shape adaptations from spherical to torpedo shape will extend the overall cell surface (or perimeter) by 40–70% in a short time (Bagge et al., 1977a), which implies that the normally ruffled cell surface changes into a smooth surface (Bagge and Brånemark, 1977; Bagge et al., 1977a). This might be beneficial for passage through a narrow capillary or sinusoid. In a small vessel of 7–9 μm, 15 to 20 WBCs pass the point of observation each minute (Schmidt-Schön-bein et al., 1980b). A further illustration of sinusoidal plugging is given by a study on the entrapment of tumour cells, which are larger (10.8 μm) and seem to be less flexible (deformation time, 10 seconds) than WBCs and these cells are mainly arrested in periportal areas (Bagge et al., 1983).

5. The sinusoidal wall

It has been demonstrated by transmission EM (TEM) in the perfusion-fixed rat liver that the endothelial lining possesses fenestrae, lacking a diaphragm. The fenestrae are arranged in clusters or sieve plates (Fig. 4) and no basal lamina is present (Burkel and Low, 1966; Wisse, 1970; Fig. 6). Fenestrae have also been described by authors using freeze etching (Orci et al., 1971; Wisse, 1970) or SEM (Brooks and Haggis, 1973). After these initial descriptions, it was found that a number of species seem to possess similar endothelial fenestrae, among which are flatfish (Tanuma et al., 1982), birds (Ohata et al., 1982) and many different mammals (Gemmell and Heath, 1972; Grubb and Jones, 1971; Itoshima et al., 1974; Oikawa, 1979; Tanuma and Ito, 1978; Tanuma et al., 1981, 1983; Vonnahme and Müller, 1981; Wisse, 1970; Wright

Figure 4. SEM photograph of the fenestrated endothelial lining. Note the arrangement of fenestrae in sieve plates interspersed by protoplasmic processes and the absence of gaps. SD, space of Disse; P, parenchymal cell.

Figure 5. Transmission EM (TEM) survey of a sinusoid (L) with bordering parenchymal cells (P). Bile capillaries (bc) are well separated from the space of Disse and parenchymal recesses.

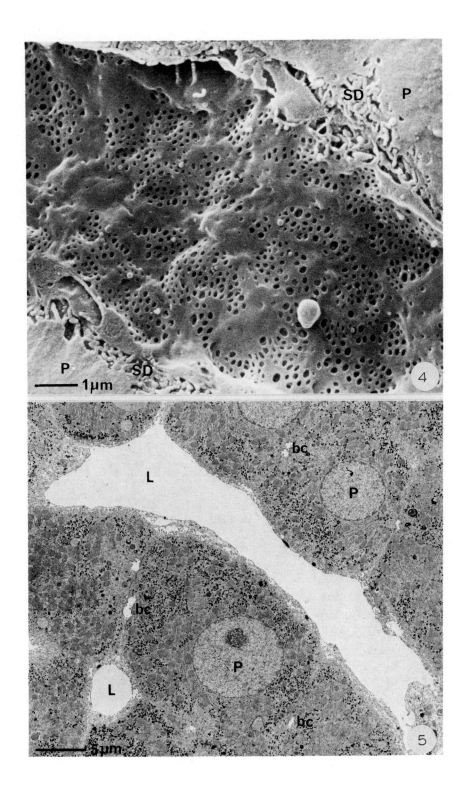

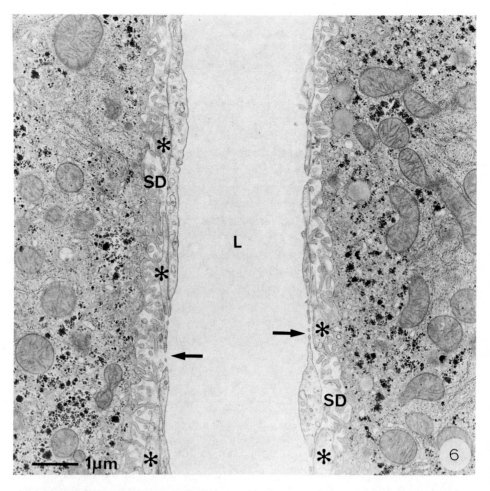

Figure 6. TEM photograph of a sinusoidal lumen (L), lined by endothelium containing fenestrae (arrows), occasionally underlined by fat-storing cell processes (asterisks). Irregular microvilli of the parenchymal cells keep the space of Disse (SD) open. A fine filamentous cytoplasm supports the microvilli.

et al., 1983), including man (Gendrault et al., 1982; Muto, 1975; Vonnahme, 1980). Open fenestrae seem to develop at the end of the fetal period, just before birth (Bankston and Pino, 1980), when fenestrae with diaphragms are changed for open ones. Fenestrae with diaphragms have been reported in sheep (Gemmell and Heath, 1972; Grubb and Jones, 1971), but a recent study clearly demonstrates the presence of open fenestrae (Wright et al., 1983a). Incidentally, small and thin fragments of basal lamina material can be seen (Wisse, 1970), especially between processes of fat-storing cells and endothelial cells. This material was immunocytochemically determined to contain fibronectin and collagen type IV (Geerts et al., 1982). The fenestrae diameter was found to increase with a number of experimental factors, such as alcohol

(Fraser et al., 1980a, 1982), pressure (Fraser et al., 1980b; Frenzel et al., 1976, 1977; Nopanitaya et al., 1976), CCl_4 (Fraser et al., 1982) and hypoxia, irradiation and endotoxin (Frenzel et al., 1977) and to decrease with serotonin and noradrenalin (Wisse et al., 1980). Lobular gradients were found to give different degrees of porosity to the endothelial lining, in periportal areas the porosity was 6% and in centrolobular areas a porosity of 8% was found. This difference was due mainly to an increase in the frequency of fenestrae (Wisse et al., 1982, 1983). The diameter of fenestrae differed only slightly in SEM preparations and was found to be 105–110 nm. It is thought that the open connection between the lumen and the space of Disse is the basis for a free exchange of fluid and solutes between the two compartments. In the case of the transport of chylomicrons or their remnants, a filtering effect of the endothelial lining has been repeatedly demonstrated (De Zanger and Wisse, 1982; Fraser et al., 1978, 1980b; Naito and Wisse, 1978). Since the relative cholesterol content increases when large chylomicrons lose their triglycerides in the peripheral tissues, the selective admission into the space of Disse of smaller remnants by endothelial fenestrae controls cholesterol uptake, which influences endogeneous cholesterol synthesis or production of bile constituents (Fraser et al., 1978). A remarkable difference in endothelial fenestrae diameter between rabbits and rats might explain the susceptibility of rabbits to atherosclerosis, since the small fenestrae in the rabbit might inhibit the admission of cholesterol into the space of Disse (Wright et al., 1983b).

Many authors report the occurrence of large gaps of about 0.5–3.0 μm in the endothelial lining (Brooks and Haggis, 1973; De Zanger and Wisse, 1982; Frenzel et al., 1976, 1977; Gemmell and Heath, 1972; Grisham et al., 1975; Ito, 1973; Montesano and Nicolescu, 1978; Motta, 1977; Muto, 1975; Muto et al., 1977; Nopanitaya et al., 1976; Oikawa, 1979; Orci et al., 1971; Tanuma and Ito, 1978; Vonnahme and Müller, 1981; Wisse et al., 1982, 1983). Gaps might occur intra- and intercellularly (Wisse et al., 1983) and the intracellular ones might be the result of a fusion or confluence of smaller fenestrae (Montesano and Nicolescu, 1978; Nopanitaya et al., 1976; Wisse et al., 1983). Sometimes, Kupffer cell processes are seen to penetrate gaps (Motta, 1977; Vonnahme and Müller, 1981). Gap frequency increases with increased portal pressure (Fraser et al., 1980b; Frenzel et al., 1976; Nopanitaya et al., 1976) and decreases when the portal pressure is lowered during perfusion fixation (De Zanger and Wisse, 1982; Wisse et al., 1983). Chylomicron remnants in the space of Disse are never larger than the largest fenestrae, indirectly proving the absence of gaps in vivo (De Zanger and Wisse, 1982; Naito and Wisse, 1978; see also Heath and Wissig, 1966). Isolated and cultured endothelial cells show beautiful fenestrations after 24 hours in culture (De Leeuw et al., 1982). For these reasons, one might assume that gaps of 250 nm or more are probably artifacts arising during fixation. In our opinion, it is essential for a better understanding of transport of fluids, solutes and particles from the blood to the parenchymal cell surface to start from the existence of an endothelial barrier with a portal to central porosity of 6–8% formed by 0.1-μm fenestrae.

6. Sinusoidal cells

Four types of sinusoidal cells have been described. These four types are endothelial cells (Wisse, 1970, 1972), Kupffer cells (Wisse, 1974), fat-storing cells or Ito cells (Ito, 1973) and pit cells (Wisse et al., 1976). These cells occupy only 6.3 volume % (Blouin et al., 1977) and 1.6% of the protein content (Knook and Sleyster, 1976) of the liver parenchymal tissue. The functions and structures of these cells have been reviewed several times (Ito, 1973; Wisse, 1977; Wisse and Knook, 1979). Since endothelial and Kupffer cells are clearly involved in transport, exchange and uptake processes, we will only briefly describe these cells here and recommend other references to interested readers for further reading.

In the sixties, many textbooks of histology and scientific articles considered endothelial cells as precursors of Kupffer cells, both being different stages of development of a single cell type. The last report on transitional stages was published in 1973 (Ogawa et al., 1973) and the generally accepted view today seems to be that endothelial (Fig. 7) and Kupffer cells (Fig. 8) are two completely different cell types (Wisse, 1972). Liver sinusoidal endothelial cells represent a unique type of endothelial cell, because they have a high pinocytotic capacity and their flat processes have open fenestrations and no basal lamina. Kupffer cells are solitary macrophages with a high phagocytotic and a considerable pinocytotic capacity. These cells are located on or within the endothelial lining and are enriched in periportal areas, where they bulge into the lumen and interfere with blood flow (McCuskey, 1966). They contain a rich population of lysosomes (Knook et al., 1977; Wisse, 1974). Kupffer cells can phagocytose enormous amounts of material, and after ingestion they swell, which might often result in occlusion of the sinusoid.

The isolation, purification and culture of different cell types from the liver, including sinusoidal cells, has provided us with many new data concerning their function (De Leeuw et al., 1982, 1983; Knook and Sleyster, 1976; Knook et al., 1977; Praaning-Van Dalen and Knook, 1982; Steffan et al., 1981; Van Berkel, 1982). One of the main functions of these cells seems to be the endocytosis and digestion of substances and the control of exchange processes between the blood and the parenchymal cells.

7. Endocytosis

Endocytosis involves three major cell types in the liver: parenchymal, Kupffer and endothelial cells. In a morphometric study on the contribution of different cell types

---

Figure 7. TEM picture of the perikaryon of rat liver endothelial cell, showing the nucleus (N), lysosomes or dense bodies, a pair of centrioles (arrow), few strands of rough endoplasmic reticulum, mitochondria and numerous small vesicles, also in the stage of pinching off from the cell membrane, as coated pits or bristle-coated micropinocytotic vesicles. Note the continuity with sieve plates (asterisks). L, sinusoidal lumen; SD, space of Disse; P, parenchymal cell.

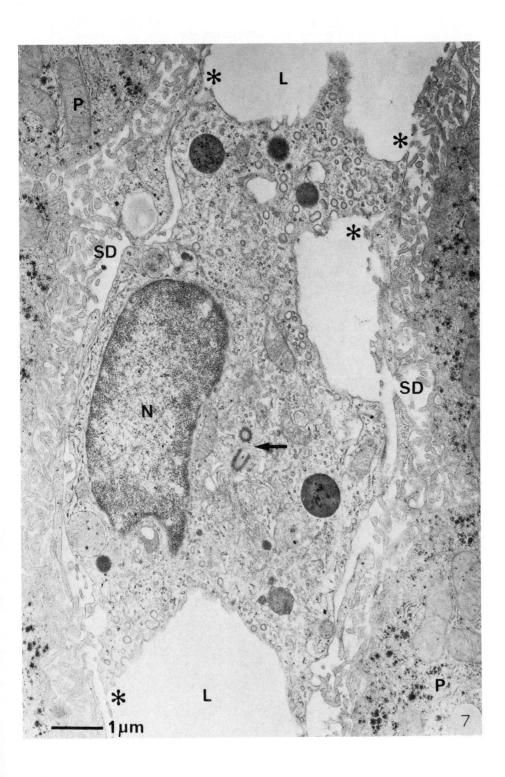

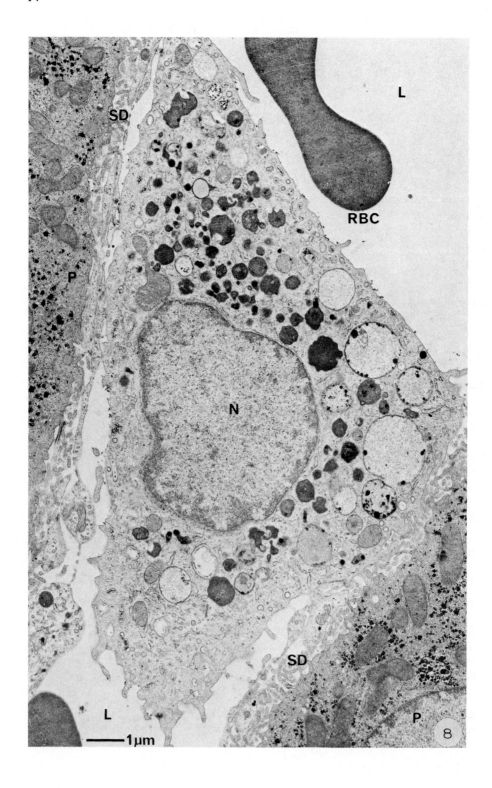

to the total hepatic volume of various organelles, it was shown that the relative contributions of the three cell types mentioned above were (Blouin et al., 1977):

	Parenchymal cell	Kupffer cell	Endothelial cell
For cell membranes	73.5%	4.3%	15.2%
For pinocytotic vesicles	47.6%	14.9%	37.0%
For lysosomes	67.6%	19.5%	12.1%

These morphometric data clearly indicate the relative importance of structures involved in pinocytosis and digestion in the different cell types.

In a survey description of morphologically recognizable endocytotic mechanisms, five structural elements were described to occur in the liver in situ after perfusion fixation (Wisse, 1977); 1, bristle-coated micropinocytosis; 2. macropinocytosis; 3, pinocytosis vermiformis; 4, pinocytosis (fuzzy coat vacuole); and 5, phagocytosis. These structures occur in endothelial cells (Nos. 1, 2), Kupffer cells (Nos. 1, 3, 4, 5) and parenchymal cells (No. 1). Recent in vitro studies on the endocytotic function of sinusoidal cells clearly indicated that the mechanism of bristle-coated micropinocytosis could be regarded as being responsible for both receptor-mediated and non-specific fluid-phase endocytosis (De Leeuw et al., 1982, 1983; Munniksma et al., 1980; Praaning-Van Dalen, 1983; Praaning-Van Dalen and Knook, 1982; Praaning-Van Dalen et al., 1981). Bristle-coated micropinocytosis and phagocytosis seem to be the most relevant mechanisms involved in endocytosis, both in situ and in vitro (De Leeuw et al., 1983; Praaning-Van Dalen, 1983; Praaning-Van Dalen et al., 1981). In endothelial and parenchymal cells, detailed studies have been performed concerning the events following the pinching off of bristle-coated vacuoles. Small tubular structures are formed and are seen to fuse with larger vacuoles (Praaning-Van Dalen, 1983) and, by the use of TEM immunocytochemistry and biochemical isolation methods, the exact way and coupling/uncoupling of ligand (asialoglycoprotein), receptor and clathrine, the bristle-coating protein, can be followed (Geuze et al., 1983; Steer et al., 1983). Pinocytosis in these cells seems to be dependent on temperature, calcium ions, the integrity of the cytoskeleton and the metabolic machinery (Praaning-Van Dalen, 1983). By using PVP solutions, it could be demonstrated that parenchymal, endothelial and Kupffer cells do pinocytose about equal amounts of fluid per day on a cellular basis, which means that together they take up about one quarter of the plasma volume per day, which might result in a contribution to the turnover of albumin of the order of 50% (Munniksma et al., 1980; Praaning-Van Dalen et al., 1981). When cellular pinocytotic activity is expressed relative to protein content, endothelial and Kupffer cells are 10–20 times more active than parenchymal

Figure 8. TEM picture of a rat liver Kupffer cell. Numerous dense bodies (lysosomes) of varying diameter, shape and density dominate the cytoplasm. N, nucleus; L, sinusoidal lumen; RBC, erythrocyte; SD, space of Disse; P, parenchymal cell.

16

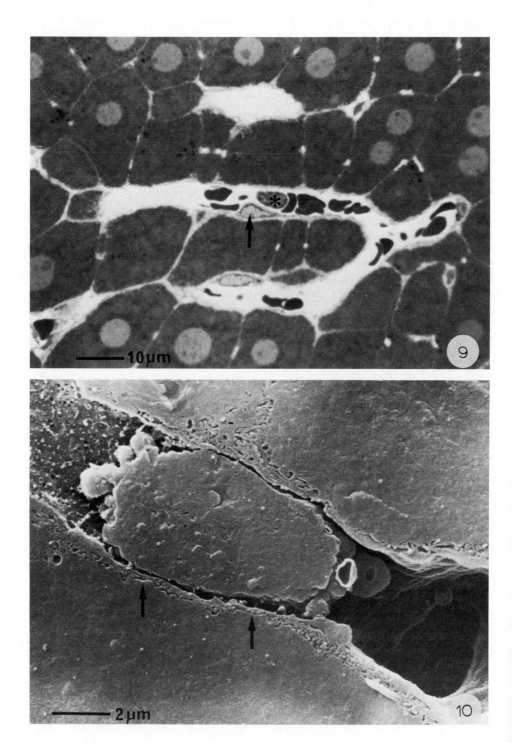

10µm

2µm

cells (Munniksma et al., 1980; Praaning-Van Dalen et al., 1981). In the case of receptor-mediated uptake of glycoproteins, lipoproteins or other substances, all kinds of
preferential uptake patterns can be obtained and expected (De Leeuw et al., 1982;
Geuze et al., 1983; Handley et al., 1983; Munniksma et al., 1980; Praaning-Van
Dalen, 1983; Praaning-Van Dalen et al., 1981; Steer et al., 1983; Van Berkel, 1982).
Surveys of literature data on compounds and particles tested for uptake by liver cells
are given (Praaning-Van Dalen, 1983; Wisse, 1977).

8. The function of the Disse space

From structural descriptions, it can be concluded that the space of Disse constitutes
a unique tissue space, bordered on the lumen side by a fenestrated endothelial lining
and on the other side by the sinusoidal surface of the parenchymal cells bearing numerous microvilli. The space of Disse takes about 5% of the total parenchymal
volume (Blouin et al., 1977). The space is considerably extended by the formation
of recesses between parenchymal cells (Heath and Wissig, 1966). About 37–42% of
the total circumference of the parenchymal cell (Heath and Wissig, 1966; Weibel et
al., 1969) borders the space of Disse, not taking into account the surface enlargement
by microvilli. Microvilli further enlarge the cell membrane locally by a factor of six
(Heath and Wissig, 1966). This means that about 70% of the parenchymal cell membrane is located in the space of Disse, illustrating the importance of the exchange
surface of parenchymal cells within the space of Disse. The microvilli are 70–120 nm
in diameter (Heath and Wissig, 1966), but their length and, therefore, the width of
the space of Disse varies. In a certain sense, it is amazing that such a tremendously
enlarged parenchymal cell surface is covered on one side by an endothelial lining with
a rather limited porosity (6–8%) available for free exchange processes. This phenomenon creates a real bottleneck situation and it is supposed that highly effective mechanisms are needed to transport, mix and pump fluids in and out the space of Disse.

As previously stated (section 4), blood cells will interact with the sinusoidal wall
(Fig. 11). Two principles are important here:
(a) RBCs fill the sinusoidal lumen, adapt to the shape of the sinusoid and they will
constantly touch and mop the wall, perhaps with the exception of a small slip layer
remaining between the surfaces of RBCs and endothelial cells. Particles, fluids and
solutes in this layer may be influenced to enter the space of Disse through the fenes-

---

Figure 9. Light microscopical picture of periportal sinusoids showing a white blood cell (asterisk) arrested
in a sinusoidal narrowing caused by the bulging perikaryon of a sinusoidal cell (arrow). Red blood cells,
including some with shapes different from the resting discoid shape, also demonstrate the local blockade
of sinusoidal blood flow in this low-pressure perfusion-fixed rat liver.

Figure 10. SEM micrograph of an elongated, longitudinally frozen-fractured white blood cell in a sinusoid.
suggesting local impression of the space of Disse (arrow).

18

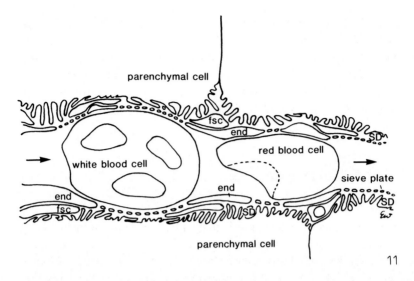

parenchymal cell

fsc

end

red blood cell

white blood cell

end

sieve plate

end

fsc

end

parenchymal cell

11

Figure 11. This diagram shows the relationship of blood cells and the sinusoidal wall. It is postulated that red blood cells deform, and form a single row of cells separating volumes of blood plasma and that white blood cells impress the space of Disse and might occasionally be stuck and interrupt blood flow. The impression on the endothelial lining is called 'endothelial massage' and is thought to represent a main mechanism of pumping fluids into and out of the space of Disse (see also Fig. 13). fsc, fat-storing cell; end, endothelium.

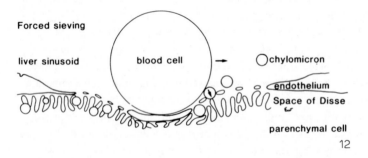

Forced sieving

liver sinusoid   blood cell   ⟶   ◯ chylomicron

endothelium

Space of Disse

parenchymal cell

12

Figure 12. This diagram illustrates the principle of forced sieving. Particles or small droplets such as chylomicrons normally show a Brownian movement in blood plasma. Due to the restriction in these movements exerted by the approaching erythrocytes and due to a possible marginating effect, chylomicrons may have an increased chance to be pressed against the endothelial wall, giving them an opportunity to meet fenestrae, which let them pass into the space of Disse.

trations by the constantly passing RBCs, resulting in a kind of *forced sieving* (Wisse et al., 1983; Fig. 12).

(b) Cells which deform because they are too large to pass freely will exert a compressing effect on the endothelial lining and the underlying space of Disse. By doing so, they will displace and mix fluids within the space of Disse, and when fenestrations

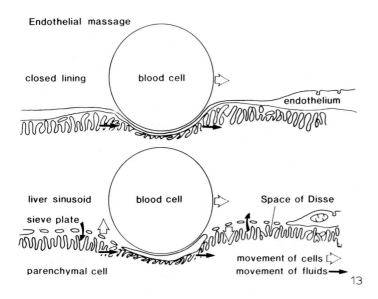

Figure 13. The endothelial massage exerted by WBCs functions in such a way that moving WBCs will move fluids downstream in the space of Disse. These fluids will escape from the space if fenestrae are present. When WBCs move on, the compressed space of Disse will resume its original width and, as a result, fluids will be drawn into the space through the nearest sieve plate. In such a way, fluids are distributed, mixed and pumped out of and into the space of Disse.

are encountered fluids can be pressed out. When a white blood cell moves on, by either its own motility or the driving forces of the small pressure gradient, impressed parts of the endothelial lining might come back into position and, as a result, fresh fluids are drawn into the space of Disse. We prefer to call this effect *endothelial massage* (Wisse et al., 1983; Fig. 13). It might be compared with the "baseball through the silk stocking" effect described earlier (Skalak, 1982).

Due to these effects, it is thought that the bottleneck aspect of endothelial porosity is not a limiting factor in a transport chain consisting of the sinusoidal lumen, the fenestrated endothelium, the fluid phase of the space of Disse and the cell membrane of the parenchymal cells. This model of transport and exchange seems to be more functional, in relation to observed and well-established fine structures and phenomena of transport and uptake, than certain physiological models, which start from the statement that "the first and only barrier that exists for substances dissolved in the plasma is the convoluted surface of the liver cells", so that there is a "free access of materials to the surface of the liver cells, in the absence of an effective barrier between the vascular space and the Disse space" (Goresky, 1982).

9. The parenchymal cell

Parenchymal cells represent about 78–83% of the total volume of the liver parenchyma (Blouin et al., 1977; Weibel et al., 1969). These cells have three surfaces: the sinusoidal surface (37–42%; without microvilli), the apposed flat lateral surfaces (50–54%) and the membranes constituting the bile canaliculi (6–13%; without microvilli) (Heath and Wissig, 1966; Weibel et al., 1969). The diameter of the cells has been determined to be about 18–20 μm (Loud, 1968; Weibel et al., 1969), without significant differences between periportal and centrolobular cells (Loud, 1968). Volume measurements resulted in values in rat livers of about 5000–5400 μm^3 for parenchymal cells (Loud, 1968; Weibel et al., 1969). Volume fractions of parenchymal cells measured in human liver biopsies showed a small difference between periportal and centrolobular cells (Hemet et al., 1983; Lemoine et al., 1982). Much more pronounced differences were described for the organelle content of periportal versus centrolobular cells: the volume percentage of mitochondria decreases (20–13%), peroxisomes increase (1.4–2.1%) and glycogen decreases (20.3–16.8%). Physiological studies indicate that cells in centrolobular areas are more sensitive to damage, ischemia, anoxia, congestion, and nutritional deficiency (Rappaport, 1973). Many substances seem to be selectively taken up in the periportal cells (Groothuis, 1982; Matsumura and Thurman, 1983; Thurman et al., 1983), with the exception of fluorescein isothiocyanate, which has been reported to be selectively taken up in centrolobular cells (Gumucio et al., 1981). Oxygen consumption is higher in periportal cells (Matsumura and Thurman, 1983; Thurman et al., 1983) and a number of other metabolic differences and gradients in enzyme activity exist (Gumucio and Miller, 1982; Jungermann and Sasse, 1978; Thurman et al., 1983).

Uptake by parenchymal cells can occur by molecular transport mechanisms in the cell membrane or by bristle-coated micropinocytosis (Geuze et al., 1983; Steer et al., 1983). Coated pits are observed at the sinusoidal cell membrane of the parenchymal cells, at the basis of and between the microvilli. In a recent study, the fate of these vesicles was described by using ultrathin frozen sections and EM immunocytochemistry (Geuze et al., 1983). It was demonstrated that ligand/receptor uncoupling occurs at the level of a newly proposed organelle, CURL, enabling receptor molecules to recycle to the cell surface, whereas ligands are transported to lysosomes after acidification of the vesicle.

10. Concluding remarks

The purpose of this chapter has been to give a brief description of structural elements involved in transport and exchange processes in the liver. From a structural point of view, the liver is a complicated organ, and this implies that studies concerning transport, uptake, exchange or secretion processes should take into account the morphological and functional aspects which might interfere in the study of fluids, solutes, macromolecules, small droplets, particles, vesicles or microspheres. Different aspects and levels of organization of the tissue should be considered:

(a) The complicated microvascular arrangement of portal veins and the arteriolar

network, peribiliary plexus and their anastomosing connections.
(b) Gradients in sinusoidal diameter, tortuosity and orientation, resulting in flow differences. The influence of bulging sinusoidal cells, sometimes acting as sphincters, and the apparent reactions to endogenous or exogenous vasoactive substances.
(c) The presence of different types of sinusoidal cells with their different reactions and their unequal distribution in the tissue, together with parenchymal cells with their functional, lobular gradients.
(d) The existence of endocytotic mechanisms, different with regard to specificity, speed and capacity and divided irregularly over the different cell types.
(e) The delicate structure of the space of Disse, with its mechanisms of forced sieving and endothelial massage and also the lobular gradient in endothelial porosity.

These morphological and functional peculiarities might each alone or in combination influence and determine the success of the uptake and handling of substances injected intravenously.

Acknowledgements

Part of this work was supported by the Belgian 'Fonds voor Geneeskundig Wetenschappelijk Onderzoek', F.G.W.O., grant No. 3.0040.80. We thank Marleen De Pauw for typing the manuscript and for bibliographic assistance, and Chris Derom for photographic assistance.

References

Bagge, U. and Brånemark, P.I. (1977) Adv. Microcirc. 7, 1–17.
Bagge, U., Johansson, B.R. and Olofsson, J. (1977a) Adv. Microcirc. 7, 18–28.
Bagge, U., Skalak, R. and Attefors, R. (1977b) Adv. Microcirc. 7, 29–48.
Bagge, U., Skobrik, G. and Ericson, L.E. (1983) J. Cancer Res. Clin. Oncol. 105, 134–140.
Bankston, P.W. and Pino, R.M. (1980) Am. J. Anat. 159, 1–15.
Blouin, A., Bolender, R.P. and Weibel, E.W. (1977) J. Cell Biol. 72, 441–455.
Brooks, S.E.H. and Haggis, G.H. (1973) Lab. Invest. 29, 60–64.
Burkel, W.E. and Low, F.N. (1966) Am. J. Anat. 118, 769–784.
De Leeuw, A.M., Barelds, R.J., De Zanger, R. and Knook, D.L. (1982) Cell Tissue Res. 223, 201–215.
De Leeuw, A.M., Brouwer, A., Barelds, R.J. and Knook, D.L. (1983) Hepatology 3, 497–506.
De Wilde, A., Van Der Spek, P., Devis, G. and Wisse, E. (1982) in Sinusoidal Liver Cells (Knook, D.L. and Wisse, E., Eds.), pp. 85–92, Elsevier, Amsterdam.
De Zanger, R.B. and Wisse, E. (1982) in Sinusoidal Liver Cells (Knook, D.L. and Wisse, E., Eds.), pp. 69–76, Elsevier, Amsterdam.
Eskelinen, S. and Saukko, P. (1983) J. Microsc. 130, 63–71.
Fraser, R., Bosanquet, A.G. and Day, W.A. (1978) Atherosclerosis 29, 113–123.
Fraser, R., Bowler, L.M. and Day, W.A. (1980a) Pathology 12, 371–376.
Fraser, R., Bowler, L.M., Day, W.A., Dobbs, B., Johnson, H.D. and Lee, D. (1980b) Br. J. Exp. Pathol. 61, 222–228.

22

Fraser, R., Bowler, L.M., De Zanger, R.B. and Wisse, E. (1982) in Connective Tissue of the Normal and Fibrotic Human Liver (Gerlach, U., Pott, G., Rauterberg, J. and Voss, B., Eds), pp. 159–160, Thieme Verlag, Stuttgart.

Frenzel, H., Kremer, B., Richter, I.E. and Hücker, H. (1976) Res. Exp. Med. 168, 229–241.

Frenzel, H., Kremer, B. and Hücker, H. (1977) in Kupffer Cells and Other Liver Sinusoidal Cells (Wisse, E. and Knook, D.L., Eds.), pp. 213–222, Elsevier, Amsterdam.

Geerts, A., Voss, B., Rauterberg, J. and Wisse, E. (1982) in Sinusoidal Liver Cells (Knook, D.L. and Wisse, E., Eds.), pp. 209–217, Elsevier, Amsterdam.

Gemmell, R.T. and Heath, T. (1972) Anat. Rec. 172, 57–70.

Gendrault, J.L., Montecino-Rodriguez, F. and Cinqualbre, J. (1982) in Sinusoidal Liver Cells (Knook, D.L. and Wisse, E., Eds.), pp. 93–100, Elsevier, Amsterdam.

Geuze, H.J., Slot, J.W., Strous, G.J.A.M., Lodish, H.F. and Schwartz, A.L. (1983) Cell 32, 277–287.

Goresky, C.A. (1982) Fed. Proc. 41, 3033–3039.

Grisham, J.W., Nopanitaya, W., Compagno, J. and Nägel, A.E.H. (1975) Am. J. Anat. 144, 295–322.

Groothuis, G.M.M. (1982) Thesis, University of Groningen.

Grubb, D.J. and Jones, A.L. (1971) Anat. Rec. 170, 75–79.

Gumucio, J.J. and Miller, D.L. (1982) in The Liver: Biology and Pathobiology (Arias, I. et al., Eds.), pp. 647–661, Raven Press, New York.

Gumucio, J.J., Miller, D.L., Krauss, M.D. and Zanolli, C.C. (1981) Gastroenterology 80, 639–646.

Handley, D.A., Arbeeny, C.M. and Chien, S. (1983) Eur. J. Cell Biol. 30, 266–271.

Hase, T. and Brim, J. (1965) Anat. Rec. 156, 157–174.

Heath, T. and Wissig, S.L. (1966) Am. J. Anat. 119, 97–128.

Hemet, J., Dubois, J.P. and Lemoine, F. (1983) Biol. Cell 47, 239–242.

Ito, T. (1973) Gunma Rep. Med. Sci. 6, 119–163.

Itoshima, T., Kobayashi, T., Shimada, Y. and Murakami, T. (1974) Arch. Histol. Jpn. 37, 15–24.

Jungermann, K. and Sasse, D. (1978) Trends Biochem. Sci. 3, 198–202.

Kardon, R.H. and Kessel, R.G. (1980) Gastroenterology 79, 72–81.

Knook, D.L. and Sleyster, E.C. (1976) Exp. Cell Res. 99, 444–449.

Knook, D.L., Blansjaar, N. and Sleyster, E.C. (1977) Exp. Cell Res. 109, 317–329.

Koo, A., Liang, I.Y.S. and Cheng, K.K. (1975) Q. J. Exp. Physiol. 60, 261–266.

Lemoine, F., Hemet, J. and Dubois, J. (1982) Biol. Cell 43, 221–224.

Loud, A.V. (1968) J. Cell Biol. 37, 27–46.

Matsumoto, T., Komori, T., Magaro, T., Ui, T., Kawakami, M., Tokuda, T., Takasaki, S., Hayashi, H., Jo, K., Hano, H., Fujino, H. and Tanaka, H. (1979) Jikeikai Med. J. 26, 1–40.

Matsumura, T. and Thurman, R.G. (1983) Am. J. Physiol. 244, G656–G659.

McCuskey, R.S. (1966) Am. J. Anat. 119, 455–478.

Miller, D.L., Zanolli, C.S. and Gumucio, J.J. (1979) Gastroenterology 76, 965–969.

Montesano, R. and Nicolescu, P. (1978) Anat. Rec. 190, 861–870.

Motta, P. (1977) Int. Rev. Cytol. 6, 347–399.

Munniksma, J., Noteborn, M., Kooistra, T., Stienstra, S., Bouma, J.M.W., Gruber, M., Brouwer, A., Praaning-Van Dalen, D. and Knook, D.L. (1980) Biochem. J. 192, 613–621.

Muto, M. (1975) Arch. Histol. Jpn. 37, 369–386.

Muto, M., Nishi, M. and Fujita, T. (1977) Arch. Histol. Jpn. 40, 137–151.

Naito, M. and Wisse, E. (1978) Cell Tissue Res. 190, 371–382.

Nopanitaya, W., Lamb, J.C., Grisham, J.W. and Carsson, J.L. (1976) Br. J. Exp. Pathol. 57, 604–609.

Nopanitaya, W., Grisham, J.W., Aghajanian, J.G. and Carsson, J.L. (1978) Scanning Electron Microsc. 2, 837–842.

Ogawa, K., Minase, T., Enomoto, K. and Onoé, T (1973) Tohoku J. Exp. Med. 110, 89–101.

Ohata, M., Tanuma, Y. and Ito, T. (1982) Okajimas Folia Anat. Jpn. 58, 325–368.

Ohtani, O., Kikuta, A., Ohtsuka, A., Taguchi, T. and Murakami, T. (1983) Arch. Histol. Jpn. 46, 1–42.

Oikawa, K. (1979) Tohoku J. Exp. Med. 129, 373–387.

Orci, L., Matter, A. and Rouiller, Ch. (1971) J. Ultrastr. Res. 35, 1–19.

Platteborse, R. (1971) Thesis, Collection 'Medico-Monographies d'Agrégés', Editions Arscia, Bruxelles.

Praaning-Van Dalen, D.P. (1983) Thesis, State University of Utrecht.

Praaning-Van Dalen, D.P. and Knook, D.L. (1982) FEBS Lett. 141, 229–232.

Praaning-Van Dalen, D.P., Brouwer, A. and Knook, D.L. (1981) Gastroenterology 81, 1036–1044.

Rappaport, A.M. (1973) Microvasc. Res. 6, 212–228.

Reilly, F.D., McCuskey, R.S. and Cilento, E.V. (1981) Microvasc. Res. 21, 103–116.

Schmid-Schönbein, G.W., Shih, Y.Y. and Chien, S. (1980a) Blood 56, 866–875.

Schmid-Schönbein, G.W., Usami, S., Skalak, R. and Chien, S. (1980b) Microvasc. Res. 19, 45–70.

Skalak, R. (1982) Blood Cells 8, 147–152.

Skalak, R. and Brånemark, P.I. (1969) Science 164, 717–719.

Steer, C.J., Wall, D.A. and Ashwell, G. (1983) Hepatology 3, 667–672.

Steffan, A.M., Lecerf, F., Keller, F., Cinqualbre, J. and Kirn, A. (1981) C. R. Acad. Sci. Paris 292, 809–815.

Tanuma, Y. and Ito, T. (1978) Arch. Histol. Jpn. 41, 1–39.

Tanuma, Y., Ohata, M. and Ito, T. (1981) Arch. Histol. Jpn. 44, 23–49.

Tanuma, Y., Ohata, M. and Ito, T. (1982) Arch. Histol. Jpn. 45, 453–472.

Tanuma, Y., Ohata, M. and Ito, T. (1983) Arch. Histol. Jpn. 46, 401–426.

Thurman, R.G., Kauffman, F.C., Ji, S., Lemasters, J.J., Conway, J.G., Belinsky, S.A., Kashiwagi, T. and Matsamura, T. (1983) Pharmacol. Biochem. Behav. 18, 415–419.

Van Berkel, T.J.C. (1982) in Metabolic Compartmentation (Sies, H., Ed.), pp. 437–482, Academic Press, London.

Vonnahme, F.J. (1980) Scanning Electron Microsc. 3, 177–180.

Vonnahme, F.J. and Müller, O. (1981) Cell Tissue Res. 215, 193–205.

Weibel, E.R., Stäubli, W., Gnägi, H.R. and Hess, F.A. (1969) J. Cell. Biol. 42, 68–91.

Wisse, E. (1970) J. Ultrastr. Res. 31, 125–150.

Wisse, E. (1972) J. Ultrastr. Res. 38, 528–562.

Wisse, E. (1974) J. Ultrastr. Res. 46, 393–426.

Wisse, E. (1977) in Kupffer Cells and Other Liver Sinusoidal Cells (Wisse, E. and Knook, D.L., Eds.), pp. 33–60, Elsevier, Amsterdam.

Wisse, E. and Knook, D.L. (1979) in Progress in Liver Diseases (Popper, H. and Schaffner, F., Eds.), Vol. VI, pp. 153–171, Grune and Stratton, New York.

Wisse, E., Van 't Noordende, J.M., Van Der Meulen, J. and Daems, W.T. (1976) Cell Tissue Res. 173, 423–435.

Wisse, E., Emeis, J.J. and Daems, W.T. (1974) in Enzyme Therapy in Lysosomal Storage Diseases (Tager, J.M., Hooghwinkel, G.J.M. and Daems, W.T., Eds.), pp. 95–109.

Wisse, E., Van Dierendonck, J.H., De Zanger, R.B., Fraser, R. and McCuskey, R.S. (1980) Proceedings Basler Liver Week 1979, pp. 195–200, MTP Press.

Wisse, E., De Zanger, R.B. and Jacobs, R. (1982) in Sinusoidal Liver Cells (Knook, D.L. and Wisse, E., Eds.), pp. 61–67, Elsevier, Amsterdam.

Wisse, E., De Zanger, R.B., Jacobs, R. and McCuskey, R.S. (1983) Scanning Electron Microsc. 3, 1441–1452.

Wright, P.L., Smith, K.F., Day, W.A. and Fraser, R. (1983a) Anat. Record 206, 385–390.

Wright, P.L., Smith, K.F., Day, W.A. and Fraser, R. (1983b) Arteriosclerosis 3, 344.

Microspheres and Drug Therapy. Pharmaceutical, Immunological and Medical Aspects
edited by S.S. Davis, L. Illum, J.G. McVie and E. Tomlinson
© *1984, Elsevier Science Publishers B.V.*

CHAPTER 2

The reticulo-endothelial system and blood clearance

John W.B. Bradfield

1. Introduction

After intravenous injection most types of microspheres tend to be cleared rapidly from the blood by cells of the reticulo-endothelial system (RES). This has important consequences. Microspheres can easily be targeting to liver, and to a lesser extent to spleen and bone marrow, which is advantageous when imaging these organs or trying to achieve the slow release of carrier-entrapped drugs after uptake into macrophages within these organs. However, if sequestration in other sites is required, then it is necessary to prevent the normal rapid reticulo-endothelial-mediated clearance.

The purpose of this chapter is to (1) update the concept of the reticulo-endothelial system, (2) review the information which is available concerning blood clearance mediated by this system and (3) draw conclusions for the use of intravenous microspheres in humans.

2. The reticulo-endothelial system — an update

For those whose reading is confined to English, the justification for collecting a population of cells together as the reticulo-endothelial system is reprinted in the Janeway Lecture given in 1924 (Aschoff, 1924). The case rests firstly on histological similarity between the various cell populations and secondly on the fact that the cells take up intra-vital dyes from the bloodstream. Mapping their distribution led Aschoff to several important conclusions. The cells were mononuclear, thereby excluding all polymorphonuclear cells; they were present in many different organs of the body; they were highly phagocytic; some were stable tissue components whereas others seemed to be wandering or migratory.

Up to that time a productive approach to the investigation of any physiological system of the body had been to excise or inactivate its components and measure any alterations in function. The widespread nature of the reticulo-endothelial system prevented excision, and therefore attempts were made by a pupil of Aschoff (Lepehne, 1921) to induce suppression of reticulo-endothelial phagocytosis using large doses of intravenous colloid metal. This, together with splenectomy, first generated the idea of reticulo-endothelial blockade. By 1924 numerous attempts had been made to achieve this, but when these were reviewed a few years later (Jaffe, 1931) it was obvious that the lack of any standardisation of either the animals or the particles injected had obscured any clear picture of what might be happening during reticulo-endothelial blockade.

Eventually one particular preparation of carbon suspension emerged as an acceptable standard* and this was mostly exploited in rats. When the results of these studies were collected and published as a symposium proceedings (Halpern, 1957) several reproducible observations had become established. The clearance of particulate matter from the blood seemed to follow an exponential first order course, but with a long tail. Many mathematical formulae were derived to describe the kinetics of uptake from blood; the validity of these is still under debate (Wagner and Iio, 1964; Drivas and Wardle, 1978). However, it was agreed that increasing doses of intravenous colloid led to decreasing rates of clearance, with eventual saturation of the clearance mechanism. In addition, the administration of a saturating dose led to a prolonged period of reduced clearance of subsequent test doses of colloid. From that time, this became the accepted definition of reticulo-endothelial blockade.

During the 1960s the emphasis of study changed as it became clear that the constituent cells of the reticulo-endothelial system were not endothelial, nor did they make reticulin. In 1969, at an international conference in Leiden, The Netherlands, a new classification was proposed, under the title of Mononuclear Phagocyte System, for which the criteria for membership were listed as mononuclear cells, being highly phagocytic and derived from bone marrow (Van Furth, 1970). This general concept has stood the test of time and the idea of this as a macrophage system is now generally accepted.

Subsequently (Van Furth, 1975, 1980), other criteria have come to be recognised as typical of macrophages. These include the presence of membrane receptors for the Fc part of the immunoglobulin molecule and for the C3b component of the complement sequence. Macrophages also characteristically express HLA-DR (Ia antigens). In general, macrophages within tissues tend to be replenished by replacement from the bone marrow, travelling in the blood as monocytes, and to have limited capacity for local proliferation. The role of the macrophage in antigen presentation has led to the study of dendritic reticulum cells and interdigitating reticulum cells in lymph nodes, Langerhans cells in the epidermis and veiled cells in afferent lymph, in order to establish how these relate to the rest of the mononuclear phagocyte system. With

---

*The standard test material for study of RES-mediated blood clearance was until very recently a type of carbon suspension made and marketed by Pelikan Ink. Corps, Hanover, under the code name of Gunther Wagner C11/1431a. This was produced especially for scientists studying the RES and comprised carbon particles stabilised in gelatin. Unfortunately, production has now been terminated, although small amounts are available on request from the author. There is a need for a new standard particle. At present, SRBCs are a convenient substitute for use intravenously in mice. Possibly a liposome or microsome preparation will eventually fulfil this need in man.

TABLE 1

The mononuclear phagocyte system

Promonocyte (bone marrow)
↓
Monocyte (blood)
↓
Macrophages (tissues) highly phagocytic:

Connective tissue	(histiocyte)
Liver	(Kupffer cell)
Lung	(alveolar macrophage)
Spleen	(free and fixed macrophages, sinusoidal lining cell)
Lymph node	(free and fixed macrophage)
Bone marrow	(macrophages, sinusoidal lining cell)
Serous cavity	(peritoneal macrophage)
Bone tissue	(osteoclast)
Nervous system	(microglia)

the advent of monoclonal antibodies specific for reticulo-endothelial cells it is becoming possible to dissect the lineage and phenotypic characteristics of the cells of this system.

3. Reticulo-endothelial-mediated blood clearance

Although much of the recent work on macrophages involves the study of these cells either in cell suspension or in tissue culture, the understanding of how macrophages clear material from the blood in vivo has also undergone rapid advance. The first important step was a re-evaluation of patterns of organ uptake as opposed to blood clearance. For this, probes such as carbon or labelled sheep red blood cells (SRBCs) in mice were used as test particles which could be taken up equally well by macrophages anywhere in the body (Bradfield, 1980b). In this type of model the pattern of organ distribution was determined solely by access to the material by the macrophages in the various organs. Thus, when SRBCs were injected intravenously into mice about 90% were cleared into the sinus-lining Kupffer cells of the liver, 5% into macrophages in the spleen and even less into macrophages in bone marrow. The clearance of material from the bloodstream is confined to those macrophages which line blood vascular channels (Bradfield, 1980b). All intravenous injections have to pass first through the lungs, but failure of clearance occurs not because there are no macrophages in lung tissue but because the large numbers of alveolar macrophages lie in the alveolar spaces in contact with inhaled air but not blood. The dominance of the liver in reticulo-endothelial blood clearance has led to one oft-quoted but mistaken statement that over 90% of the body macrophages are situated in the liver. In

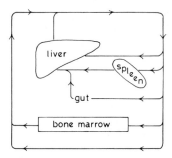

Figure 1. Sites of reticulo-endothelial-mediated blood clearance.

fact, the pattern of uptake from blood reflects the fact that although there are large populations of macrophages elsewhere in the body (see Table 1), unless they line blood channels they cannot contribute to blood clearance. Demonstration of their clearance potential would require administration of the test particles by other routes, such as air-borne or directly into tissues.

Similar physical factors dictate the partition of clearance between liver, spleen and bone marrow. Each of these three sites of blood clearance must be considered independently and only their net effect is revealed by study of blood clearance. A further complication is that the liver and the spleen lie in series, whereas the bone marrow lies in parallel with the other clearance sites (Fig. 1).

Partition of an intravenous substance between these three sites depends on their relative blood flow, the local kinetics of uptake at each site and the capacity of each site. This is dramatically revealed if the normally predominant hepatic clearance is depressed using an intravenous blockading agent. In this case there is slowing of the rate of clearance of a subsequent intravenous test particle, but organ uptake studies reveal that, far from being decreased, the total uptake into spleen and bone marrow is greatly increased. This is because the blood sinus-lining macrophages in these latter sites now have better access to blood-borne material, previously denied them by overwhelming competition from the liver. This experiment also shows that although the intravenous route can readily be used to achieve blockade of the hepatic site of clearance with a prolonged circulation time, removal is still RE-mediated. Blockade of splenic clearance has never been convincingly demonstrated by this technique, unless failure of clearance is dependent on depletion of serum factors. If microspheres are to be used intravenously for targetting to sites other than liver, spleen and bone marrow, then the desired sites of uptake may still have to compete with RE-mediated blood clearance even in the presence of so-called reticulo-endothelial blockade.

Not all intravenous particles distribute competitively between liver, spleen and bone marrow. Particles can be designed which are taken up preferentially into either liver or spleen. The best documented examples are own red cells whose surface has been altered in vitro before reinfusion. This type of study has been performed in a number of ways (see section 4.2 below). Because organ uptake studies using intravenous exogenous particles have provided the most direct information about mechanisms of RE-mediated blood clearance in humans, these studies will be reviewed next.

4. Organ distribution of exogenous particles after intravenous injection

Most of these agents were developed in order to investigate the nature of RE-mediated blood clearance.

4.1. Albumin

In many respects, heat-aggregated albumin seemed to be the ideal agent to study RE clearance in man. After intravenous injection the particles are cleared into liver, spleen and bone marrow (Benacerraf et al., 1957) and the material is non-antigenic. Unfortunately the mechanism of clearance is not known. Aggregated particles can attract a coating of plasma constituents (Molnar et al., 1979). It is probably not lectin-mediated. In dogs and man, Wagner and his colleagues showed that there was a Lineweaver-Burke double reciprocal relationship between the administered dose of albumin and the rate of removal from the circulation (Iio and Wagner, 1963; Wagner et al., 1963). Others disagree (Drivas and Wardle, 1978). Standardised albumin microspheres are now available commercially for studies in humans but the clearance of these is not always the same as that for heat-aggregated albumin. For instance, preliminary experiments in rats and mice have failed to demonstrate any saturation phenomena when using albumin microspheres compared with those seen after large doses of heat-aggregated albumin (Scheffel and Bradfield, unpublished results). Similar preparations of aggregated albumin have been made using glutaraldehyde cross-linkage as the aggregating agent (Berghem et al., 1976). Reticulo-endothelial blockade has been induced in man using heat-aggregated albumin intravenously, with no apparent ill effects (Wagner and Iio, 1964), although studies in animals and man suggest that the blockade may have been specific for albumin only (Iio and Wagner, 1963; Wagner and Iio, 1964).

4.2. Altered own red cells

Own red cells provide readily available, non-toxic particles which can be easily labelled and reinjected. They have the advantage that if specific changes can be made in the membrane such that RE-mediated clearance is induced, then this provides a very precise probe for the investigation of mechanisms of recognition and clearance by the reticulo-endothelial system.

4.2.1. Heat treatment

After mild heat treatment in vitro the re-injection of red cells in humans results in their sequestration in the spleen (Harris et al., 1957; Wagner et al., 1962b; Pettit, 1977). Previous splenectomy results in prolonged circulation with slow accumulation in the liver (Wagner et al., 1962a; Marsh et al., 1966). More severe heat treatment, still short of haemolysis, produces further membrane change. After reinfusion these cells are removed rapidly from the circulation due to sequestration in the liver (Wagner et al., 1962b). The kinetics of blood clearance and organ uptake can be quantitated using a dynamic data accumulation system (Wagner et al., 1962b; Bowring et al., 1976).

4.2.2. Sulphydryl reagents

A similar organ distribution to either spleen or liver can be achieved by treating the person's own red cells with a sulphydryl reagent, such as N-ethylmaleimide. Gentle treatment results in splenic sequestration after reinjection; more severe treatment leads to hepatic uptake (Wagner et al., 1962b).

4.2.3. Antibody or complementing coating

Studies in animals initially showed that when autologous red cells were coated with a low concentration of non-complement-fixing IgG and reinjected, the main site of clearance was into the spleen, whereas coating with complement-fixing IgM caused sequestration in the liver (Schreiber and Frank 1972a, b). A similar sequence holds for humans, and spleen-seeking (Jandl, 1955; Hughes-Jones et al., 1957; Jaffe et al., 1978; Frank et al., 1979; Lockwood et al., 1979) or liver-seeking (Jaffe et al., 1978; Frank et al., 1977) altered red cells have been produced in this way. Spleen sequestration appears to be mediated via Fc receptors whereas liver sequestration seems to be complement-mediated. This seems to be in contrast to the removal of soluble immune complexes, which is mainly into liver by an Fc-mediated, complement-independent mechanism (Arend and Mannik, 1971). The role of complement in blood clearance of immune complexes is further complicated by the observation that complement may prevent removal at some sites (Skogh and Stendahl, 1983).

From these studies it is clear that the use of monoclonal or polyclonal antibodies to target microspheres to sites other than the reticulo-endothelial system requires exposure of the Fab portion without allowing Fc recognition (see later parts of this volume).

4.2.4. Alteration of surface sugars

Own red cells have formed an important probe for investigating the role of surface sugars in the removal of material from the blood. When animal autologous red cells are treated in vitro with neuraminidase, to remove sialic acid, and reinfused, there is rapid sequestration in the liver and spleen (Gregoriadis et al., 1974; Aminoff et al., 1977). In the liver this appears to be due to ingestion by Kupffer cells (Jancik et al., 1978). Subsequently, it has been shown that the removal of sialic acid to expose terminal galactosyl residues will result in hepatocyte uptake, whereas the further sequential removal of the surface galactose to reveal N-acetylglucosamine or mannose results in uptake by Kupffer cells and endothelial cells. These results considerably complicate the interpretation of data concerning the clearance of immunoglobulin-coated particles since the latter are glycoproteins. The increasing literature on carbohydrate-mediated clearance of immune complexes on the one hand (Day et al., 1980; Thornburg et al., 1980) and Fc-mediated clearance of desialated particles on the other (Rosenberg and Rogentine, 1972; Winchester et al., 1975) shows that this relationship is far from simple.

4.3. Lipids and lipoproteins

Many types of lipid emulsion are removed from the circulation by sinus-lining macrophages, although sieving through pores in the fenestrated endothelium is a second well-documented mechanism of removal in the liver (Wisse et al., 1980; and see this volume). A gelatinised glycerol corn oil has been used to measure RE-mediated blood clearance in man (Salky et al., 1964). Other preparations based on cotton seed oil (Biozzi et al., 1963) and soya bean oil (Lemperle and Denk, 1970; Lemperle et al., 1971) have also been used. More recently the commercially available product 'Intralipid' has attracted increasing interest, but it is unclear whether or not this agent is removed from the blood by RE-mediated blood clearance (Di Luzio, 1972; Jarstrand et al., 1978). In animals clearance is stimulated by treatment with *Corynebacterium parvum*, which causes enhancement of Re-mediated clearance. There is controversy as to whether overload by Intralipid can lead to reticulo-endothelial blockade (Jarstrad et al., 1978; Bradfield, 1980a; Fischer et al., 1980a).

The clearance of lipoproteins by Kupffer cells of the liver has been reviewed recently (Van Berkel et al., 1982). Using in vivo clearance and uptake studies plus in vitro experiments, at least three types of receptor have been identified. There is considerable evidence for independent lipid- and apoprotein-mediated uptake by Kupffer cells.

4.4. Polyvinylpyrrolidone (PVP)

Polyvinylpyrrolidone is a rather heterogenous preparation which has been used as a plasma substitute. In mice (Morgan and Soothill, 1975a) and rats (Regoeczi, 1976) blood clearance is into the liver and spleen, and this can be slowed by pretreating the animals with carbon or PVP. These results prompted a study which showed a relationship between PVP clearance and affinity of anti-protein antibody in several different strains of mice (Passwell et al., 1974; Morgan and Soothill, 1975b). However, there is considerable doubt as to whether clearance is RE-mediated and, if so, whether this is by phagocytosis or fluid phase pinocytosis (Minniksona et al., 1980).

4.5. Liposomes

Liposomes are uni- or multilamella spherules. Their fate after intravenous injection depends mainly on the lipid composition of the outermost layer (Richardson et al., 1978). The main sites of uptake after intravenous injection are liver and spleen (Gregoriadis and Ryman 1972; McDougall et al., 1975; Dunnick and Kriss, 1977; Hinkle et al., 1978; Finkelstein and Weissman, 1978), where they can be vizualised within macrophages (Segal et al., 1974; Tanaka et al., 1975). In man, uptake of one liposome preparation was into liver and spleen (Richardson et al., 1979), although liver uptake may have been into hepatocytes (Gregoriadis et al., 1974). The problems of designing liposomes which will escape clearance by the reticulo-endothelial system (Hnatowich and Clancy, 1980) will not be reviewed comprehensively in this chapter.

4.6. Sulphur colloid

After intravenous injection in humans ^{99}Tc-sulphur colloid is rapidly taken up into liver, spleen and bone marrow. It has been suggested (Dornfest and Lipp, 1975; Rai et al., 1977) that as this agent is removed by reticulo-endothelial clearance it might constitute a good test agent of this function. However, there are doubts (Chanduri et al., 1973) as to whether the material is cleared by RE-phagocytosis, since clearance can be relatively normal in the presence of blockade (Quinones, 1973; Haibach et al., 1975; Bradfield and Wagner, 1977). Possibly the uptake into Kupffer cell is by fluid-phase pinocytosis (George et al., 1980).

5. Serum factors in the blood clearance of exogenous particles

Serum factors which promote phagocytosis are called opsonins, and these will enhance the clearance of blood-borne material by RE-mediated uptake. It has become traditional to divide opsonins into immune and non-immune. The first major assessment of serum factors in clearance and in the phenomenon of reticulo-endothelial blockade was by Saba (1970), and since then their role has received increasing attention.

5.1. Immune opsonins

The effects of immunoglobulin and complement on RE-mediated blood clearance have been discussed above, in relation to the clearance of particulate complexes in the form both of immunoglobulin-coated own red cells and soluble immune complexes. In animals, Kupffer cells have been isolated and studied in culture. Their membranes express receptors for the Fc component of immunoglobulin and/or for the C3 component of complement (Munthe-Kaas 1976; Munthe-Kaas et al., 1976; Steer et al., 1979; Seljelid, 1980). Using Kupffer cells from animals, scanning electron microscopy suggests that phagocytosis mediated by Fc receptors differs in appearance from that mediated by complement (Munthe-Kaas et al., 1976; Seljelid, 1980). Failure of clearance of blood-borne immune complexes due to complement deficiency has been documented in both animals (Brown et al., 1970; Schreiber and Frank, 1972b) and man (Atkinson and Frank, 1974). Ia antigens are also expressed on Kupffer cells in animals (Widman et al., 1978; Forsum et al., 1979; Richman et al., 1979; Rogoff and Lipsky, 1979; Rogoff et al., 1979), but it is not known whether this is important for immune clearance. After adherence mediated by C3b there may be cleavage of this component on the surface of the particle so that the latter, now coated with C3d, is released back into the blood for prolonged circulation (Atkinson and Frank, 1974).

5.2. Non-immune opsonins

Of the possible other circulating factors which contribute to opsonic blood clearance the best documented is plasma fibronectin. This long-chain glycoprotein is found within cells, on cell surfaces and in plasma, where it circulates as a dimer of 450,000 molecular weight (McDonagh, 1981). In animals RES blockade correlates with depletion of plasma fibronectin and recovery is associated with return to normal levels (Blumenstock et al., 1977). Patients with sepsis or trauma have reduced levels of circulating fibronectin (Scovill et al., 1977), which can be corrected by infusing a cryoprecipitate containing this opsonin (Saba et al., 1978). The physiological role of plasma fibronectin is not known, although its ability to opsonise fibrin monomers and microaggregates and its affinity for collagen (Kaplan, 1980) plus its depletion during disseminated intravascular coagulation (Stathakis et al., 1981) all suggest that it is important in the clearance of products of thrombosis.

Many substances, when introduced into the bloodstream, cause thrombus formation on their surface, either as aggregated platelets or as deposition of fibrin. These adherent products can then act as opsonins by enhancing clearance, although it is unclear whether this is fibronectin-mediated, or is even a function of reticulo-endothelial cells (for reviews, see Bradfield, 1974; Jones and Summerfield, 1982).

6. Strategies in the design of microspheres for intravenous injection in man

There are two completely opposing reasons for wanting to inject particulate agents intravenously into humans. The first is to concentrate the material in the liver, spleen and bone marrow. For this, effective and rapid reticulo-endothelial-mediated blood clearance is an advantage. Potential uses of such agents include the following:

(a) The delivery of imaging agents to the liver, spleen and bone marrow. Effective and ethically acceptable agents, such as labelled sulphur colloid, tin sulphur colloid and particulate preparations of albumin, are in widespread use in diagnostic departments of nuclear medicine. Microspheres have not, so far, been widely exploited for this.

(b) The delivery of therapeutic agents to the reticulo-endothelial cells of the liver. Recently it has been shown, in animals, that if anti-leishmanial drugs are enclosed within liposomes for intravenous injection, the concentration of drug achieved in the reticulo-endothelial cells carrying the parasites is more than 100 times that found after the injection of the drugs alone (New et al., 1978; Alving et al., 1978).

(c) The assessment of RES function in blood clearance. Several methods for doing this have been covered in the present chapter, and the subject has been reviewed fully elsewhere (Bradfield, 1980c; Jones and Summerfield, 1982; Bradfield, 1984).

(d) The slow release of active agents by allowing breakdown of the carrier microsphere after uptake into lysosomal phagosomes in macrophages.

(e) The delivery of enzymes to macrophages in order to provide replacement of cell deficiencies.

The second reason for wanting to inject particulate agents intravenously in humans is to achieve enhanced uptake in a site or sites other than the reticulo-endothelial system, for instance in a tumour. For this type of agent to be effective it is necessary to abrogate the reticulo-endothelial-mediated clearance in order to achieve prolonged circulation in the blood and thence opportunity for adequate sequestration in the target tissue. Several approaches are possible and these include the following:

(a) Attempts can be made to suppress RE clearance by pretreating the host with an RE-blockading agent. In animal models, substances such as carbon, methyl palmitate, latex beads, dextran sulphate and unlabelled liposomes (Gregoriadis and Neerunjun, 1974; Tanaka et al., 1975; Caride et al., 1976; Souhami et al., 1981; Proffitt et al., 1983) have been used to keep subsequently injected liposomes out of the liver. Similarly, heat-aggregated albumin has been used to cause RE blockade in man (Wagner and Iio, 1964), although it is not known whether this would lead to prolongation of the clearance time of microspheres injected thereafter.

(b) The surface conformation of the proposed particles can be modified in order to make them less susceptible to RE clearance. Important variables include size, surface charge and the exact nature of the exposed surface groups including sugars. Attempts to reduce the attractiveness of particles to the cells of the RES forms the basis of other presentations in this volume. If the injected particles acquire a coating of certain serum factors then these can act as opsonins and lead to accelerated RE-mediated clearance. The testing of microspheres for their propensity to become coated by immunoglobulin, complement, fibronectin and fibrin is an important stage in the assessment of new agents. Because a coating of sialic acid is known to inhibit the clearance of red cells from blood, erythrocyte membrane sialoglycoprotein has been incorporated into liposomes in order to enhance their prolonged circulation in blood (Utsumi et al., 1983). This system has not, as yet, been tested in vivo, and its applicability to microspheres is not known.

(c) Specific uptake of particles in the required target tissue can be enhanced by incorporating target-specific antibody into the surface membrane of the injected agent, or trapping can be accentuated by applying an appropriately arranged local magnetic field during the intravenous injection of magnetically responsive microspheres.

7. Conclusions

There are often great advantages to be gained by incorporating active agents into carrier microspheres for injection into the bloodstream, compared with the injection of the agents themselves. However, once in the blood the fate of any particles is dominated by the ability of the RE system to clear such material rapidly into liver, spleen and bone marrow. Recent increase in the understanding of how this clearance is mediated is allowing manipulation of both particles and host so as to enhance or prevent reticulo-endothelial-mediated blood clearance to suit the objectives of the injection.

35

References

AlvingAlving, C.R., Steck, E.A., Chapman, W.E., Waits, V.B., Hendricks, L.D., Swartz, G.M. and Hanson, W.L. (1978) Proc. Natl. Acad. Sci. U.S.A. 75, 2959–2963.

Aminoff, D., Vorder Bruegge, W.F., Bell, W.C., Sarpolis, K. and Williams, R. (1977) Proc. Natl. Acad. Sci. U.S.A. 74, 1521–1524.

Arend, W.P. and Mannik, M. (1971) J. Immunol. 107, 63–75.

Aschoff, L. (1924) Lectures on Pathology, pp. 1–33, Paul Hoeber Inc, New York.

Atkinson, J.P. and Frank, M.M. (1974) J. Clin. Invest. 54, 339–348.

Benacerraf, B., Biozzi, G., Halpern, B.N., Stiffel, C. and Mouton, C. (1957) Br. J. Exp. Pathol. 38, 35–48.

Berghem, L., Denker, L., Hoglund, S. and Schildt, B. (1976) Scand. J. Clin. Lab. Invest. 36, 849–856.

Biozzi, G., Stiffel, C. and Mouton, D. (1963) Rev. Franc. Etude. Clin. Biol. 8, 341.

Blumenstock, F.A., Weber, P., Saba, T.M. and Laffin, R. (1977) Am. J. Physiol. 232, R80–R87.

Bowring, C.S., Glass, H.I. and Lewis, S.M. (1976) J. Clin. Pathol. 29, 852–854.

Bradfield, J.W.B. (1974) Lancet 2, 883–886.

Bradfield, J.W.B. (1980a) Lancet 2, 1138.

Bradfield, J.W.B. (1980b) Br. J. Exp. Pathol. 61, 617–623.

Bradfield, J.W.B. (1980c) in The Reticulo-endothelial System and the Pathogenesis of Liver Disease (Liehr, H. and Grun, M., Eds.), pp. 309–316, Elsevier, Amsterdam.

Bradfield, J.W.B. (1984) in The Reticulo-endothelial System: A Comprehensive Treatise. Vol. 7B, Physiology (Reichard, S. and Filkins, J., Eds.), pp. 189–222, Plenum Press, New York.

Bradfield, J.W.B. and Wagner, H.N. (1977) J. Nucl. Med. 18, 620.

Brown, D.L., Lachmann, P.J. and Dacie, J.W. (1970) Clin. Exp. Immunol. 7, 401–421.

Caride, V.J., Taylor, W., Cramer, J.A. and Gottschalk, A. (1976) J. Nucl. Med. 17, 1067–1072.

Chauduri, T.K., Evans, T.C. and Chauduri, T.C. (1973) Radiology 109, 633–637.

Day, J.F., Thornburg, R.W., Thorpe, S.R. and Baynes, J.W. (1980) J. Biol. Chem. 255, 2360–2365.

Di Luzio, N.R. (1972) Adv. Lipid. Res. 10, 43–88.

Dornfest, B.S. and Lipp, C. (1975) J. Reticuloendothel. Soc. 17, 274–281.

Drivas, G. and Wardle, E.N. (1978) Metabolism 27, 1533–1538.

Dunnick, J.K. and Kriss, J.P. (1977) J. Nucl. Med. 18, 183–186.

Finkelstein, M. and Weissman, G. (1978) J. Lipid. Res. 19, 289–303.

Fischer, G.W., Hunter, K.W., Wilson, S.R. and Mease, A.D. (1980a) Lancet 2, 819–820.

Fischer, G.W., Hunter, K.W. and Wilson, S.R. (1980b) Lancet 2, 1300.

Forsum, U., Klareskog, L. and Peterson, R.A. (1979) Scand. J. Immunol. 9, 343–349.

Frank, M.M., Schreiber, A.D., Atkinson, J.P. and Jaffe, C.J. (1977) Ann. Int. Med. 87, 210–222.

Frank, M.M., Hamburger, M.I., Lawley, T.J., Kimberley, R.P. and Plotz, R.M., (1979) N. Engl. J. Med. 300, 518–523.

George, E.A., Henderschott, L.R., Klos, D.J. and Donati, R.M. (1980) Eur. J. Nucl. Med. 5, 241–245.

Gregoriadis, G. and Neerunjun, D.E. (1974) Eur. J. Biochem. 47, 179–185.

Gregoriadis, G. and Ryman, B.E. (1972) Eur. J. Biochem. 24, 485–491.

Gregoriadis, G., Swain, C.P., Willis, E.J. and Tavill, A.S. (1974) Lancet 1, 1313–1316.

Haibach, H., George, E.S., Hendershott, L.R. and Donati, R.M. (1975) J. Nucl. Med. 16, 532.

Halpern, B.N. (1957) Physiopathology of the Reticulo-endothelium: A Symposium. Blackwell Scientific Publications, Oxford.

Harris, I.M., McAlister, J.M. and Prankerd, T.A.J. (1957) Clin. Sci. 16, 223–230.

Hinkle, G.M., Born, G.S., Kessler, W.V. and Shaw, S.M. (1978) J. Pharm. Sci. 67, 795–798.

Hnatowich, D.J. and Clancy, B. (1980) J. Nucl. Med. 21, 662–669.

Hughes-Jones, N.C., Mollison, P.L. and Veall, N. (1957) Br. J. Haematol. 3, 125–133.

Iio, M. and Wagner, H.N. (1963) J. Clin. Invest. 42, 417–426.

Jaffe, C.J., Vierling, J.M., Jones, E.A., Lawley, T.J. and Frank, M.M. (1978) J. Clin. Invest. 62, 1069–1077.

36

Jaffe, R.H. (1931) Physiol. Rev. 11, 277–327.

Jancik, J.M., Schauer, R., Andres, K.H. and Von Düring, M. (1978) Cell Tissue Res. 186, 209–226.

Jandl, J.H. (1955) J. Clin. Invest. 34, 912.

Jarstrand, C., Berghem, L. and Lahnborg, G. (1978) J. Parenternal. Enteral Nutrition. 2, 663–670.

Jones, E.A. and Summerfield, J.A. (1982) in The Liver: Biology and Pathobiology (Arias, I., Popper, H., Schachter, D. and Shafritz, D.A., Eds.), pp. 507–523, Raven Press, New York.

Kaplan, J.E. (1980) in The Reticulo-endothelial System and Liver Disease (Liehr, H. and Grun, M., Eds.), pp. 55–67, Elsevier, Amsterdam.

Lemperle, G. and Denk, S. (1970) Therapie Woche 20, 1266–1268.

Lemperle, G., Reichelt, M. and Denk, S. (1971) in The Reticulo-endothelial System and Immune Phenomena (Di Luzio, N.R., Ed.), pp. 137–143, Plenum Press, New York.

Lepehne, G. (1921) Ergels. Inn. Med. u. Kinderkeilk 10, 221–228.

Lockwood, C.M., Worlledge, S., Nicholas, A., Cotton, C. and Peters, D.K. (1979) N. Engl. J. Med. 300, 524–530.

Marsh, G.W., Lewis, S.M. and Szur, L. (1966) Br. J. Haem. 12, 161–166.

McDonagh, J. (1981) Arch. Pathol. Lab. Med. 105, 393–396.

McDougall, I.R., Dunnick, J.K., Goris, D.M. and Kriss, J.P. (1975) J. Nucl. Med. 16, 48.

Minniksona, J., Noteborn, M., Kooistra, T., Steinstra, S., Bouna, J.M.W., Gruber, M., Brouwer, A., Praaning-Van Dalen, D. and Knook, D.L. (1980) Biochem. J. 192, 613–621.

Molnar, J., Mclaín, S., Allen, C., Laga, H., Gara, A. and Gelder, F. (1977) Biochim. Biophys. Acta. 493. 37–54.

Morgan, A.G. and Soothill, J.F. (1975a) Clin. Exp. Immunol. 20, 489–498.

Morgan, A.G. and Soothill, J.F. (1975b) Nature 254, 711;712

Munthe-Kaas, A.C. (1976) Exp. Cell. Res. 99, 319–327.

Munthe-Kaas, A.C., Kaplan, C. and Seljelid, R. (1976) Exp. Cell. Res. 103, 201–212.

New, R.R.C., Chance, M.L., Thomas, S.C. and Peters, W. (1978) Nature 272, 55–56.

Passwell, J.H., Steward, M.W. and Soothill, J.F. (1974) Clin. Exp. Immunol. 17, 159–167.

Pettit, J.E. (1977) Clin. Haematol. 6, 639–656.

Proffitt, R.T., Williams, L.E., Presant, C.A., Tin, G.W., Uliana, J.A., Gamble, R.C. and Baldeschwieler, J.D. (1983) Science 220, 502–505.

Quinones, J.D. (1973) J. Nucl. Med. 14, 443–444.

Rai, G.S., Haggith, J., Fenwick, J. and James, O. (1977) Gut 18, 417.

Regoeczi, E. (1976) Br. J. Exp. Pathol. 57, 431–442.

Richardson, V.J., Jeyasingh, K., Jewkes, R.F., Ryman, B.E. and Tattersale, M.N.H. (1978) J. Nucl. Med. 19, 1049–1054.

Richardson, V.J., Ryman, B.E., Jewkes, R.F., Jeyasingh, K., Tattersall, M.N.H., Newlands, E.S. and Kaye, S.B. (1979) Br. J. Cancer 40, 35–43.

Richman, L.K., Klingenstein, R.J., Richman, J.A., Strober, W. and Berkofsky, J.A. (1979) J. Immunol. 123, 2602–2609.

Rogoff, T.M. and Lipsky, P.E. (1979) J. Immunol. 123, 1920–1927.

Rogoff, T.M., Vitetta, E.S. and Lipsky, P.E. (1979) Gastroenterology 77, A35.

Rosenberg, S.A. and Rogentine, G.N. (1972) Nature New Biol. 239, 203–204.

Saba, T.M. (1970) Arch. Int. Med. 126, 1031;1052.

Saba, T.M., Blumenstock, F.A., Scovill, W.A. and Bernard, H. (1978) Science 201, 622–624.

Salky, N.K., Di Luzio, N.R., P'Bool, D.B. and Sutherland, A.J. (1964) J. Am. Med. Assoc. 187, 744–748.

Schreiber, A.D. and Frank, M.M. (1972a) J. Clin. Invest. 51, 575–582.

Schreiber, A.D. and Frank, M.H. (1972b) J. Clin. Invest. 51, 583–589.

Scovill, W.A., Saba, T.M., Kaplan, J.E., Bernard, H. and Powers, S.R. (1977) J. Surg. Res. 22, 709–716.

Segal, A.W., Willa, E.J., Richmon, J.E., Slavin, G., Black, C.D.V. and Gregoriadis, G. (1974) Br. J. Exp. Pathol. 55, 320–327.

Seljelid, R. (1980) in Mononuclear Phagocytes (Van Furth, R., Ed.), pp. 157–202, Martinus Nijhof, The Hague.

Skogh, T. and Stendahl, O. (1983) Immunology 49, 53–59.

Souhami, R.L., Patel, H.M. and Ryman, B.E. (1981) Biochim. Biophys. Acta. 674, 354–371.

Stakhakis, N.E., Fountas, A. and Tsianos, E. (1981) J. Clin. Pathol. 34, 504–508.

Steer, C.J., Richman, L.K., Hague, N.E. and Richman, J.A. (1979) Gastroenterology 75, 988 (Abstr.).

Tanaka, T., Taneda, K., Kobayashi, H., Okumura, K., Muramishi, S. and Sesaki, H. (1975) Chem. Pharm. Bull (Tokyo) 23, 3069–3074.

Thornburg, R.W., Day, J.F., Baynes, J.W. and Thorpe, S.R. (1980) J. Biol. Chem. 255, 6820–6825.

Utsumi, S., Shinomiya, H., Minami, J. and Sonoda, S. (1983) Immunology 49, 113–120.

Van Berkel, T.J.C., Nagelkirke, K.P. and Harkes, L. (1982) in Sinusoidal Liver Cells (Knook, D.L. and Wisse, E., Eds.), pp. 305–318, Elsevier Biomedical, Amsterdam.

Van Furth, R. (1970) Mononuclear Phagocytes, Blackwell Scientific Publications, Oxford. Later editions were published in 1975 and 1980.

Wagner, H.N. and Iio, M. (1964) J. Clin. Invest. 43, 1525–1532.

Wagner, H.N., McAfee, J.G. and Winkelman, J.W. (1962a) Arch. Int. Med. 109, 673–684.

Wagner, H.N., Razzak, M.A., Gaertner, R.A., Caine, N.P. and Feagin, O.T. (1962b) Arch. Int. Med. 110, 90–135.

Wagner, H.N., Iio, M. and Hornick, R.B. (1963) J. Clin. Invest. 42, 427–434.

Widman, K., Curman, B., Forsum, H., Klareskog, L., Malmnas-Tjernlund, U., Rask, L., Tragardh, L. and Peterson, P.A. (1978) Nature 276, 711–713.

Winchester, R.J., Fu, S.M., Winfeld, J.B. and Kunkel, H.G. (1975) J. Immunol. 114, 410–414.

Wisse, E., Van Dierendonck, J.H., De Zanger, R.B., Fraser, R. and McCuskey, R.S. (1980) in Communications of Liver Cells. Falk Symposium 27 (Popper, H., Bianchi, L., Gudad, F. and Reutter, W., Eds.), pp. 195–200, MTP Press Ltd., Lancaster.

Microspheres and Drug Therapy. Pharmaceutical, Immunological and Medical Aspects
edited by S.S. Davis, L. Illum, J.G. McVie and E. Tomlinson
© *1984, Elsevier Science Publishers B.V.*

39

CHAPTER 3

Physicochemical aspects of the behaviour of biological components at solid/liquid interfaces

Willem Norde

1. Introduction

A synthetic material brought into a biological environment induces various surface phenomena. First, if the material contacts a biofluid, biological components may be transferred from the solution, to accumulate at the surface. Second, if the material is supplied as a dispersion of fine particles, the particles may deposit at the phase boundaries they encounter. These interfacial phenomena are of great importance, not only in the application of synthetic microspheres in drug therapy but also in various other branches of (medical) biology and technology, such as cardiovascular surgery, dental plaque formation, opthalmology (dry spot formation on contact lenses), serological tests, etc.

The physical binding of molecules on a surface is referred to as *adsorption*. For the interfacial accumulation of particles the terms *deposition* and *adhesion* are used. Deposition refers to the settling of the particles at the surface, whereas adhesion is defined by the force to remove the particles. The processes of deposition and adhe-

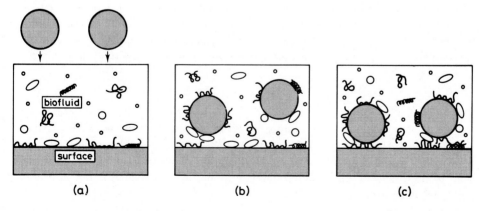

Figure 1. (a) Injection of particles in a biofluid contacting a surface that is covered with a layer of adsorbed material. (b) Adsorption of (macro)molecules from the fluid onto the particles. (c) Deposition of the particles on the surface.

sion are in most cases not similarly reversible, because after deposition has occurred short-range interactions may affect the adhesive bond.

The diffusion of (macro)molecules proceeds much faster than that of the larger particles, so that the rate of adsorption of the molecules on the particles is much higher than the deposition rate of the particles themselves. As a consequence, particles that are placed in a biological environment are usually covered with an adsorbed layer before they deposit at any surface that is also loaded with an adsorbed layer. Therefore, the adhesion characteristics may be largely determined by the properties of the adsorbed layer. This sequence of events is shown in Figure 1.

With respect to the application of microspheres in drug therapy, the special requirements of drug availability and biodegradability of the carrier material may be largely affected by the formation of the adsorbed layer.

However, it is clear that the systems under consideration are far too complex and too ill-defined to allow a quantitative analysis of the interfacial events. Nevertheless, the application of physicochemical theories that have been developed for much simpler, well-defined, model systems is helpful in providing some insight into the interactions at biosurfaces.

2. The interfacial behaviour of biological molecules

Biofluids contain dissolved molecules that range from the simple and small, such as low-molecular-weight ions, to the large, complicated macromolecules. It is the last-mentioned group, i.e. polymeric material, that is particularly surface-active. In discussing polymer adsorption we shall distinguish between two limiting cases: (i) flexible, highly solvated polymers and (ii) polymers that have a rigid, compact structure due to their strong internal coherence. Such a sharp distinction is only made to facilitate the discussion. In reality, many biopolymers adopt an intermediate structure. For instance, glycoproteins consist of a compact protein part and a flexible polysaccharide part. The present paper is aimed only at indicating trends. Comprehensive treatment of this subject has been given by Miller and Bach (1973), Vincent and Whittington (1981), MacRitchie (1978), Fleer and Lyklema (1983), Hesselink (1983) and Norde (1985).

2.1. Flexible polymers

The polymers belonging to this category adopt a loose, random coil-like structure. However, at a submolecular level local ordering such as α-helices or β-sheets may exist. Examples of such polymers are various polysaccharides, such as amylose, dextran, hyaluronic acid, etc., non-globular proteins, such as β-casein, and also denatured, unfolded proteins.

A general characteristic of polymer adsorption is the relatively large amount that can be accomodated at the sorbent surface. The reason is that only a fraction of the polymer is actually attached at the surface (trains), whereas the remainder protrudes

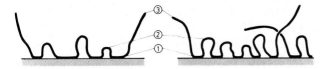

Figure 2. Possible conformations of adsorbed, flexible, highly solvated polymer molecules, 1, Trains; 2, loops; 3, tails. Note that the fraction of the polymer that is attached to the sorbent surface decreases with increasing amount of polymer adsorbed.

into the solution (loops and tails). Thus, depending on the surface concentration, the adsorbed polymer may attain a conformation such as that illustrated schematically in Figure 2.

Unlike low-molecular-weight materials, polymers do not readily desorb on rinsing with the pure solvent. This is because the polymer molecule is attached to the surface at several contact points. Desorption would imply the simultaneous detachment of all these contacts, which is statistically highly improbable. However, individual segments of the polymer chain attach and detach reversibly, involving a free energy of adsorption that may be only little more than that of their thermal motion. For that reason, polymers can be displaced by other (macro)molecules that adsorb with a larger segmental free energy. Such competitive adsorption processes are especially relevant in biological systems where, as a rule, various surface-active species are mutually present. It is likely that in these systems the population at the sorbent surface and, hence, in the solution changes with time, leading to a final state in which the component having the highest *molar* adsorption free energy resides at the surface. Transferring a polymer molecule from solution to an interface often affects its conformation, and on subsequent displacement of that molecule from the surface it may not (fully) rearrange into its original structure. This has been observed to different extents with various proteins (Soderquist and Walton, 1980; Chan and Brash, 1981).

In view of the structure-function relation, biopolymers that are adsorbed and eventually desorbed may have altered biological properties. A drug that is bound to a microsphere by physical adsorption will, after administration to the patient, be subjected to displacement by other substances. This is a crucial aspect in the design of controlled release systems.

As a result of the large number of attached segments, polymer molecules generally show a high affinity for surfaces, even if the adsorption free energy for the individual segments is low. The high affinity is reflected in the adsorption isotherm, where the adsorbed amount Γ is plotted against the polymer concentration c_p in the solution at equilibrium. A typical isotherm is given in Figure 3. At low polymer dosage all the material is adsorbed, until the surface is fully covered; the initial part of the isotherm merges with the ordinate axis. At higher polymer concentrations, where Γ increases slightly, a smaller part of the molecule is attached to the surface and, hence, a larger part is dangling in the solution (see Fig. 2). In the semi-plateau region of the isotherm Γ usually attains a few mg per m^2 sorbent surface. This region is further

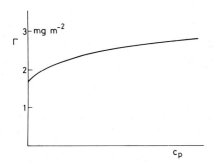

Figure 3. Typical adsorption isotherm for a flexible polymer. The values at the ordinate axis have only a qualitative meaning.

characterized by an attached fraction of 0.5–0.1 and an adsorbed layer of a thickness of 5–50 nm.

It is virtually impossible to describe the exact structural arrangement in the adsorbed layer due to the continuous motion of the segments. Moreover, such an 'instant' picture has little practical value. It is more realistic to find a statistical average for the distribution of the segments over the trains, loops and tails. Such statistical theories have been developed over the last two decades (e.g., Hoeve, 1966, 1970, 1971; Silberberg 1968; Roe, 1974; Scheutjens and Fleer, 1979, 1980). For uncharged homopolymers (polymers of only one type of monomer) the most recent theories give satisfactory predictions.

Most biopolymers are less simple. For instance, they usually carry charged groups. With such polyelectrolytes the adsorption mechanism is much more complex because, in addition to chemical interactions, electrostatic interactions must be taken into account. Recently, some attempts have been made to incorporate electrostatic interactions in polymer adsorption theories (Hesselink, 1977; Van der Schee and Lyklema, 1984).

As mentioned above, most biological polymers are electrically charged and the same is true for the surfaces to which they are exposed. Then, both *inter*molecular and *intra*molecular electrostatic interactions play a role in the adsorption process. Intramolecular interactions refer to interactions between charged groups within the same polymer molecule and intermolecular to those between different molecules and between a polyelectrolyte molecule and the sorbent surface. The range of the interaction between two charges is twice the Debye length, κ^{-1}, which, in turn, is determined by the composition of the medium

$$\kappa = \left(\frac{e^2}{\varepsilon \varepsilon_0 k T} \sum_i c_i z_i^2 \right)^{1/2} \qquad \{1\}$$

where e is the elementary charge, $\varepsilon \varepsilon_0$ the dielectric permittivity of the medium, k the Boltzmann constant, T the absolute temperature, c_i and z_i the concentration and

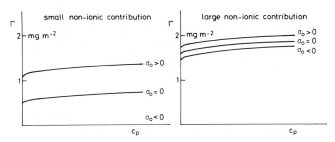

Figure 4. Adsorption of a negatively charged polyelectrolyte on surfaces of different charge densities, σ_0. Values at the ordinate axis are only qualitative indications.

valency, respectively, of the ionic species, i. Thus, the range of the electrostatic interaction decreases with increasing ionic strength. For instance, in blood, having an ionic strength of approximately 0.15 M, it is less than 1 nm.

It is obvious that adsorption is promoted by charges of opposite sign on the polyelectrolyte and the sorbent. When electrostatic factors dominate, the amount adsorbed decreases with increasing ionic strength (Froehling et al., 1977), leading to desorption if the non-ionic contributions oppose the adsorption process. However, if the main driving force for adsorption is of a non-ionic nature, the adsorbed mass tends to increase with increasing ionic strength (Lipatov et al., 1978) due to reduced lateral repulsion between the adsorbed polyelectrolyte molecules. In those cases where the charged polymer and the sorbent have the same sign adsorption only occurs if the electrostatic repulsion is outweighed by non-ionic attraction. Increasing the ionic strength again results in larger amounts adsorbed (Peyser and Ullmann, 1965; Böhm, 1974). The effects of the electrostatic and the chemical contributions are illustrated in Figure 4. Note that the influence of electrostatic interactions is less pronounced if the energy of chemical adsorption is relatively large.

Another important variable in polyelectrolyte adsorption is the degree of ionization of the polymer. As a rule, the amount adsorbed decreases with increasing ionization. This is caused by a stronger intermolecular repulsion. With ambivalent polyelectrolytes, like proteins, the plateau value of the adsorption isotherm is often found to be at a maximum in the isoelectric region of the molecule (e.g., Maternaghan and Ottewill, 1974) (for further discussion, see section 2.2). Furthermore, if the charged polyelectrolyte and the sorbent have the same charge, attachment of polymer segments is more difficult to realize at higher ionizations. This may ultimately result in desorption (Pavlovic and Miller, 1971; Joppien, 1978). The interpretation of the influence of ionization on the adsorption behaviour may be complicated by structural transitions in the polymer molecule. At low charge densities many polyelectrolytes attain a compact structure that changes into an extended conformation at high degrees of ionization. For example, various polyamino acids dissolved in an aqueous medium show charge-induced helix-to-coil transitions. In the adsorbed state such structural alterations may be more or less hampered (e.g., Bonekamp, 1984).

Finally, it should be mentioned that, in addition to the general effect of the ionic strength, polyelectrolyte adsorption may be drastically influenced by the type of small ions that are present in solution. More specifically, unlike monovalent ions, divalent and multivalent ions may form bridges between like charges on the polyelectrolyte and the sorbent surface, thus stabilizing the adsorptive bond.

2.2. Rigid compact polymers

The main examples in this group are the globular proteins. Special attention will be paid to their adsorption behaviour since in biological fluids these proteins are abundant.

The compact structure of proteins is stabilized by hydrogen bonds, ion pairs and, in an aqueous medium, hydrophobic interaction. As a result of the hydrophobic interactions the inner part of the dissolved protein molecule contains a large number of apolar amino acid residues whereas the exterior is relatively hydrophilic. The most favourable distribution of the polar and apolar residues over the protein molecule may be constrained by various other structure-determining factors. Moreover, the aqueous periphery is often partly hydrophobic for geometric reasons, especially with smaller molecules where the surface/mass ratio is large. If a protein molecule is transferred from an aqueous to an non-aqueous medium hydrophobic interaction ceases to exist. The molecule may then change its structure into an expanded coil or, as is likely in an aprotic solvent, into a rod-like helix or β-sheet. Proteins contain both positively and negatively charged groups. If the numbers of the positive and negative groups are equal the protein is called isoelectric. Thus, changing the pH away from the isoelectric point implies an increase of the net charge on the molecule, resulting in intramolecular repulsion. If this electrostatic repulsion exceeds the attractive forces the protein molecule expands.

Protein molecules are of amphiphilic nature since they contain both polar and apolar amino acids. Therefore, proteins have a strong tendency to adsorb at interfaces. As with flexible polymers, globular proteins generally show a very poor desorbability towards dilution. High-affinity adsorption isotherms would be anticipated but, for unknown reasons, more rounded isotherms are often obtained. Influenced by this observation, various authors have interpreted their data using models that assume reversibility; Langmuir's model being the most frequently used. However, if the real system does not fulfill the assumptions of the model the fit of the experimental data is only fortuitous and the reported values for the adsorption free energy are without any physical meaning. Although desorption usually cannot be achieved by dilution, exchange of protein molecules between the adsorbed and the dissolved state is a rule rather than an exception (Brash and Samak, 1978; Chan and Brash, 1981; Chuang et al., 1978; Vroman, 1980). By the same principle, proteins may be displaced by other types of surface-active agents (Meijer and Norde, 1984). Furthermore, desorption, especially from hydrophilic surfaces, may occur by exposing the system to extreme conditions of pH (Dillman and Miller, 1973) or ionic strength (Armstrong and Chesters, 1964).

Since the three-dimensional structure of a protein molecule is to a large extent determined by its interactions with the environment, the transfer from solution to a phase boundary may be accompanied by changes in that structure. As an alternative for intramolecular hydrophobic interactions, apolar parts of the protein may be exposed to the sorbent surface, thus shielded from water. A schematic illustration is given in Figure 5. This kind of structural rearrangement is more probable if the compact structure in aqueous solution is stabilized by intramolecular hydrophobic interactions, whilst the sum effect of the other structure determining factors favours a more expanded conformation. Intramolecular hydrophobic interactions stabilize secondary structures as α-helices and β-sheets. A loss of intramolecular hydrophobic bonds may, therefore, cause a decrease in secondary structure which involves more rotational freedom along the polypeptide chain. The resulting entropy gain could be an important factor in driving the adsorption process (Norde and Lyklema, 1979) (see below). Thus, many proteins undergo structural changes upon adsorption, but a compact structure usually persists in the adsorbed state (Cuypers et al., 1978; Uzgiris and Fromageot, 1976; Morrissey and Han, 1978). Surface-induced structural changes are likely to affect the physiological activity of the protein. Moreover, as discussed in section 2.1, even after displacement from the sorbent surface the biological functioning may not be (fully) regained. This could have implications in medical applications, such as artificial kidney dialysis, controlled drug release, etc.

As a rule, adsorption isotherms for proteins develop well-established plateau values that amount to a few mg per m^2 of sorbent surface. The values correspond to a monolayer of more or less structurally perturbed molecules. At extreme conditions, such as high protein concentration, high ionic strength, temperature, etc., the proteins may coagulate at the interface, yielding a load of more than 10 mg m^{-2}.

The role of charged groups in the adsorption mechanism of proteins is complex. First, the relatively long range of interaction between charges may affect the rate of arrival of the protein at the sorbent surface. The rate is reduced in the case of like charges on the protein and the sorbent (Van Dulm and Norde, 1983). Slower adsorption leaves the protein molecules more time for structural rearrangements before ad-

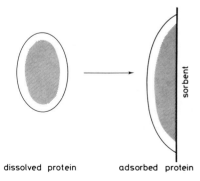

dissolved protein   adsorbed protein

Figure 5. Possible rearrangement in the structure of an adsorbing protein molecule. Shaded areas indicate hydrophobic regions.

jacent sites are occupied by newly arriving molecules. This, of course, has consequences for the final conformation of the adsorbed layer. Second, lateral repulsion between adsorbed protein molecules having the same charge may further reduce the amount adsorbed. The extent of this effect depends on the strength of the interactions between the protein molecules on the one hand and between the protein and the sorbent on the other. Third, the stability of a compact protein structure depends, amongst other things, on intramolecular electrostatic interactions. In the isoelectric region where the numbers of positive and negative groups are about equal the net electrostatic interaction is attractive, supporting a compact protein structure. Excess of either positive or negative charge causes intramolecular repulsion, which favours an expanded structure. Therefore, when the structure in solution is to a large extent stabilized by intramolecular hydrophobic bonding, the susceptibility of proteins to structural rearrangements induced by adsorption is expected to increase with increasing net charge on the protein molecule.

Some of the general features discussed above will be illustrated by experimental data obtained with human plasma albumin (HPA) and ribonuclease (RNAase) from bovine pancreas (Norde and Lyklema, 1978a,b,c,d). HPA and RNAase are both globular, but otherwise they differ in many respects. HPA is a much larger molecule than RNAase; the molecular masses are 66,408 and 13,680 g mol^{-1}, respectively. The isoelectric point of HPA is in the region between pH 4.2 and 5.0 and that of RNAase between 9.0 and 9.5. Under most conditions the RNAase molecule is more densely charged than the HPA molecule. The compact structure of HPA is much less stable than that of RNAase (Tanford et al., 1955; Foster, 1977; Tanford and Hauenstein, 1956). The stability of the compact structure can be expressed by the change of free energy ΔG on altering the structure from an expanded state (i.e., reference state) into the compact state. The more stable the compact structure the more negative is the value of ΔG. Thus,

$$\Delta G^{HPA} = (G^{HPA}_{compact} - G^{HPA}_{expanded}) > \Delta G^{RNAase} = (G^{RNAase}_{compact} - G^{RNAase}_{expanded})$$

ΔG is the net result of all structure determining factors, so that

$$\Delta G^{HPA}_{h.i.} + \Delta G^{HPA}_{other factors} > \Delta G^{RNAase}_{h.i.} + \Delta G^{RNAase}_{other factors}$$

(h.i. = hydrophobic interaction).

The hydrophobicity is larger and, hence, $\Delta G_{h.i.}$ is much more negative for HPA than for RNAase (Bigelow, 1967; Eisenberg et al., 1983). Consequently,

$$\Delta G^{HPA}_{other factors} > \Delta G^{RNAase}_{other factors}$$

For this reason it is expected that HPA is more inclined to change its structure upon adsorption.

The plateau values, Γ_p, of the adsorption isotherms for HPA and RNAase on various substrates are shown in Figures 6 and 7. The sorbents are (in decreasing order of hydrophobicity): negatively charged polystyrene (PS), uncharged, crystalline poly(oxy methylene) (POM) and hematite (α-Fe$_2$O$_3$), which is positive at pH < 6.2 and negative beyond that value. All sorbents are supplied as colloidal dispersions in water. With each substrate Γ_p^{HPA} passes through a maximum in the isoelectric region of the protein. This is a very common trend in protein adsorption. The maximum value of 2–3 mg m^{-2} corresponds to a complete monolayer of adsorbed native HPA molecules in a side-on configuration. From additional data (Norde and Lyklema, 1978a, b) it can be inferred that the decrease in Γ_p^{HPA} at either side of the isoelectric point is due to structural rearrangements in the protein molecule rather than to increased intermolecular separation at the sorbent surface. It is important to realize that HPA adsorbs at both hydrophobic and hydrophilic surfaces, even if the charge on the protein and the sorbent have the same sign. In other words, HPA adsorption is dominated neither by sorbent dehydration nor by electrostatic interaction. Yet, electrostatic interactions exert some influence on the plateau adsorption: for each sorbent Γ_p^{HPA} increases with increasing charge difference between the protein and the sorbent.

RNAase adsorbs readily at the hydrophobic PS surface, but, in contrast to HPA, Γ_p^{RNAase} is more or less constant over the entire pH region studied. The value of approximately 1 mg m^{-2} can be accounted for by assuming a complete monolayer of hydrated structurally unperturbed RNAase molecules. The comparable value for Γ_p^{RNAase} suggests that RNAase does not change its structure considerably upon adsorption, not even at pH values where the protein has reached a high charge densi-

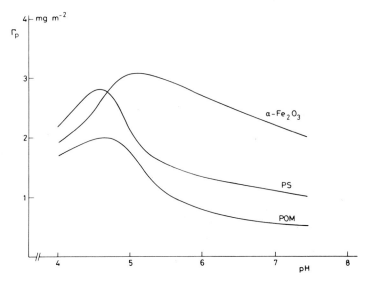

Figure 6. Plateau values of adsorption isotherms for HPA on various surfaces. Ionic strength, 0.05 M. $T = 22°C$.

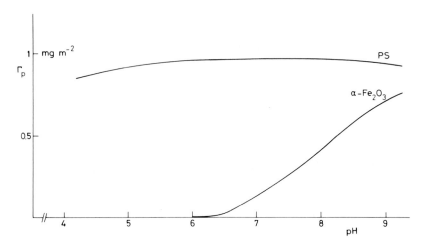

Figure 7. Plateau values of adsorption isotherms for RNAase on different surfaces. Ionic strength, 0.05 M. $T = 22°C$.

ty. With POM, which is uncharged and less hydrophobic than PS, no significant adsorption of RNAase can be detected. Adsorption of RNAase at α-Fe$_2$O$_3$ occurs beyond pH $\approx$ 6.2, the isoelectric point of the sorbent. The different patterns for adsorption of HPA and RNAase are summarized in Table 1 in relation to their structural stability.

RNAase adsorbs by virtue of dehydration of a hydrophobic sorbent surface and/ or favourable charge-charge interactions. Contributions from the RNAase molecule itself, for instance by changing its structure or hydration, are not sufficient for adsorption to occur. However, with HPA the contribution associated with structural changes exceeds the opposing effects of dehydration of a hydrophilic surface and of electrostatic repulsion. These differences between the adsorption behaviour of HPA and RNAase follow from the differences between the stabilities of their structure. The considerations concerning the relation between structural properties and adsorption characteristics, as outlined above, may therefore have a more general validity.

Recent experiments revealed that HPA molecules displaced from α-Fe$_2$O$_3$ surfaces show a decrease in α-helix content from 53 to 43% (Meijer and Norde, 1984). It implies that approximately 60 amino acid residues are transferred from a helical into a randomly coiled state. Since in the helix two bonds per peptide unit are blocked for rotation, the helix-coil transition involves increasing rotational freedom for 120 bonds, each gaining an entropy of maximally $R\ln2$ J K^{-1} (R is the general gas constant which equals 8.31 J K^{-1} mol^{-1}). The maximum entropy increase due to the reduced helix content in HPA then amounts to $120 \times R\ln2 = 691$ J K^{-1}. Calorimetric measurements on the adsorption of HPA on α-Fe$_2$O$_3$ (Koutsoukos et al., 1983) and also on other substrates (Norde and Lyklema, 1978e) revealed that the change in energy is positive, which would oppose the adsorption process. Hence, sponta-

TABLE 1

Protein-sorbent interactions. Influence of charge, hydrophobicity and structural properties of the protein

	Structural properties of the protein molecule	
	Contribution of intra-molecular hydrophobic inter-action to the stability of a globular structure in solution	Structure stability towards charge density at the protein molecule
HPA	Large	Small
RNAase	Small	Large

Sorbent	Adsorption of	
	HPA	RNAase
Hydrophobic		
Opposite charge	+	+
Same charge	+	+
Hydrophilic		
Opposite charge	+	+
Uncharged	+	−
Same charge	+	−

+, Adsorption; −, no adsorption.

neous adsorption must be driven by an increase of entropy. As mentioned above, structural rearrangements in the protein molecule could be a major source for the increase in entropy.

Finally, the role of charged groups in the overall adsorption process deserves attention. After the formation of a compact protein layer the medium of the charged groups at the sorbent surface changes from an aqueous into a non-aqueous, proteinaceous one. The charged groups of the protein that in the adsorbed state are oriented towards the sorbent surface undergo a similar change of medium. For adsorbed layers of HPA and RNAase on PS surfaces it has been shown that a large fraction of the negatively charged protein carboxyl groups become located adjacent to the negatively charged PS surface (Norde and Lyklema, 1978b). This would result in an accumulation of net negative charge in the contact region of protein-sorbent. The dielectric permittivity in this region is relatively low, so that the presence of net charge leads to a high electrostatic potential, which is energetically very unfavourable. Accumulation of net charge could be avoided by the concomittant incorporation of low-molecular-weight ions. For the HPA-PS and RNAase-PS systems co-adsorption of ions has indeed been found (Van Dulm et al., 1981). The chemical effect of ion transfer from an aqueous to a non-aqueous medium is unfavourable (Abraham, 1973; Abra-

50

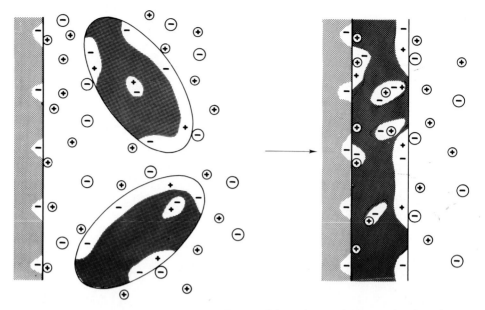

Figure 8. Schematic representation of the redistribution of charged groups in the protein adsorption process. $+/-$ refer to the proton charge of the protein and the surface charge of the sorbent. $\oplus/\ominus$ refer to low-molecular-weight ions. Shaded areas indicate hydrophobic regions.

ham et al., 1978; Danil de Namor et al., 1983) and an alternative way to avoid high electrostatic potentials is the unfolding of the adsorbed protein molecules so that a loosely structured layer is formed in which the dielectric constant is not much different from that in the surrounding aqueous medium. In such a layer hydrophobic amino acid residues would be exposed to water, implying hydrophobic hydration. The observation that globular proteins generally form compact layers suggests that the change of medium of the transferred ions is less unfavourable than the exposure of the hydrophobic parts of the protein to water. The protein adsorption process is schematically represented in Figure 8, with particular reference to the redistribution of charged groups.

In view of the subtle interplay between the various kinds of interactions that determine the specific structures that proteins adopt, a general theory describing protein adsorption still seems far away. Nevertheless, the present discussion has indicated some general principles that govern the interfacial behaviour of proteins. A more detailed, thermodynamic analysis can be found in Norde and Lyklema (1979).

3. Particle adhesion

The 'particles' considered in this section are much larger than single (macro)molecules, that is, of the order of 100 to 10,000 nm. This range includes most particles that are used as drug carriers, and biological cells such as bacteria and erythrocytes.

In section 1 it was mentioned that both the particle and the interface at which the particle may attach are probably covered with adsorbed biopolymers before the particle actually deposits. However, to obtain a better understanding of the factors that control particle adhesion the interaction between a clean particle and a clean surface will be discussed. In this context 'clean' means the absence of adsorbed material. Thereafter, the influence of adsorbed layers on the adhesion process will be considered.

3.1. Clean surfaces

The surfaces of most particles accomodate charged groups. Biological particles are usually negatively charged. Synthetic microspheres, including those used in drug therapy, may also contain charged groups. The sign and the magnitude of the surface charge can be chosen at will by controlling the chemical composition and the preparation procedure. In therapeutic application the surface at which the particles are collected is a biosurface. Most biosurfaces are negatively charged and in order to maintain overall electroneutrality in the system, the charge on the particle and on the collector surface is balanced by the charge on the counterions that are diffusely distributed in the surrounding fluid. The surface charge, together with its counter charge, is called the electrical double layer. The most common picture of the charge distribution in the electrical double layer is that developed by Gouy (1910) and Chapman (1913). This distribution is shown in Figure 9, together with the corresponding gradients in the electrostatic potentials.

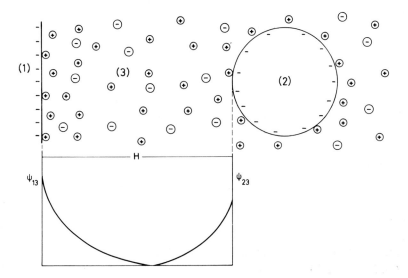

Figure 9. The electrical double layers at a planar surface (1) and around a spherical particle (2) with their corresponding gradient in the electrostatic potential. H is the particle-surface separation across a medium (3).

3.1.1. Long range interactions

When the two charged bodies approach each other the electrical double layers overlap. This results in repulsion if the charges on the particle and the collector are of the same sign and in attraction if the charges are of opposite sign. The classical theory describing the long-range interactions between charged bodies is the DLVO theory, developed by Derjaguin and Landau (1941) and Verwey and Overbeek (1948).

At a given separation, H, between the collector surface (1) and the particle (2) across a medium (3), G_E is determined by the electrostatic surface potentials, ψ, the particle radius, R, the dielectric permittivity, $\varepsilon\varepsilon_o$, and the ionic strength of the medium. The surface potentials are usually approximated by the experimentally accessible electrokinetic potentials (i.e., the potential at the hydrodynamic plane of shear). In most systems the potential does not exceed a value of more than a few tens of millivolts. Under this condition G_E is given by (Hogg et al., 1966; Visser, 1976):

$$G_E = \kappa\, \varepsilon\varepsilon_o R \,(\psi_{13}^2) + \psi_{23}^2) \left\{ \frac{2\psi_{13}\psi_{23}}{\psi_{13}^2 + \psi_{23}^2} \ln\left[\frac{1 + \exp(-\kappa H)}{1 - \exp(-\kappa H)}\right] \right.$$

$$\left. + \ln\left[1 - \exp(-2\kappa H)\right] \right\} \qquad \{2\}$$

The subscripts indicate the boundary between the phases 1, 2 and 3. The ionic strength exerts its influence through ψ and κ. The absolute value of ψ decreases and, according to equation 1, κ increases by increasing the ionic strength of the bulk solution. Both effects reduce the value of G_E.

In addition to electrostatic interaction, the two bodies interact with each other through dispersion forces. The resulting free energy, G_A, may in the case of a sphere and a planar surface be approximated by (Visser, 1976)

$$G_A = -\frac{A}{6}\left[\frac{2R(H+R)}{H(H+2R)} - \ln\left(\frac{H+2R}{H}\right)\right] \qquad \{3\}$$

A is the so-called Hamaker constant of the system. It is composed of the Hamaker constants for the individual components

$$A = (A_1^{1/2} - A_3^{1/2})(A_2^{1/2} - A_3^{1/2}) \qquad \{4\}$$

For various materials values of Hamaker constants have been listed (e.g., Visser, 1976; Nir, 1977). In aqueous media usually $A_1 > A_3$ and $A_2 > A_3$, yielding $A > 0$ and, hence, $G_A < 0$, which implies attraction.

According to the DLVO theory, the total free energy G_{tot} of interaction equals the sum of G_E and G_A. In Figure 10 G_E, G_A and G_{tot} are represented graphically as a function of the particle-surface separation. In this example the particle and collector surface have the same charge, so that G_E is positive (repulsive). From the previous discussion it follows that $G_E(H)$ decreases with increasing ionic strength. However, G_A

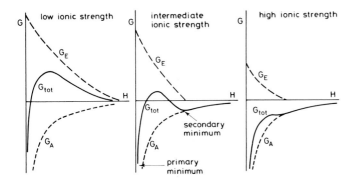

Figure 10. Free energy of interaction between two bodies having the same charge. For further explanation see the text.

is insensitive to this property. As a result, $G_{tot}(H)$ is reduced by increasing the ionic strength of the system. At lower ionic strengths the maximum in $G_{tot}(H)$ reaches a positive value. The more positive this maximum, the more it constitutes a barrier for contact between the particle and the surface. At intermediate ionic strengths the maximum in $G_{tot}(H)$ is sufficiently low so that a fraction of the particles contains sufficient thermal energy to pass the barrier. At higher ionic strengths, where the maximum in $G_{tot}(H) \leqslant 0$, all particles can attach freely at the collector surface. In this case they become trapped in the 'primary minimum' of G_{tot}, which is adjacent to the collector surface where, due to a dominant contribution of G_A, G_{tot} is largely negative. Deposition in the primary minimum implies a strong permanent contact between the particle and the surface. At somewhat larger separation a secondary minimum exists. It is most pronounced at intermediate ionic strengths. The secondary minimum is deeper for materials having large Hamaker constants and/or for relatively large particles, such as many biological cells. Particles captured in the secondary minimum are not actually attached to the collector surface and the binding is much weaker than in the primary minimum. The particles may be removed by rinsing, shaking, etc. In the context of this discussion, in biofluids the ionic strength is sometimes high (seawater, 0.7 M), often intermediate (blood plasma and lachrymal fluid, 0.15 M; urine, 0.15–0.20 M; milk, 0.07 M) and seldomly low (saliva, 0.03–0.07 M).

It is necessary to state that in the case of opposite charges on the particle and the collector, G_{tot} is attractive at all separations, which results in irreversible attachment.

As the collector surface becomes covered, lateral interactions between adhered particles play an increasingly important role. These lateral interactions determine the crowding of the particles at the surface (Vincent et al., 1978, 1980). Usually the particles have the same charge sign, and therefore the lateral interaction is repulsive. Since electrostatic interaction is screened by the surrounding ions, the maximum surface coverage will increase with increasing ionic strength. This is illustrated in Figure 11. In the same figure the influence of the charge sign on the affinity between an isolated particle and the collector surface is indicated, as reflected by the initial slope of the

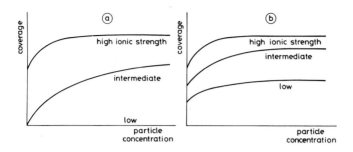

Figure 11. Isotherms for particle adhesion in the cases of (a) the same charge, and (b) opposite charge on the particles and the collector surface.

isotherm. In the case of the same charge the affinity increases with increasing ionic strength due to a progressive reduction of the maximum in $G_{tot}(H)$. With opposite charge signs high-affinity isotherms are derived at each ionic strength.

It must be realized that the principles outlined in the foregoing discussion are based on model systems. Reality, especially in biological environments, is much more complex. Nevertheless, the observations made for natural systems, such as the deposition of marine bacteria (Fletcher and Loeb, 1979) and of oral streptococci (Ørstavik, 1977), qualitatively follow the predictions from the model.

3.1.2. Short-range interactions

At very short separations, for example, under 0.5 nm, other interactions also become effective. It is primarily these short-range interactions that determine the strength of the adhesive bond, that is, the force required to remove the particle from the surface. Examples of such short-range interactions are hydrogen bonds, ion pair formation, dipole-dipole interaction and covalent bonding. In aqueous systems in particular, short-range interactions are significant. This is related to the uniqueness of the three-dimensional structure of liquid water. Intermolecular hydrogen bonding and dipole interactions lead to the formation of dynamic aggregates of water molecules. A phase boundary induces local order in the vicinal water. At hydrophilic surfaces the water structure has a lower free energy than that of bulk water but at hydrophobic surfaces the free energy is higher. Consequently, dehydration of a hydrophilic surface is repulsive and that of a hydrophobic surface is attractive. Hence, the adhesion at a hydrophobic surface is in general stronger than at a hydrophilic surface.

3.2. Polymer-covered surfaces

The presence of an adsorbed (polymer) layer may have a drastic effect on particle adhesion. Coating the particle and/or the collector surface with an adsorbed layer implies the introduction of a fourth (and fifth, if the coatings on the particle and the collector are different) component in the model (Fig. 9). In discussing the effect of the adsorbed layer(s) on particle adhesion, we have to distinguish between a compact layer, which is usually formed by globular proteins (see Fig. 8), and a loosely structured layer formed by random coil-like polymers (see Fig. 2). The effect of a compact layer will be considered first.

G_A may still be calculated using Equation 3, but the value of A should account for the adsorbed layer(s) as well. Hence, Equation 4 has to be modified to include the Hamaker constant A_4 and, eventually, A_5. In applying Equation 2 to calculate G_E, the electrokinetic potentials of the polymer-coated surfaces must be determined. Furthermore, the addition of G_A and G_E, to obtain G_{tot}, is only possible at separations wider than the sum of the adsorbed layer thicknesses on the particle and the collector, respectively. Thus, polymers that adsorb in a compact or a flat conformation will affect particle adhesion mainly through a change in the surface potentials of the interacting bodies. If the adsorbed layers cause a larger charge contrast the free energy barrier to deposition will be reduced.

In addition to the modifications mentioned above, one often has to account for other factors for loosely structured layers. The loose structure allows the free penetration of low-molecular-weight material so that the counterions are partly distributed within the adsorbed polymer layer (see Fig. 12). If the loops and tails of the adsorbed polymer molecules protrude into the solution over a distance greater than the electrical double layer thickness κ^{-1} (Debye length), the adsorbed layers of the two approaching bodies start to interfere at a separation, $(\delta_{pa} + \delta_{co})$, which is larger than the separation $2\kappa^{-1}$, where double layer overlap becomes effective. For example, in blood, which has an ionic strength of approximately 0.15 M, double layer overlap occurs at approximately 1.5 nm, whereas the extension of a loosely structured adsorbed polymer layer is usually in the range of 5–20 nm.

The interference of the polymer layers gives rise to a steric repulsion, G_S, which increases steeply at $H \lesssim (\delta_{pa} + \delta_{co})$ (Napper, 1977). In Figure 13 it is shown how, under these conditions, G_{tot} is composed of G_E, G_A and G_S. G_{tot} attains a minimum

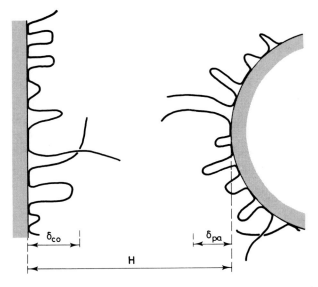

Figure 12. Polymer-coated surfaces. Steric repulsion at $H \lesssim (\delta_{co} + \delta_{pa})$.

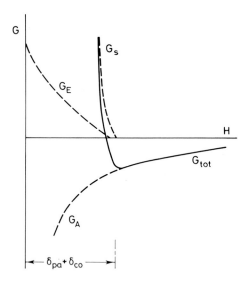

Figure 13. Interaction free energy for two similarly charged, polymer-coated, bodies.

at $H = (\delta_{pa} + \delta_{co})$. The depth of the minimum at that separation is determined by G_A. For layers that are not too thick, about 10 nm or less, the minimum is usually sufficiently deep to cause weak, reversible particle adhesion.

If only one of the interacting surfaces is loaded with polymer or if both surfaces are no more than partly covered, a totally different situation may arise. Then, one and the same polymer molecule may attach to both the particle and the collector surfaces (Vincent, 1974). This phenomenon, known as 'polymer bridging', is illustrated in Figure 14. With a particle and a collector that have the same charge bridging can occur only if the extension of the adsorbed polymer layer outdistances the electrostatic repulsion: $\delta \gtrsim 2 \kappa^{-1}$. Since κ increases with increasing ionic strength, bridging is more probable in the presence of added electrolyte.

The formation of new polymer-surface bonds involves a negative free energy effect, G_{br}, at $H \approx \delta$. Closer approach of the two bodies would squeeze the polymer layer and, hence, G_{br} would become positive. Figure 15 shows the various contributions to $G_{tot}(H)$ for similarly charged species. If the adsorption free energy of the newly attached polymer segments is not too small, the depth of the minimum in $G_{tot}(H)$ is determined primarily by G_{br}. The minimum may attain rather large values, resulting in a strong irreversible adhesion at a finite separation between the particle and the collector.

4. Conclusions

Adsorption and adhesion are complex phenomena, governed by electrostatic, disper-

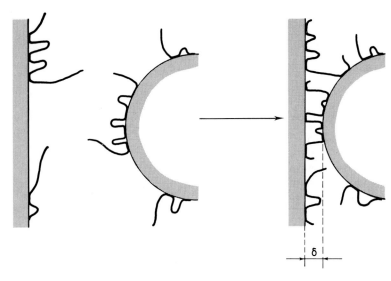

Figure 14. Polymer bridging between a sphere and a planar surface.

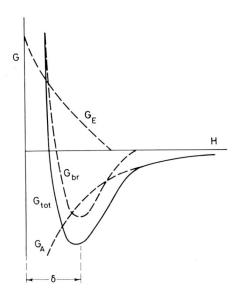

Figure 15. Interaction free energy for two similarly charged bodies between which polymer bridging occurs.

whether or not interfacial accumulation of material occurs is dependent on a delicate balance of forces. Under certain conditions the binding is weak and reversible, under other conditions it is strong and irreversible. In nature many specific interactions are involved which are not accounted for in the present discussion. Nevertheless, a thorsion and steric forces, by hydration and other short-range interactions. Thus,

58

ough knowledge of the physicochemical principles of the adsorption and adhesion processes provides the general basis for the understanding of interfacial phenomena in biological systems.

References

Abraham, M.H. (1973) J. Chem. Soc. Faraday Trans. I 69, 1375–1388.

Abraham, M.H., Ah-Sing, E., Danil de Namor, A.F., Hill, T., Nasehzadeh, A. and Schulz, R.A. (1978) J. Chem. Soc. Faraday Trans I 74, 359–365.

Armstrong, D.E. and Chesters, C. (1964) Soil Science 98, 39–52.

Bigelow, C.C. (1967) J. Theor. Biol. 16, 187–211.

Böhm, J.T.C. (1974) Thesis, Agricultural University, Wageningen, The Netherlands.

Bonekamp, B.C. (1984) Thesis, Agricultural University, Wageningen, The Netherlands.

Brash, J.L. and Samak, Q.M. (1978) J. Colloid Interface Sci. 65, 495–504.

Chan, M.B.C. and Brash, J.L. (1981) J. Colloid Interface Sci. 84, 263–265.

Chapman, D.L. (1913) Phil. Mag. 25, 475–481.

Chuang, H.Y.K., King, W.F. and Mason, R.G. (1978) J. Lab. Clin. Med. 92, 483–496.

Cuypers, P.A., Hermens, W.T. and Hemker, H.C. (1978) Anal. Biochem. 84, 56–67.

Danil de Namor, A.F., Contreras, E. and Sigstad, E. (1983) J. Chem. Soc. Faraday Trans. I 79, 1001–1007.

Derjaguin, B.V. and Landau, L. (1939) Acta Physico Chem. U.S.S.R. 10, 333–346.

Dillman, W.J. and Miller I.F. (1973) J. Colloid Interface Sci. 44, 221–241.

Eisenberg, D., Weiss, R.M., Terwilliger, T.C. and Wilcox, W. (1983) Faraday Symp. 17, 109–120.

Fleer, G.J. and Lyklema, J. (1983) in Adsorption from Solution at the Solid-Liquid Interface (Parfitt, G.D. and Rochester, C.H., Eds.), pp. 153–220, Academic Press, New York.

Fletcher, M. and Loeb, G.I. (1979) Appl. Environm. Microbiol. 37, 67–72.

Foster, J.F. (1977) in Albumin Structure, Function and Uses (Rosenoer, V.M., Oratz, M. and Rothschild, M.A., Eds.), pp. 53–84, Pergamon Press, Oxford.

Froehling, P.E., Bantjes, A. and Kolar, Z. (1977) J. Colloid Interface Sci. 62, 35–39.

Gouy, G. (1910) J. Phys. 9, 457–468.

Hesselink, F.T. (1977) J. Colloid Interface Sci. 60, 448–466.

Hesselink, F.T. (1983) in Adsorption from Solution at the Solid-Liquid Interface (Parfitt, G.D. and Rochester, C.H., Eds.), pp. 377–412, Academic Press, New York.

Hoeve, C.A.J. (1966) J. Chem. Phys. 44, 1505–1509.

Hoeve, C.A.J. (1970) J. Polymer Sci. C 30, 361–367.

Hoeve, C.A.J. (1971) J. Polymer Sci. C 34, 1–10.

Hogg, R., Healy, T.W. and Fuerstenau, D.W. (1966) Trans Faraday Soc. 62, 1638–1651.

Joppien, G.R. (1978) J. Phys. Chem. 82, 2210–2215.

Koutsoukos, P.G., Norde, W. and Lyklema, J. (1983) J. Colloid Interface Sci. 95, 385–397.

Lipatov, Y.S., Fedorko, V.F., Zakordonskii, V.P. and Soltys, M.N. (1978) Colloid J. U.S.S.R. 40, 31–34.

MacRitchie, F. (1978) Adv. Protein Chem. 32, 283–326.

Maternaghan, T.J. and Ottewill, R.H. (1974) J. Photograph. Sci. 22, 279–285.

Meijer, D. and Norde, W. (1984) in preparation.

Miller, I.R. and Bach, D. (1973) in Surface and Colloid Science (Matijević, E., Ed.), Vol. 6, pp. 185–260, Wiley & Sons, New York.

Morrissey, B.W. and Han, C.C. (1978) J. Colloid Interface Sci. 65, 423–431.

Napper, D.H. (1977) J. Colloid Interface Sci. 58, 390–407.

Nir, S. (1977) Prog. Surface Sci. 8, 1–58.

Norde, W. (1985) Adv. Colloid Interface Sci., in press.

Norde, W. and Lyklema, J. (1978a) J. Colloid Interface Sci. 66, 257–265.

Norde, W. and Lyklema, J. (1978b) J. Colloid Interface Sci. 66, 266–276.

Norde, W. and Lyklema, J. (1978c) J. Colloid Interface Sci. 66, 277–284.

Norde, W. and Lyklema, J. (1978d) J. Colloid Interface Sci. 66, 285–294.

Norde, W. and Lyklema, J. (1978e) J. Colloid Interface Sci. 66, 295–302.

Norde, W. and Lyklema, J. (1979) J. Colloid Interface Sci. 71, 350–366.

Ørstavik, D. (1977) Acta Path. Microbiol. Scand. Sect. B 85, 38–46.

Pavlović, O. and Miller, I.R. (1971) J. Polymer Sci. C. 34, 181–200.

Peyser, P. and Ullmann, R. (1965) J. Polymer Sci. A 3, 3165–3173.

Roe, R.J. (1974) J. Chem. Phys. 60, 4192–4207.

Scheutjens, J.M.H.M. and Fleer, G.J. (1979) J. Chem. Phys. 83, 1619–1635.

Scheutjens, J.M.H.M. and Fleer, G.J. (1980) J. Chem. Phys. 84, 178–190.

Silberberg, A. (1968) J. Chem. Phys. 48, 2835–2851.

Soderquist, M.E. and Walton, A.G. (1980) J. Colloid Interface Sci. 75, 386–397.

Tanford, C., Swanson, S.A. and Shore, W.S. (1955) J. Am. Chem. Soc. 77, 6414–6421.

Tanford, C. and Hauenstein, J.D. (1956) J. Am. Chem. Soc. 78, 5287–5291.

Uzgiris, E.E. and Fromageot, H.P.M. (1976) Biopolymers 15, 257–263.

Van der Schee, H.A. and Lyklema, J. (1984) J. Phys. Chem., submitted.

Van Dulm, P. and Norde, W. (1983) J. Colloid Interface Sci. 91, 248–255.

Van Dulm, P., Norde, W. and Lyklema, J. (1981) J. Colloid Interface Sci. 82, 77–82.

Verwey, E.J. and Overbeek, J.T.G. (1948) The Theory of the Stability of Liophobic Colloids, Elsevier Publishing Co, Amsterdam.

Vincent, B. (1974) Adv. Colloid Interface Sci. 4, 193–277.

Vincent, B. and Whittington, S. (1981) in Surface and Colloid Science, (Matijević, E., Ed.), Vol. 12, pp. 1–117, Wiley & Sons, New York.

Vincent, B., Young, C.A. and Tadros, T.F. (1978) Faraday Disc. Chem. Soc. 65, 296–305.

Vincent, B., Young, C.A. and Tadros, J.F. (1980) J. Chem. Soc. Faraday Trans. I 76, 665–673.

Visser, J. (1976) in Surface and Colloid Science (Matijević, E., Ed.), Vol. 8, pp. 3–84, Wiley & Sons, New York.

Vroman, L. (1980) Blood 55, 156–159.

Microspheres and Drug Therapy. Pharmaceutical, Immunological and Medical Aspects
edited by S.S. Davis, L. Illum, J.G. McVie and E. Tomlinson
© *1984, Elsevier Science Publishers B.V.*

CHAPTER 4

Interactions of polyamide microcapsules with blood components

Tamotsu Kondo

1. Introduction

Hemolysate-loaded poly($N^{\alpha},N^{\varepsilon}$-L-lysinediylterephthaloyl) (PPL) microcapsules have been studied as a possible substitute for mammalian red blood cells in this laboratory (Kondo et al., 1976; Arakawa and Kondo, 1977, 1980). These hemolysate-loaded PPL microcapsules (artificial red blood cells) have been found to be comparable, in their ability to absorb oxygen, their carbonic anhydrase activity and their rheological properties, to natural mammalian red blood cells. However, their interactions with blood components are not yet fully understood. Knowledge in this area is important and useful in predicting the behaviour and fate of the artificial cells in the blood stream.

This chapter deals with the interaction of carboxylated polyamide (CPA) micro-capsules, as a prototype of artificial cells, with various blood components.

2. Preparation of microcapsules

Preparation of CPA microcapsules with diameters larger than 5 μm was carried out by making use of the interfacial polycondensation reaction between diamines and ter-ephthaloyl dichloride according to the method described previously (Arakawa and Kondo, 1977; Kondo, 1978).

10 ml of 0.2 M aqueous diamine solution were mechanically dispersed in 50 ml of a mixed organic solvent (chloroform/cyclohexane, 1:3, v/v) containing 15%, v/v, sor-bitan trioleate as an emulsifier with a constant speed stirrer at 1360 rpm for 10 min-utes to yield a water-in-oil emulsion. Then, without stopping the stirring, 50 ml of 0.04 M terephthaloyl dichloride solution in the mixed organic solvent was quickly added to the emulsion and the stirring was continued for another 10 minutes. At the end of this period, 75 ml of cyclohexane was added to the dispersion to stop the poly-condensation reaction. The dispersion was centrifuged to separate the newly formed microcapsules and they were transferred into water with the aid of polyoxyethylated sorbitan monolaurate. Then, the aqueous dispersion was centrifuged to remove fine capsules and excess surfactant, and the separated microcapsules were washed repea-

tedly with deionized water, followed by dispersion in a buffer solution. When the microcapsules were used for studying the interaction with platelets they were treated with glutaraldehyde to reinforce the membrane prior to dispersion into buffer solution.

The diamines employed were L-lysine and mixtures of L-lysine and piperazine in different molar ratios. PPL is a special preparation of CPA, in which L-lysine alone is used as the diamine.

CPA microcapsules having diameters of 1 μm or less were prepared by a previously reported method (Arakawa and Kondo, 1980). Into 100 ml of the mixed organic solvent containing 0.04 M terephthaloyl dichloride, 1.5×10^{-4} M tetraethylammonium chloride, and 5% sorbitan trioleate in a beaker surrounded by ice was added 1.5 ml of a sheep haemolysate containing L-lysine and piperazine, in a given molar ratio, and sodium carbonate through a needle at a constant rate of 0.0042 ml/min by means of a microfeeder. A platinum wire as the cathode was immersed in the organic solvent and an electric potential of 1000 volts was applied between this wire and the needle as the anode during the addition of the hemolysate. Then, spontaneous emulsification occurred and a shower of very fine haemolysate droplets was formed. The quaternary ammonium salt served to give electroconductivity to the organic solvent. A polycondensation reaction took place between the diamine mixture and terephthaloyl dichloride on the surface of each haemolysate droplet, to form a carboxylated polyamide membrane. Hydrogen chloride generated in the reaction was neutralized with the alkali in the aqueous phase. After stirring the system for 30 minutes, 100 ml of cyclohexane were added to stop the interfacial polycondensation reaction. The microcapsules thus prepared were separated by centrifugation and washed three times with cyclohexane, followed by dispersion in a small volume of 50%, v/v, aqueous polyoxyethylated sorbitan monolaurate solution under stirring with a magnetic stirrer.

The haemolysate-loaded microcapsules were fractionated into three fractions of different capsule sizes by centrifugation using sucrose gradients. After 10 ml each of 1.0, 0.6, and 0.2 M sucrose solutions and microcapsule suspension had been layered upon one another in a centrifuge tube, the contents of the tube were centrifuged at 2500 rpm for 20 minutes. The microcapsules that gathered at the interfaces between the sucrose solutions of different concentration were collected separately. Then, carbon monoxide gas was passed through suspensions of the fractionated microcapsules for 3 hours to convert haemoglobin into carboxyhaemoglobin, which is unable to react with oxygen. The microcapsule concentration in each suspension was determined turbidimetrically after the suspension had been dialyzed against isotonic phosphate buffer solution (pH 7.4) for 3 days.

3. Interactions with plasma proteins

The interactions of PPL microcapsules (mean diameter, 5 μm) with bovine serum albumin and bovine serum γ-globulin were investigated by Suzuki and Kondo (1979) as a function of the pH and ionic strength of the medium. It was found that the interactions depend strongly on the pH of the medium while the ionic strength has little or no effect. When the pH was 2.0, the proteins with a high positive net charge were adsorbed on the negatively charged surface of PPL microcapsules, so lowering the surface potential of the microcapsules, leading to their aggregation. Since the proteins bore only a very low positive net charge at pH 4.0, the electrostatic interaction with the microcapsules was weak. Both protein adsorption and capsule aggregation were much lower than at pH 2.0. No appreciable protein adsorption and capsule aggregation were observed at pH 7.0, where both the capsules and the proteins were negatively charged.

Sumida et al. (1983) found that PPL microcapsules (mean diameter, 10 μm) undergo disintegration by the action of fibrinogen molecules at high ionic strengths of the medium, irrespective of the pH. Treatment of the microcapsules with glutaraldehyde prevents the disintegration. The effect of the ionic strength on the disintegration of PPL microcapsules by bovine fibrinogen is shown in Figure 1, where the degree of capsule disintegration is plotted against the concentration of bovine fibrinogen at pH 7.4. The degree of capsule disintegration was defined by the equation

$$\text{degree of disintegration} = \frac{N_0 - N_f}{N_0} \times 100$$

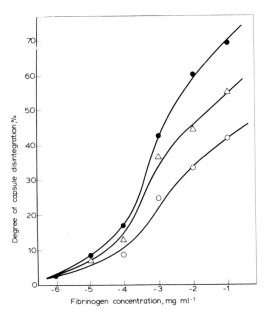

Figure 1. Effect of ionic strength on the disintegration of PPL microcapsules by fibrinogen. Ionic strength: $\bigcirc$, 0.01; $\triangle$, 0.1; $\bullet$, 0.2. Reproduced from Sumida et al. (1983), with permission.

where N_0 and N_f are the total number of PPL microcapsules in unit volume of the control suspension without fibrinogen and that of the sample suspension remaining unbroken after reacting with fibrinogen, respectively. An optical microscope was used to count the capsule number in a suspension placed in a haemocytometer.

Microcapsule disintegration became significant when the concentration of fibrinogen reached a value of 10^{-4} mg/ml. This value can be regarded as the minimum amount of fibrinogen needed to cause capsule disintegration and it corresponds to a number of fibrinogen molecules of about 1.4×10^5 per capsule, as the suspension contained approximately 10^6 capsules in unit volume. The degree of capsule disintegration was strongly dependent on the ionic strength of the medium, increasing with increasing ionic strength. This suggests that the interaction of PPL molecules constituting the microcapsules with fibrinogen molecules is of a hydrophobic nature rather than an ionic one since it is well known that a high concentration of salt screens the electrostatic interaction between charged particles. In view of this, it is not unreasonable to predict that disintegration of PPL microcapsules by fibrinogen is affected by the presence of those ions which produce disturbance of the water structure around the hydrophobic moieties of the microcapsules.

The prediction was confirmed as shown in Figure 2, which shows how anions with sodium ion as the common counterion affect the phenomenon of capsule disintegration. Thiocyanate ion significantly enhances disintegration of PPL microcapsules by fibrinogen, probably because the anion breaks down extensively the hydrophobic hydration around the microcapsules and fibrinogen molecules, so making their direct contact possible. A similar disrupting effect of thiocyanate ion has been reported on the hydrophobic hydration surrounding the hydrocarbon moieties of polypeptides and lipids at an interface (Shibata et al., 1982). Good (1961) suggested that this prop-

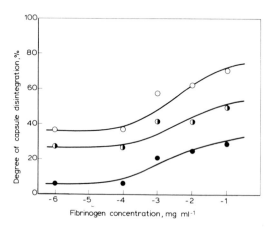

Figure 2. Effect of the anion species of added salts on the disintegration of PPL microcapsules by fibrinogen. Anion: ○, thiocyanate; ◑, chloride; ●, citrate. Reproduced from Sumida et al. (1983), with permission.

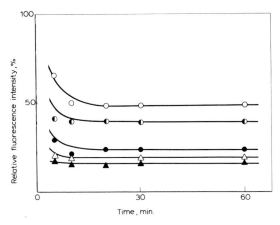

Figure 3. Rate of fibrinogen adsorption to PPL microcapsules as revealed by the change with time in the fluorescence intensity of the supernatant solution. Fibrinogen concentration (mg/ml): ▲, 0.02; △, 0.04; ●, 0.06; ◑, 0.08; ○, 0.10. Reproduced from Sumida et al. (1983), with permission.

erty of the thiocyanate ion of breaking water structure is due to its linear shape, which distorts the water lattice to a great extent.

In contrast, citrate ion, a maker of water structure, seems to suppress capsule disintegration owing, presumably, to its strong tendency to form a Coulombic hydration atmosphere around the particle. It is possible that the citrate ion strengthens the hydrated structure surrounding the hydrophilic moieties of the microcapsules without affecting the hydrophobic hydration of the hydrophobic moieties. By virtue of its moderate water structure-breaking ability, the chloride ion assumes an intermediary position between thiocyanate and citrate ions.

Earlier papers from this laboratory (Suzuki and Kondo, 1978, 1980) have suggested that cationic and amphionic polyelectrolyte molecules of molecular weights higher than 5000 can act on PPL microcapsules at high ionic strengths in such a way as to cause an intermingling with the PPL molecules constituting the microcapsules. Similarly, in the present case, fibrinogen molecules are likely to intermingle with PPL molecules after being adsorbed by the microcapsules, with liberation of water molecules from the hydrophobic moieties of the polyions involved in such interaction. In this sense, disintegration of PPL microcapsules by fibrinogen would be an entropically driven process rather than an energetically driven phenomenon. Treatment of PPL microcapsules with glutaraldehyde would increase the chain length of the PPL molecules of the microcapsules, thereby making it difficult for the polymers to intermingle with fibrinogen molecules.

Adsorption of fibrinogen molecules to PPL microcapsules is demonstrated in Figure 3, where changes with time in fluorescence intensity are shown for the supernatant solutions of mixtures of the microcapsule suspension and solutions of various concentrations of dansylated fibrinogen at constant pH and ionic strength. The fluorescence intensity decreases rapidly with time and levels off within 15 minutes, indicating a rapid adsorption of dansylated fibrinogen molecules to the microcapsules.

66

4. Interaction with platelets

A series of studies has been performed in this laboratory on the adhesion of platelets to CPA microcapsules (Muramatsu and Kondo, 1980, 1983a; Muramatsu et al., 1982a,b).

When CPA microcapsules (mean diameter, 10 μm) having different membrane compositions but approximately the same surface potential were added to platelet-rich plasma (PRP) from rabbit, the platelets adhered rapidly to the microcapsules and obvious differences were seen in platelet adhesion among microcapsules of different membrane composition. The membrane composition was varied by substituting either L-histidine, L-arginine or L-ornithine for L-lysine in the equimolar diamine mixture of L-lysine and piperazine used in the preparation of the microcapsules. In contrast, platelet adhesion was not affected by membrane composition in the absence of plasma, suggesting that platelet adhesion is strongly influenced by plasma components.

On the other hand, if polyamide microcapsules with the same surface composition but different surface potentials were used, platelet adhesion to PRP was found to be facilitated by an increase in the surface potential of the microcapsules. No effect of surface potential was observed on adhesion of washed platelets to the bare microcapsules. Coating of the microcapsules with plasma caused no change in this trend of facilitated platelet adhesion, though the difference in surface potential of the microcapsules disappeared after plasma coating. Hence, it can be concluded that the surface potential of the microcapsules does not affect the platelet adhesion directly but influences the adsorption of plasma components on the microcapsules, thereby producing changes in platelet adhesiveness. In this case, the surface potential was varied by encapsulating different amounts of dextran sulfate, an anionic polyelectrolyte,

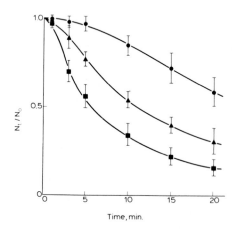

Figure 4. Platelet adhesion to microcapsules in PRP: ●, MC-1; ▲, MC-2; ■, MC-3. Each point shows the mean value of six experiments and each bar the standard deviation. Reproduced from Muramatsu and Kondo (1983b), with permission.

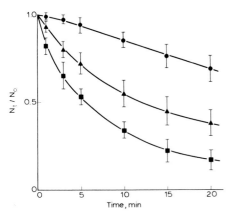

Figure 5. Platelet adhesion to plasma-coated microcapsules in PRP. Symbols are the same as those in Figure 4. Each point shows the mean value of six experiments and each bar the standard deviation. Reproduced from Muramatsu and Kondo (1983b), with permission.

into poly(1,4-piperazinediylterephthaloyl) membranes prepared using piperazine and terephthaloyl dichloride.

The effects of plasma components on platelet adhesion to CPA microcapsules were investigated in detail. Figure 4 shows the decrease with time of the number of single rabbit platelets remaining unadhered after adding the microcapsules to PRP. The number of single platelets was counted using a Coulter Counter. As is indicated in the figure, rabbit platelets adhered more readily to the microcapsules having a high surface potential (prepared using a high molar ratio of L-lysine to piperazine in the diamine mixture) than to those of a low surface potential (prepared using a low proportion of the amino acid in the diamine mixture). This is in complete accordance with the findings on the platelet adhesion to poly(1,4-piperazinediylterephthaloyl) microcapsules in PRP and suggests again that plasma proteins rapidly adsorb on the microcapsule capsule surface in advance of platelet adhesion.

Treatment of CPA microcapsules with plasma was found to diminish the difference in electrophoretic mobility among the bare microcapsules and to give a nearly identical mobility value, indicating that considerable amounts of plasma components are adsorbed on the microcapsule surface to screen the original negative surface charge. Single platelet number versus time curves obtained with the plasma-coated microcapsules in PRP were quite similar to those in Figure 4, as shown in Figure 5. These results imply that the surface potential of microcapsules affects platelet adhesion not directly but indirectly through the adsorbed plasma layer. In fact, no clear dependence of platelet adhesion on the surface potential was observed when the bare microcapsules were added to a suspension of washed rabbit platelets. However, adhesion of the washed platelets to the plasma-coated microcapsules was remarkably dependent on the surface potential of the bare microcapsules. This is shown in Figure 6. Platelet washing was carried out on the centrifuge and this process was found to produce no serious damage to platelets.

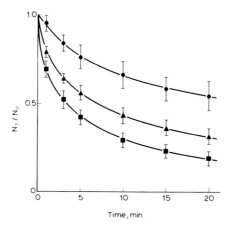

Figure 6. Adhesion of washed platelets to plasma-coated microcapsules. Symbols are the same as those in Figure 4. Each point shows the mean value of six experiments and each bar the standard deviation. Reproduced from Muramatsu and Kondo (1983b), with permission.

TABLE 1

Adhesion of washed rabbit platelets to CPA microcapsules coated with plasma components

Microcapsule plasma component	% adhered		
	MC-1	MC-2	MC-3
Plasma	45	69	82
Serum	78	84	85
Albumin	53	52	52
γ-Globulin	5	6	3
Fibrinogen	7	9	6
Serum			
Heat-inactivated before coating	1	2	4
Heat-inactivated after coating	80	86	91

Table 1 shows the results on adhesion of washed rabbit platelets to CPA microcapsules coated with various rabbit plasma components. The figures in the table give the ratios of the number of adhered platelets to the total number of platelets in the original platelet suspension 20 minutes after mixing platelet and microcapsule suspensions. MC-1, MC-2 and MC-3 refer to CPA microcapsules prepared using molar ratios of L-lysine to piperazine in the diamine mixture of 0, 0.2 and 0.6, respectively. Serum coating enhanced platelet adhesion, irrespective of the surface potential of the microcapsules, suggesting the presence of certain components in the serum which are adsorbed to the microcapsule surface, thereby affecting platelet adhesion. The major plasma proteins, albumin and γ-globulin, exhibited an inhibitory action on platelet adhesion, while the serum heated at 56°C for 30 minutes almost completely inhibited platelet adhesion. Hence, it was suggested that certain complement components would be involved in the platelet adhesion to the microcapsules. In this connection, it is worthwhile to cite papers (Hakin and Lowrie, 1980; Herzlinger and Cumming, 1980) describing complement activation when it comes into contact with synthetic polymer surfaces, thereby affecting the response of leucocytes and platelets with the polymer. It is assumed that certain complement components are rapidly adsorbed to the microcapsule surface and platelets adhere to the microcapsules through the adsorbed complement components. As platelet adhesion was not inhibited even when the microcapsules were heated at 56°C for 30 minutes after being coated with fresh serum, the adsorption of complement is strong and the adsorbed complement is heat-resistant.

Although certain complement components would be regarded as the factors in the serum facilitating the adhesion of platelets, the adsorption of the complement components alone may not explain the fact that the platelet adhesion is dependent on the surface potential of the bare microcapsules in the presence of plasma. The major difference between serum and plasma is the presence of fibrinogen in the latter. Inspection of Table 1 reveals that coating with fibrinogen prevents rabbit platelets from adhering to the microcapsules. In view of this, it can be argued that an opposing effect of the complement components and fibrinogen may operate in platelet adhesion to PRP, which depends on the surface potential of the bare microcapsules. Figure 7 shows the effect of competitive adsorption of the complement components and fibrinogen on the adhesion of rabbit platelets to the microcapsules. In the absence

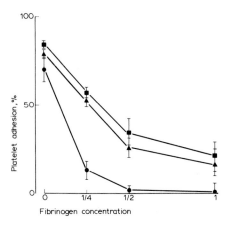

Figure 7. Effect of competitive adsorption of complement and fibrinogen: ●, MC-1; ▲, MC-2; ■, MC-3. Each of the microcapsules was treated with mixtures of equal volumes of fresh serum and a series of diluted solutions of fibrinogen. Each point shows the mean value of three experimental runs and each bar the standard deviation. Reproduced from Muramatsu and Kondo (1983b), with permission.

of fibrinogen, washed rabbit platelets adhered noticeably to the microcapsules, while adhesion decreased as the amount of fibrinogen added to fresh plasma increased. Moreover, the inhibitory effect of fibrinogen on platelet adhesion was more pronounced for MC-1 than for MC-2 and MC-3. Muramatsu and Kondo (1983b) have recently reported that the velocity and amount of fibrinogen adsorption are greater for microcapsules having a low surface potential than for those having a high surface potential. Accordingly, fibrinogen is likely to be adsorbed more readily to MC-1 than to MC-2 and MC-3 to prevent the adsorption of complement components, and this would probably be the primary cause for the observed difference in platelet adhesion in PRP among the microcapsules with different surface potentials.

Although it is still uncertain which component or components of the complement are responsible for enhanced adhesion of rabbit platelets to the microcapsules, C3b would be the most probable candidate because the platelets are known to have C3b receptors on their surface (Nelson, 1953).

5. Interaction with leucocytes

Phagocytosis by human polymorphonuclear leucocytes (PMNs) of haemolysate-loaded CPA microcapsules with diameters less than 1 μm was studied by Watanabe et al. (1983), who found that, regardless of capsule size, the extent of phagocytosis increases with increasing difference in surface potential between the microcapsules and PMNs in the absence of plasma proteins while it is affected greatly by the presence of the proteins, depending on the protein species present and the surface potential of the bare microcapsules.

Figure 8 shows the effect of electrophoretic mobility (which is parallel with surface potential) on the rate of oxygen consumption (an index of phagocytosis) in the phagocytosis by PMNs of haemolysate-loaded CPA microcapsules prepared using different molar ratios of L-lysine to piperazine in the diamine mixture. The rate of oxygen consumption increased as the difference in electrophoretic mobility increased between the microcapsules and PMNs, whose electrophoretic mobility was 1.0 μm/sec/volt/cm.

According to the theory of heterocoagulation based on the DLVO theory of colloid stability (Hogg et al., 1966), the interaction between two colloidal particles is dependent on electrostatic repulsive forces and Van der Waals attractive forces. Although much care should be taken in applying this theory to the interaction between microcapsules and PMNs the theory would still be useful, at least in the early stages of phagocytosis of microcapsules by PMNs. Microcapsules having surface potentials much higher or lower than that of PMNs will adhere easily to the surface of PMNs due to the attractive force operating between them, while those having surface potential equal or very close to that of the leucocytes will be less adhesive. Since adhesion of microcapsules to the surface of PMNs is a prerequisite for phagocytosis to occur, it is reasonable to assume that the more microcapsules adhere to the surface

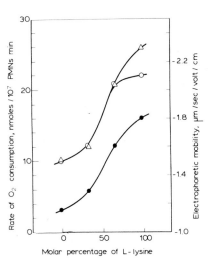

Figure 8. Effect of surface potential on the rate of oxygen consumption in phagocytosis of haemolysate-loaded CPA microcapsules by PMNs: ○, initial oxygen consumption rate; △, maximum oxygen consumption rate; ●, electrophoretic mobility. Reproduced from Watanabe et al. (1983).

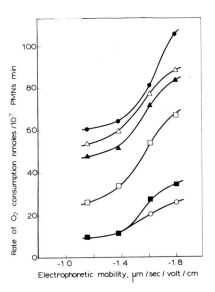

Figure 9. Effects of plasma proteins on the maximum rate of oxygen consumption in phagocytosis by PMNs of haemolysate-loaded CPA microcapsules with different surface potentials: ●, human plasma; △, human serum; ▲, human inactive serum; □, human γ-globulin; ■, human serum albumin; ○, buffer. Reproduced from Watanabe et al. (1983).

of PMNs the more the rate of oxygen consumption increases. Thus, it is suggested that the surface potential of foreign particles plays an important role in phagocytosis by PMNs. The same argument may be applied to the interaction of microcapsules with platelets in its early stages.

When microcapsules come into contact with blood they should adsorb some components of plasma before they are phagocytosed by PMNs. In view of this, the effects of plasma proteins on phagocytosis of microcapsules by PMNs are very important. The effects of plasma proteins on the phagocytosis of haemolysate-loaded CPA microcapsules with various surface potentials are shown in Figure 9, where the rate of oxygen consumption is plotted against the electrophoretic mobility of the bare microcapsules.

All plasma proteins except serum albumin enhanced phagocytosis of haemolysate-loaded CPA microcapsules by PMNs. The electrophoretic mobilities of CPA microcapsules were reduced by the presence of those plasma proteins which enhanced phagocytosis, indicating adsorption of these proteins on the microcapsule surface. Serum albumin was not adsorbed to the microcapsules and it had no enhancing effect on the phagocytic activity of PMNs. Although these data clearly suggest the existence of a certain relationship between phagocytosis and protein adsorption the details are still unknown.

References

Arakawa, M. and Kondo, T. (1977) Can. J. Physiol. Pharmacol. 55, 1378–1382.

Arakawa, M. and Kondo, T. (1980) Can. J. Physiol. Pharmacol. 58, 183–187.

Good, W. (1961) Biochim. Biophys. Acta 49, 397–399.

Hakin, R.M. and Lowrie, E.G. (1980) Trans. Am. Soc. Artif. Int. Organs 26, 159–164.

Herzlinger, G.A. and Cumming, R.D. (1980) Trans Am. Soc. Artif. Int. Organs 26, 165–170.

Hogg, R., Healy, T.W. and Fuerstenau (1966) Trans. Faraday Soc. 62, 1638–1654.

Kondo, T. (1978) in Colloid and Surface Science (Matijevic, E., Ed.), Vol. 10, pp. 1–43, Plenum Press, New York.

Kondo, T., Arakawa, M. and Tamamushi, B. (1976) in Microencapsulation (Nixon, J.R., Ed.), pp. 163–172, Marcel Dekker, New York.

Muramatsu, N. and Kondo, T. (1980) J. Biomed. Mater. Res. 14, 211–224.

Muramatsu, N. and Kondo, T. (1983a) J. Biomed. Mater. Res 17, 959–971.

Muramatsu, N. and Kondo, T. (1983b) Chem. Pharm. Bull. 31, 4517–4523.

Muramatsu, N., Yoshioka, T. and Kondo, T. (1982a) Chem. Pharm. Bull. 30, 257–265.

Muramatsu, N., Goto, Y. and Kondo, T. (1982b) Chem. Pharm. Bull. 30, 4562–4565.

Nelson, R.E., Jr. (1953) Science 118, 733–735.

Shibata, A., Yamashita, S. and Yamashita, T. (1982) Bull. Chem. Soc. Jpn. 55, 2814–2819.

Sumida, S., Jomura, A., Arakawa, M. and Kondo, T. (1983) Progr. Colloid Polym. Sci. 68, 133–138.

Suzuki, S. and Kondo, T. (1978) J. Colloid Interface Sci. 67, 441–447.

Suzuki, S. and Kondo, T. (1979) Kobunshi Ronbunshu (Polym. Rep.) 36, 197–201.

Suzuki, S. and Kondo, T. (1980) J. Colloid Interface Sci. 77, 280–282.

Watanabe, Y., Kondo, T., Miyamoto, M. and Sasakawa, S. (1983) unpublished data.

Microspheres and Drug Therapy. Pharmaceutical, Immunological and Medical Aspects
edited by S.S. Davis, L. Illum, J.G. McVie and E. Tomlinson
© *1984, Elsevier Science Publishers B.V.*

The adsorption of plasma proteins and poly-L-lysine on polystyrene latex, and the effects on phagocytosis

T.L. Whateley and G. Steele

The effect of particle size in phagocytosis is relatively well understood (Illum et al., 1982); however, the role of particle charge, nature of the surface, adsorption of plasma proteins and the possibility of particle aggregation in vivo has been less well studied. The effect of particle charge in vivo has been studied using polystyrene latex particles modified with complex coacervates of oppositely charged macromolecules (Wilkins and Myers, 1966). It was found that positively charged particles had a significant initial accumulation in the lung and spleen whereas negatively charged particles were mostly found in the liver. In vitro studies using polymorphonuclear leukocytes (Deierkauf et al., 1977) found that latex carrying a bound negatively charged macromolecule, such as albumin, inhibited phagocytosis, whereas bound polylysine stimulated phagocytosis. Further experiments by Beukers et al. (1980) showed that the electrophoretic mobility of polystyrene latex could be altered from negative to positive by altering the amount of polylysine added. The adsorption of human plasma albumin on polystyrene latex has been extensively studied by Norde and Lyklema (1978), whilst studies involving the adsorption of γ-globulin have been carried out by Morrissey and Han (1978).

Investigations into the binding of poly-L-lysine (M_r 70,000), HSA and γ-globulin onto negatively charged polystyrene latex (0.497 μm diameter) were carried out using

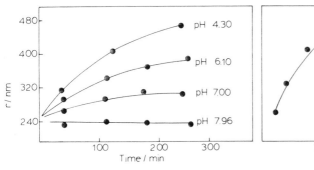

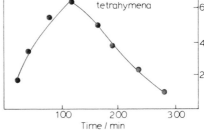

Figure 1   Figure 2

microelectrophoresis and photon correlation spectroscopy. The charge modification reported by Beukers et al. (1980) was confirmed and extended to show that the modification was dependent not only on the molecular weight of the polylysine but also on the amount of latex that was present. As Morrissey and Han (1978) have found for the adsorption of γ-globulin on polystyrene latex, poly-L-lysine also causes flocculation which is pH-dependent (Fig. 1).

Phagocytosis experiments were initially carried out by counting microscopically the number of food vacuoles formed when the fresh water ciliate *Tetrahymena pyriformis* was fed with 0.497 μm diameter latex. The uptake of the latex beads is shown in Figure 2. In order to get a more quantitative estimate of the uptake of polystyrene latex by *T. pyriformis* the microspheres were radioactively labelled with ^{125}I using the method described by Huh et al. (1974): excess ^{125}I was removed by dialysis. This has facilitated the study of the influence of adsorbed poly-L-lysine, HSA and γ-globulin on uptake by phagocytosis.

References

Beukers, H., Deierkauf, F.A., Blom, C.P., Deierkauf, M., Scheffers, C.C. and Riemersma, J.C. (1980) Chem-Biol. Interac. 33, 91–100.

Deierkauf, F.A., Beukers, H., Deierkauf, M. and Riemersma, J.C. (1977) J. Cell Physiol. 92, 169–176.

Huh, Y. (1974) Rad. Res. 60, 42–53.

Illum, I., Davis, S.S., Wilson, C.G., Thomas, N.W., Frier, M. and Hardy, J.G. (1982) Int. J. Pharmacol. 12, 135–146.

Morrissey, B.W. and Han, C.C. (1978) J. Colloid Interface Sci. 65, 423–431.

Norde, W. and Lyklema, J. (1978) J. Colloid Interface Sci. 66, 257–302.

Wilkins, D.J. and Myers, P.A. (1966) Br. J. Exp. Pathol. 47, 568–576.

Section 2

Pharmaceutical and pharmacodynamic aspects

Microspheres and Drug Therapy. Pharmaceutical, Immunological and Medical Aspects
edited by S.S. Davis, L. Illum, J.G. McVie and E. Tomlinson
© 1984, Elsevier Science Publishers B.V.

Human serum albumin microspheres for intraarterial drug targeting of cytostatic compounds. Pharmaceutical aspects and release characteristics

E. Tomlinson, J.J. Burger, E.M.A. Schoonderwoerd and J.G. McVie

1. Introduction

The clinical effectiveness of a cytotoxic compound is often reduced due to its non-ideal pharmaceutical and pharmacokinetic properties (Table 1). Targeting of such agents to tumour areas by liposomes, nanoparticles and microspheres is intended to increase the specific distribution of a drug and to reduce its side effects. Figure 1 (Tomlinson, 1983) illustrates the biological fate of particles in the size range 50 nm to 40 μm, showing that size, route of administration and accessorising of particles are all of critical importance. Our own studies in the cancer chemotherapy area (Tomlinson et al., 1982, 1984a) have been based on the intraarterial delivery of drug-

TABLE 1

Reasons for targeting of drugs

Pharmaceutical
    Drug instability in conventional formulation
    Solubility
Biopharmaceutical
    Low absorption
    High membrane binding
    Biological instability
Pharmacokinetic/pharmacodynamic
    Short half-life
    Large volume of distribution
    Low specificity
Clinical
    Low therapeutic index
    Anatomical and/or cellular barriers
Commercial
    Drug presentation

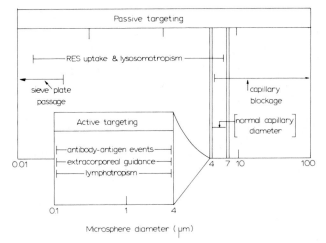

Figure 1. Passive and active targeting of colloidal particles (Tomlinson, 1983).

bearing colloidal particles in the size range 15–25 μm. As shown in Figure 1, systemic delivery of this size of particle results in their entrapment in the first capillary bed that they encounter. After intravenous delivery this leads to first-order targeting (Widder et al., 1979) of the lungs; with intraarterial targeting, this leads to entrapment in, for example, the liver, and for tumour-bearing organs can lead to selective (i.e., second-order) targeting to the tumour capillaries (Blanchard et al., 1965). It is probable that this latter effect is due to a qualitative and quantitative difference in capillary networks of tumours compared to those of the host organ (Lindell et al., 1977). Apart from the potential use of these particles as carriers of cytostatics, experience at the Netherlands Cancer Institute has shown that intraarterial injection of radioactively labelled colloidal particles in this size range does lead to excellent imaging of tumours due to selective blockage of their capillaries. Although the literature contains information on particular aspects of microsphere production and characteristics, no comprehensive study on the pharmaceutical and biopharmaceutical aspects of microspheres exists. Here we describe the pharmaceutical aspects and drug-release characteristics of albumin microspheres intended for intraarterial delivery to tumours. Much of the information can be used with regard to human serum albumin microspheres intended for other therapeutic rôles (Tomlinson, 1983).

2. Pharmaceutical aspects

Elsewhere in this volume, authors have alluded to the characteristics of an ideal microsphere carrier. Basically, they refer to a selectivity for the target, coupled with a controllable and sustained release of drug, as well as to non-damage of the host. To achieve many of these ideals, the pharmaceutical aspects of a microsphere delivery system need to be considered first. Table 2 (Tomlinson, 1983) lists these, and it is

TABLE 2

Pharmaceutical and biopharmaceutical considerations in the development of a microsphere product

1.	Core material
2.	Route of preparation with respect to (3–7)
3.	Size, related to (13)
4.	Drug incorporation
5.	Payload
6.	Drug release (in vitro and in vivo)
7.	Drug stability during (2) and (9)
8.	TDS[a] stability (in vitro and in vivo)
9.	Effect of storage on (6–8)
10.	Surface properties as they relate to (4), (6) and (11)
11.	Presentation (e.g., free-flowing, freeze-dried powder or emulsified suspension)
12.	Antigenicity
13.	Biofate and TDS toxicity
14.	Drug and TDS biokinetics

[a]TDS refers to a targetable delivery system.

apparent that many are interrelated and sometimes opposing. For example, although a smaller size of microsphere may be desired for targeting reasons, this leads to a much faster release of drug, necessitating a change in manufacturing conditions (and hence microsphere stability). A number of these aspects will now be considered.

2.1. Manufacture

Human serum albumin microspheres are generally manufactured by one of two routes. The first involves either thermal denaturation or chemical cross-linking in a water-in-oil emulsion. Second, non-drug-bearing albumin microspheres intended for diagnostic imaging may be prepared using either a single one-step procedure with thermal denaturation of protein aerosol in a gas medium (Przyborowski et al., 1982), or an aerosol step followed by denaturation in oil (Millar et al., 1982). In this chapter, preparative routes involving chemical stabilization of microspheres, using 2,3-butadione and 1,5-glutaraldehyde as cross-linking agents, will be described.

Well-defined human serum albumin (HSA) microspheres can be prepared with diameters in the range 0.2–100 μm using the following procedures (Tomlinson et al., 1984b). In all cases, microsphere formation occurs within a water-in-oil emulsion placed in a flat-bottomed glass beaker (diameter, 60 mm; height, 110 mm) equipped with four baffles (4 mm depth) positioned against the sides. Although the use of a cell having no baffles leads to poorly defined spheres, equipping the cell with baffles results in microspheres having a well-defined size maximum and a Gaussian size distribution (Figs. 2a and 3).

Highly purified olive oil (125 ml) is added to the mix-cell, and a motor-driven, four-bladed axial-flow impeller is positioned two thirds into the oil, such that there is a distance of 3 mm between the baffles and the impeller blades. After stirring the

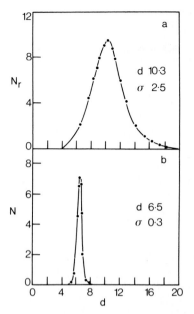

Figure 2. (a) Relative number of 2,3-butadione-stabilized HSA microspheres per milligram ($N_r \times 10^{-2}$) versus sphere diameter (d, μm), for spheres manufactured in a cell fitted with baffles, and at a stirring speed of 1120 rpm. (b) Number of microspheres per milligram ($N \times 10^{-4}$) versus sphere diameter for HSA microspheres prepared at 1350 rpm and subsequently sieved between 5- and 10-μm sieves.

oil for 30 minutes at the desired speed, an aqueous solution of HSA and drug in isotonic buffer (pH 7) is added dropwise from a syringe to the olive oil. This aqueous phase has a final volume (including additions of cross-linker) of 0.5 ml. The resulting water-in-oil emulsion is stirred for a further period of time depending upon the method of stabilization. Calculation of the Reynolds number for the above described system, using a stirring speed of 1800 rpm, gives that streaming within the cell lies in the transitional phase between laminar flow and fully developed turbulence. Clearly, for large-scale manufacture such considerations need to be studied further. For microspheres manufactured under these conditions, the speed of mixing has been found to be the most critical factor with regard to mean diameter of sphere produced. For example, using an aqueous disperse phase volume of 0.4 ml 25% HSA, the following relationship has been found (Tomlinson et al., 1982):

$$\bar{d} = -33\,\text{rpm} + 112 \quad (n = 8; r = 0.94) \tag{1}$$

where the mean diameter, $\bar{d}$, refers to freeze-dried spheres. Figure 4 gives this relationship also for microspheres suspended in isotonic saline containing 0.1% Tween 80. These relationships are valid using olive oil as the continuous phase and a size range of spheres from 1 to 50 μm. For smaller albumin microspheres (diameter, 0.1–1 μm) much more viscous oils have to be employed (Tomlinson and Burger, 1984).

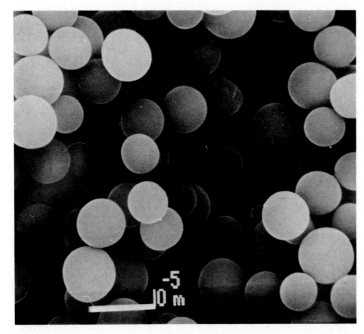

Figure 3. Scanning electron microscope picture of freeze-dried HSA microspheres sieved between 5- and 10-μm microsieves.

Table 3 gives the influence of other manufacturing variables on microsphere size.

2.1.1. Non-stabilized microspheres

These are prepared at room temperature by addition of 0.5 ml of a 25% HSA solution

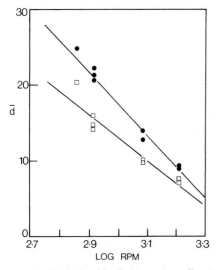

Figure 4. Relationships between mean diameter ($\overline{d}$, μm) of HSA microspheres and stirring speed. Open (□) and closed (●) points are for freeze-dried spheres in the dry state and after suspension for 18 hours in 0.1% Tween 80 phosphate buffer, respectively.

TABLE 3

Effect of manufacturing variable on the mean diameter of human serum albumin microspheres[a]

Factor	Change	Mean diameter[b]
Oil viscosity[c]	decrease	increase
Oil amount	increase	increase
Protein amount	increase	increase
Aqueous phase[d]	increase	increase
Stirring speed	increase	decrease
Surfactant[e]	addition	no effect

[a] Estimated using microscopy.
[b] Standard factors were 125 ml olive oil and 0.5 ml of a 25%, w/v, HSA solution.
[c] The viscosity of the oil was varied by addition of petroleum ether (100–140 °C) to give an end volume of 125 ml.
[d] Addition of 1 ml of a 12.5%, w/v, HSA solution.
[e] Addition of 0.1% sodium dodecyl sulphate to the aqueous HSA solution.

containing dissolved drug to the oil. After stirring for 90 minutes, 60 ml of diethyl ether are added to the emulsion, and stirring is continued for a further 10 minutes, after which the formed microspheres are isolated by centrifugation for 5 minutes at 2000 rpm, followed by decanting of the supernate. After resuspending the microspheres in diethyl ether, and collecting them on a 0.8-μm polycarbonate filter, residual oil is removed by further washing with diethyl ether.

2.1.2. Stabilization with 2,3-butadione
This is similar to the above method, except that after stirring for 90 minutes the emulsion is then transferred to a sealed beaker where stirring is continued at 40 rpm and 2,3-butadione is added in either a 3 ml or 15 ml volume (the sealed beaker is to prevent loss of cross-linker through evaporation). After reaction for the desired time, the stabilized spheres are centrifuged, washed and collected as above.

2.1.3. Stabilization with 1,5-glutaraldehyde
To 125 ml of olive oil is added 0.4 ml of 25% aqueous HSA solution containing dissolved drug. After stirring for 15 minutes at the desired speed, 0.1 ml of an aqueous glutaraldehyde solution is added, so as to produce a final (aqueous) concentration of glutaraldehyde of between 1 and 5%. Stirring is continued for the required time, after which the stabilized spheres are centrifuged and washed as above.

2.2. Microsphere fractionation
Figure 2a shows that the size distribution of HSA microspheres produced in a cell fitted with baffles have a size standard deviation of approximately 25%. Although this may be satisfactory with some areas of therapy, a narrower size distribution range may be necessary. This can be achieved using microsieves (Veco Inc., Eerbeek, The Netherlands). These are produced at any specific mesh size in 1-μm steps from

1 μm upwards, although the standard sizes are from 5 μm in 5-μm steps,. Fractionation is achieved by sieving approximately 80 mg of freeze-dried microspheres suspended in 50 ml of chloroform. After sieving, microspheres are freeze-dried and stored. Figures 2b and 3 exemplify the approximate monodispersivity of product that can be achieved.

2.3. Storage

After collection, microspheres are lyophilized at 10–20 mtorr and –60°C for 18 hours. Upon freeze-drying, sample vials are sealed with an air-tight seal, and stored at 4°C in the dark. At no stage during manufacture are attempts made to quench the cross-linking process.

2.4. Sizing

Microspheres are generally sized in a 0.1% Tween 80 saline solution using a Coulter Counter (model Z_B) fitted with a Channelyser (type C-1000). Sizing can also be performed using a scanning electron microscope, using sputter coating with a 35-nm layer of Au/Pd. Also, for larger microspheres, a light microscope fitted with a calibrated graticule can be used. An advantage of scanning electron microscopy is that the appearance of the microsphere surface may be examined. Results indicate that at levels of drug incorporation above 25% (by weight), crennelations in the surface begin to appear.

2.5. Surface charge

The colloidal and surface characteristics of a microsphere delivery system are of importance to its presentation, injection and biofate. Microspheres intended for intraarterial delivery should be presented for clinical use as a free-flowing, lyophilized drug-containing sterile powder, which is to be suspended in a sterile solution of 0.1% Tween 80 in isotonic saline. Thus, although these present microspheres are unlikely to be taken up by the reticulo-endothelial system, it is still of interest to know what the surface charge characteristics of drug-bearing HSA microspheres are, since this can affect platelet adhesion (Murumatsu et al., 1982) and aggregation of the spheres prior to injection. Table 4 gives the measured Zeta potentials for some different microsphere systems in different media. Although all spheres have a negative charge, the magnitude of this depends upon both the medium and the presence of (ionised) drug. Results with plasma indicate an adsorption of plasma components (Wilkins and Myers, 1966) which leads to all spheres having a similar surface charge.

2.6. Swelling

Freeze-dried HSA microspheres swell in an aqueous environment. Thus, such spheres, when exposed to the moisture of the atmosphere, take up approximately 9% of water (by weight) after 24 hours exposure (Tomlinson et al., 1984b), this uptake being equal to the weight loss upon freeze-drying. When placed into a 0.1% Tween 80 saline solution at 20°C, HSA microspheres swell between 20 and 80% in diameter,

TABLE 4

Zeta potentials of human serum albumin microspheres[a] at 25°C

Microsphere	Zeta potential at 25°C (mV)			Mean diameter (μm)
	Suspension medium			
	0.1% Tween 80 in physiological salt solution	0.1% Tween 80 in plasma	Plasma	
0.1 mol dm^{-3} SCG, ultrasonicated[b]	−18.5	−9.5	−8.9	21.7
0.1 mol dm^{-3} SCG	−8.7	−7.2	−6.9	23.0
Non-drug containing, ultrasonicated	−18.9	−7.1	−8.2	21.7
Non-drug containing	−13.0	−5.3	−7.5	21.7

[a] Stabilised by cross-linking for 4 hours with 5% glutaraldehyde.

[b] Approximately 40 mg freeze-dried microspheres suspended in 15 ml 0.1% Tween 80 physiological salt solution, followed by ultrasonication for 5 minutes, filtration, washing with water, ethanol and ether, and then freeze-dried.

a phenomenon that, with glutaraldehyde, is independent of amount of cross-linker above 1%, though it is dependent upon the level of drug incorporated. For example, we have found that 30-μm lyophilized microspheres containing approximately 25% by weight of the highly water-soluble drug sodium cromoglycate (SCG) — and prepared using cross-linking with glutaraldehyde for 18 hours — increased in diameter on average by 75% when placed in saline, whereas similarly prepared non-drug-containing microspheres increased in diameter by approximately 40%. In cases where size of microspheres is critical for targeting (Fig. 1) this will be an important feature of microsphere manufacture and product presentation.

3. Drug incorporation

Yapel (1979) has studied the incorporation of more than 40 drugs and drug types into HSA microspheres denatured by heat or chemically stabilized. A recent survey (Tomlinson, 1983) has shown that for all microsphere systems, over 90 drugs have been incorporated. Incorporation is highly dependent upon the aqueous solubility of the drug. Figure 5 gives the incorporation of several water-soluble compounds, including doxorubicin and 5-fluorouracil. A number of features are evident. First, for water-soluble drugs the extent of incorporation is dependent upon both drug solubility in the aqueous phase, and the amount of protein used. These factors are intimately interrelated with the size of the formed microsphere (Table 3), and hence

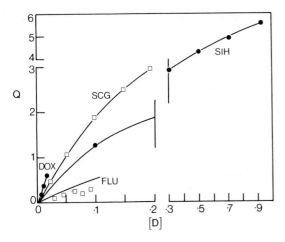

Figure 5. Incorporation of water-soluble compound into 10–20-μm HSA microspheres, showing the relationship between the amount (mg) of compound incorporated per 10 mg of formed sphere (Q) and the original disperse-phase compound concentration ([D], M). SIH, SCG, DOX and FLU refer to sodium iodohippurate, sodium cromoglycate, doxorubicin and 5-fluorouracil, respectively. Drawn lines are for a theoretical 100% incorporation. (Microspheres manufactured with 25%, w/v, HSA in the disperse phase of the emulsion.)

(as shown later) the subsequent release of drug from the sphere. For SCG and sodium iodohippurate (SIH), incorporation is 100% of compound originally present in the aqueous disperse phase of the emulsion, whereas for doxorubicin and 5-fluorouracil this is 95 and 50%, respectively. As the aqueous solubility of the compound (in the presence of protein) is approached, the size of the microspheres changes (Tomlinson and Burger, 1984). For example, as the concentration of SCG rises from 0.05 to 0.19 M, HSA microspheres manufactured at 1215 rpm and using 25% w/v HSA increase in diameter from approximately 8 μm to almost 14 μm. Similar effects are observed with SIH. This appears to be due to a microsuspension being formed, which then becomes incorporated into the matrix of the microsphere. Indeed, Lee et al. (1982) showed that water-insoluble drugs can be incorporated into monolithic HSA microspheres using a suspension/emulsion technique, although the size of the formed particles approached 100 μm. Clearly, if larger spheres are acceptable, then a microsuspension preparative technique is of use. Other features of Figure 5 are (a) that the relationships between amount of compound incorporated are not linear — since the high levels of incorporation possibly mean that the weight of the drug contributes significantly to the weight of the formed microsphere, and (b) that compounds with a reasonably high solubility in oil (e.g., 5-fluorouracil), are not totally incorporated due to loss of compound upon distribution into both the continuous phase of the emulsion and the diethyl ether used for washing.

Figure 5 shows that, using a 25%, w/v HSA solution, incorporation of, for example, sodium iodohippurate can be as high as 54% (by weight) of the formed microsphere. By altering the amount of HSA, much higher levels of drug incorporation may be achieved. For example (Tomlinson and Burger, 1984), using a 0.1 M concentration of SCG results in 100% incorporation of drug, such that at 25%, w/v, HSA this leads to 16% (by weight) of the formed microsphere being drug, and with 15%, w/v, and 5%, w/v, HSA to 35% (by weight) and 50% (by weight), respectively. Although this can be a most attractive way of increasing the drug dose per unit weight of microsphere, it may be seen from Table 3 that a reduction in the amount of protein leads to a reduction in the size of the microspheres. Thus, to maintain the original size of spheres, changes in the speed of stirring (for example) are necessary (Fig. 4).

To summarise, drug incorporation can affect (i) the route of microsphere manufacture, (ii) the appearance and (iii) surface charge of the spheres, (iv) extent of swelling, (iv) size of spheres, and (v), as shown in the following section, rate of release.

4. Drug release

The release of drugs which are associated with microsphere carriers has been found to be dependent upon a large number of constitutional and environmental factors. These include (Tomlinson, 1983) (i) the position of drug in the microsphere, (ii) size and (iii) density of the sphere, (iv) the extent and nature of cross-linking, denaturation or polymerization, (v) the physicochemical type and molecular weight of the drug, (vi) its incorporation level in the sphere, (vii) the presence of adjuvants in the microsphere, (viii) physicochemical and physical interactions between the drug and the matrix material, (ix) the type and amount of the matrix material, and (x) the release environment (including the presence of enzymes). Here we shall examine in particular the influence of drug concentration, microsphere size and extent of chemical denaturation on the release rates of highly water-soluble model compounds from HSA microspheres.

4.1. Biexponential release

Except for release from ion-exchange resins (Tomlinson 1983), in vitro passive release of drugs from monolithic microspheres is characteristically biphasic, with an initital large and fast release (i.e., the 'burst effect'), followed by a much slower release. Although it is possible to manipulate both phases of release, the very large burst effect, which is often complete within 5 minutes, means that alterations in the characteristics of drug-bearing HSA microspheres result in therapeutically significant changes in drug release being obtained only for the second (slow) phase of release. The normally found release profile for a highly water-soluble compound is seen in Figure 6, which shows the release of SCG from HSA microspheres into isotonic buffer. For this, microspheres are packed with glass beads into a short stainless-steel column, through which eluent is passed at a constant rate (generally 15–20 ml/hour, which ensures sink conditions), and the appearance of drug in the eluent is constantly monitored. Mass balance calculations show that for the example shown 88% of drug

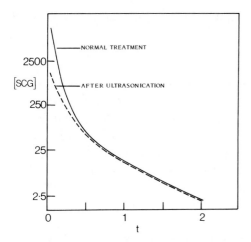

Figure 6. Release of sodium cromoglycate (SCG) into phosphate buffer (pH 7) from HSA microspheres stabilized by cross-linking with 5% glutaraldehyde for 18 hours. The mean diameter of the microspheres was 15–20 μm and the original concentration of SCG in the disperse phase was 0.1 M. Graph gives the concentration of SCG appearing in the eluent (ng/ml) with time (hours).

originally incorporated is released within 10 minutes. After this burst, release continues to be first-order, but is much slower.

It should be appreciated with Figure 6 that the area under the curve gives the total amount of drug being released, and that both the height and the steepness of the second portion of the release profile gives the *amount* of drug being released *from* the microspheres per unit of time. These release profiles may be modelled using a simple biexponential function (Tomlinson et al., 1984b), i.e.

$$Q_1 = Ae^{-\alpha t} + Be^{-\beta t} \qquad \{2\}$$

where the amount remaining in the microspheres at time t (Q_t) is given by the two constants A and B and the two (mixed) rate constants α and β. A, B, α and β can be used to characterize drug release so that, for example, the time for total emptying of the spheres is known, etc. Thus, calculations for the microspheres shown in Figure 6 give that all SCG will have left the spheres after 50 hours.

4.2. Reducing the burst effect

It is possible to reduce the burst effect for water-soluble compounds by first ultrasonicating the spheres in isotonic saline for 2 minutes. Figure 6 shows that this has the result of reducing the amount of SCG released in the first 10 minutes, without affecting the second phase of release. For this example, ultrasonication has removed approximately 70% of drug originally released during the burst period; presumably because this amount was to be found on or near the surface of the sphere. These findings reinforce the view that the slower phase of release is due to a combination of swelling of the spheres, solution of drug and diffusion of drug out of the matrix of the spheres.

4.3. Effect of microsphere size on drug release

Release of drug from microspheres of smaller size results in a much greater and faster release of drug during the second release phase. This is shown in Figure 7, and presumably is due to (a) the much larger surface area available for release, and (b) the shorter path length necessary for drug to diffuse through. Fitting these results to Equation 2, gives, for example, that spheres of 7.5 μm manufactured using 5% glutaraldehyde for 4 hours will empty totally in 12.5 hours, whereas those made under the same conditions but being of 10 μm diameter will still have 6% of their payload in them after 24 hours. Thus, alteration in microsphere size will dramatically slow down the second phase of drug release. We consider that this is attractive not only for our cancer chemotherapy project, where sizes may be spread between 15 and 25 μm, but particularly when larges sizes of spheres may be acceptable, for example with intra-articular use.

Conversely, these data indicate that release of highly water-soluble drugs from HSA particles of less than 1 μm in diameter will be so fast as to render their therapeutic rôle insignificant without recourse to either a different sort of linking (e.g., covalent) between drug and microsphere, or the use of a completely different means of drug entrapment.

4.4. Effect of stabilization on release

A priori one expects that as the microspheres become more stabilized (i.e., there is a greater degree of cross-linking or heat denaturation), release of drug becomes slower. However, Figure 8 shows that the release profiles are somewhat more complicated than this.

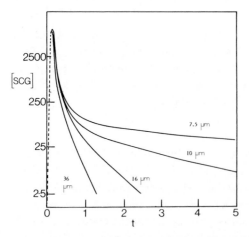

Figure 7. Influence of sphere diameter on SCG release from HSA microspheres manufactured using 5% glutaraldehyde for 4 hours. (Units as for Fig. 6.)

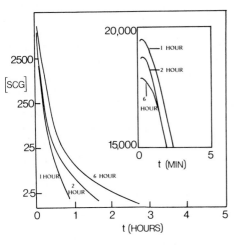

Figure 8. Appearance of SCG (ng/ml) in phosphate buffer eluent with time, showing the influence of time of cross-linking with 1% glutaraldehyde (given next to the curves) on release. The detail shows release over the first 5 minutes. The microspheres had a mean diameter of 15–20 μm — other conditions as Fig. 6.

Thus, for HSA microspheres stabilized by cross-linking with 1% glutaraldehyde for differing periods of time, both the burst phase and the second phase of release are altered. That is, an increase in time of stabilization *reduces* the burst effect for sodium cromoglycate, but for the second phase of release, greater amounts of SCG are released into the eluent with HSA spheres that have been stabilized for longer periods of time. The detail of Figure 8 shows that this effect arises because more drug remains associated with the microspheres after the burst phase with longer stabilized spheres, so that there is more compound available for release in the second phase. These results also suggest that longer periods of stabilization do not greatly affect the diffusion of drug from within the microspheres to the outside. These findings are verified by the observation (Tomlinson and Burger, 1984) that incorporation of greater amounts of drug into the microspheres, up to levels of 45% (by weight), results in more drug being released into the eluent at a faster rate, though still exhibiting biexponential release. Yapel (1979) has shown that for epinephrine at levels of 30% (by weight) release becomes monoexponential. None of our data for water-soluble compounds such as sodium cromoglycate, sodium iodohippurate, rose bengal, alizarin red, doxorubicin and 5-fluorouracil show this trend towards monoexponential release, and it seems that this is dependent upon the compound under study.

Similar alterations in release can be obtained using higher concentrations of cross-linker. Also, 2,3-butadione has the same effect on drug release as glutaraldehyde does, although the longer times needed for effective cross-linking are a problem. Glutaraldehyde appears to be the cross-linker of choice, although with, for example, methotrexate, its use does lead to drug instability.

5. Concluding remarks

There appear to be few pharmaceutical reasons why HSA microspheres cannot be formulated to produce a targetable, and controlled and sustained drug release delivery system for cancer chemotherapy. The freeze-dried microspheres prepared by us are free-flowing, and may be resuspended in isotonic saline containing 0.1% Tween 80. This results in discretely suspended spheres, which do not aggregate in vivo upon injection (Tomlinson et al., 1984a). Although these present spheres are not sterile, aseptic techniques should ensure a sterile product. (Gamma ray sterilization and autoclaving may result in alterations in the extent of protein denaturation, and hence drug release.)

For highly water-soluble compounds our results show that even with high degrees of HSA microsphere stabilization the loss of drug in the burst phase can be between 40 and 93% of the amount of drug originally incorporated. Pre-treatment by ultrasonication will reduce this, but the results appear to indicate that for these compounds a covalent linkage between drug and microsphere matrix material is required. For less water-soluble compounds, and for compounds that specifically interact with serum albumin, the described form of drug incorporation may be satisfactory, since release is much more delayed (unpublished data). Drug release in vitro is biphasic, with release being affected by (a) microsphere size, (b) the extent of chemical cross-linking or heat denaturation, (c) the level of drug incorporation, (d) microsphere swelling, and (e) drug physicochemical structure. It is probable that in vivo microsphere breakdown due to enzyme attack will affect the rate of drug release. Our present studies are directed towards confirming this.

Acknowledgement

This project was largely funded by the Queen Wilhelmina Cancer Fund (project GU 82-8), which is gratefully acknowledged by us.

References

Blanchard, R.J.W., Grotenhuis., I., LaFavre, J.W. and Perry, J.F. (1965) Proc. Soc. Biol. Med. 118, 465–468.

Lee, T.K., Sokoloski, T.D. and Royer, G.P. (1982) Science 213, 233–235.

Lindell, B., Aronsen, K.F., Rothman, U. and Sjoegren, H.O. (1977) Res. Exp. Med. 171, 63–70.

Millar, A.M., McMillan, L., Hannan, W.J., Emmett, P.C. and Aitken, R.J. (1982) Int. J. Appl. Radiat. Isot. 33, 1423–1426.

Muramatsu, N., Goto, Y. and Kondo, T. (1982) Chem. Pharm. Bull. 30, 4562–4565.

Przyborowski, M., Lachnik, E., Wiza, J. and Licińska, I. (1982) Eur. J. Nucl. Med. 7, 71–72.

Tomlinson, E. (1983) Int. J. Pharm. Technol. Prod. Manuf. 4, 49–58.

Tomlinson, E. and Burger, J.J. (1984) in Drug and Enzyme Targeting (Widder, K.J. and Green, R., Eds), Academic Press, New York, in press.

Tomlinson, E., Burger, J.J. Schoonderwoerd, E.M.A., Kuik, J., Schlötz, F.C., McVie, J.G. and Mills, S.N. (1982) J. Pharm. Pharmacol. 34, 88P.

Tomlinson, E., Burger, J.J., Schoonderwoerd, E.M.A. and McVie, J.G. (1984a) in Recent Advances in Drug Delivery Systems (Anderson, J.M. and Kim, S.W., Eds.), Plenum Press, New York, in press.

Tomlinson, E., Burger, J.J., Schoonderwoerd, E.M.A. and McVie, J.G. (1984b) Int. J. Pharmaceutics, submitted.

Widder, K.J., Senyei, A.E. and Ranney, D.F. (1979) Adv. Pharmacol. Chemotherap. 16, 213–271.

Wilkins, D.J. and Myers, P.A. (1966) Br. J. Exptl. Pathol. 47, 568–576.

Yapel, A.F. (1979) U.S. Patent, No. 4,147,767.

Microspheres and Drug Therapy. Pharmaceutical, Immunological and Medical Aspects
edited by S.S. Davis, L. Illum, J.G. McVie and E. Tomlinson
© *1984, Elsevier Science Publishers B.V.*

CHAPTER 2

Stability and release kinetics of drugs incorporated within microspheres

J.P. Benoît, S. Benita, F. Puisieux and C. Thies

1. Introduction

Parenteral controlled release systems, which can be targeted to tissue sites to deliver their active ingredients for a prolonged period, are of considerable interest (Widder et al., 1982). Biodegradable polymers are prime candidates for fabricating such systems. The polymers include gelatin (Yoshioka et al., 1981), albumin (Hashida et al., 1980; Sugibayashi et al., 1977; Friedman and Groves, 1983), polylactide (PLA) (Mason et al., 1976; Beck et al., 1979a; Wakiyama et al., 1982; Gurny et al., 1981) and lactide glycolide copolymer (PGA/PLA) (Wise et al., 1979). Since PLA microspheres have given promising prolonged action in vivo (Beck et al., 1979b), the present study was carried out to show how various process parameters affect the preparation and properties of PLA microspheres. Two drugs were used: progesterone and lomustine (CCNU). The effect of some of the process parameters on the properties of the microspheres formed has been reported recently (Benoît et al., 1983, Benita et al., 1984b). The present work is an examination of the kinetics of in vitro release of drugs from such microspheres. It should be emphasized that little is known about drug release from microspheres, probably as a result of the lack of information concerning the morphology and internal structure of the drug-loaded microspheres. Therefore, a differential thermal analysis and various transmission electron microscopy studies were performed on these microspheres to determine the nature of the internal structure.

2. Materials and methods

2.1. Materials

Poly(($\pm$)-lactide), having a mean molecular weight of 61,000, was supplied by Dr. N. Mason (Biological Transport Laboratory, Washington University, Saint Louis, MO). The poly(vinyl alcohol) used (Vinol 205, Air Products and Chemicals, Allentown, PA) had an average molecular weight of 22,000–31,000, and was 88% hydrolysed. The methylcellulose (Methocel, Dow Chemical Company, Midland, MI) grades used were specified as 10,400 and 8,000 cps. Progesterone and CCNU were supplied by Sigma Chemical Company, Saint Louis, MO, and Roger Bellon Laboratories, Neuilly sur Seine, France, respectively. Methylene chloride (analar grade; J.T. Baker Chemical Company, Phillipsburg, NJ) was used as received.

2.2. Methods

2.2.1. Microsphere preparation

Microspheres were formed at 22°C and atmospheric pressure by a solvent evaporation process (Beck et al., 1979b). The standard procedure used involved placing 250 ml of deionized water in a 400-ml glass beaker. The water contained 0.27 wt% poly(vinyl alcohol) or methylcellulose. An organic solution consisting of 20 ml CH_2Cl_2 and 927 mg ($\pm$)-PLA, with a known weight of drug (280 mg), was poured rapidly into the aqueous phase whilst it was being stirred at a constant rate (Heidolph RZR-2000 stir motor, Heidolph Elektro, Kelheim, F.R.G.). The resulting emulsion was agitated at 22°C for a known period of time, during which the CH_2Cl_2 evaporated. In a few cases, the system was agitated continuously until CH_2Cl_2 evaporation was complete. In most cases, agitation was stopped before CH_2Cl_2 evaporation was complete. The partially dried microspheres were allowed to settle and the aqueous phase containing the polymeric dispersing agent was replaced by deionized water. This was accomplished by three washing and decanting steps. Once the microspheres had been resuspended in emulsifier-free water, they were agitated for 7–17 hours so that CH_2Cl_2 evaporation could proceed to completion. Removal of the polymeric emulsifier from the aqueous phase before completion of CH_2Cl_2 evaporation minimized the formation of free drug crystals in the aqueous phase or on the surface of the microspheres (Bissery et al., 1983).

When CH_2Cl_2 evaporation was judged to be complete, the microspheres were isolated by filtration, washed, and dried in vacuo at 22°C for 20 hours. The dried microspheres were sieved, and stored with a desiccant until required for use. Each microsphere sample was at least triplicated. The drug content did not vary beyond 5% for different batches of the same formulation.

2.2.2. Microsphere evaluation

2.2.2.1. Progesterone content. Progesterone-loaded microspheres (30 mg) were dissolved in 2 ml of CH_2Cl_2. Ethanol (23 ml) was added until precipitation of ($\pm$)-PLA occurred. The resulting suspension was centrifuged at 20,000 rpm for 10 minutes. The clear supernatant was diluted (5 ml) with ethanol and 10 μl of this solution were injected into an HPLC (SP 8000 model, Spectra Physics, Santa Clara, CA). The chromatograph operating conditions were the following: C-8 reverse-phase column (10-μm spheres), methanol as eluent, 2 ml/min eluent flow rate, 254 nm detector. The progesterone content of the sample solutions was obtained from a progesterone calibration curve.

2.2.2.2. CCNU content. CCNU microspheres (30 mg) were dissolved in 2 ml of acetone. Ethanol was added until the ($\pm$)-PLA precipitated. After centrifugation at 20,000 rpm for 10 minutes, a portion of the clear supernatant was diluted with 0.1

N HCl solution containing 5% polysorbate 20. The CCNU content of the diluted solution was determined by high-pressure liquid chromatography. HPLC was carried out under the same operating conditions used for progesterone, except that the eluent was a 50/50 (v/v) acetonitrile/water mixture.

2.2.2.3. Microsphere characterization. Microsphere morphology was characterized by optical, scanning and transmission electron microscope. The latter was carried out on 600-Å thick, microtomed slices obtained from microspheres embedded in epoxy resin. Microsphere size distribution was performed according to the method previously described (Benoît et al., 1983).

Differential thermal analysis of the microspheres was carried out in order to evaluate the internal structure after drug incorporation. This was achieved by means of a Rigaku simultaneous differential thermal and thermal gravimetric analyzer (Rigaku, Tokyo, Japan).

2.2.2.4. Microsphere release studies. Since progesterone and CCNU are poorly soluble in water, the in vitro kinetic experiments were carried out by suspending a given amount of progesterone and CCNU microspheres in different release media, which ensured the maintenance of sink conditions during the overall release process. Progesterone microspheres were suspended in 1000 ml of an aqueous isopropanol solution (30%, v/v), whereas CCNU microspheres were suspended in 500 ml of a Tris buffer solution (pH 7.2) containing 5% (v/v) polysorbate 20. The resulting suspensions were agitated (200 rpm) at 37°C and small filtered portions of the release solutions were withdrawn at different time intervals. The sink solution volumes were maintained constant during the entire kinetic process. Progesterone release was measured spectrophotometrically (242 nm), and CCNU release was determined using the HPLC method already described. Alternatively, the CCNU fraction released was determined after complete decomposition in acidic conditions by the Griess colorimetric method (Loo and Dion, 1965).

3. Results and discussion

The effects of the preparative parameters, such as emulsifier type and concentration, amount of drug incorporated, rate and length of agitation on the various properties of the microspheres formed, have been reported previously (Benita et al., 1984b). It should be noted that the microsphere formation depended to a large extent on the nature of the emulsifier used. Poly(vinyl alcohol) and methylcellulose, two nonionic polymers, produced non-aggregated spherical microspheres. Both emulsifiers acted as protective polymers by being adsorbed at the oil/water interface of the droplets to produce a steric barrier which prevented the coalescence of the droplets (Sabet et al., 1982). Poly(vinyl alcohol) and methylcellulose formed stable methylene chloride in water emulsions, even when progesterone or CCNU and (±)-PLA were dissolved in the methylene chloride phase. However, both drugs tended to crystallize spontaneously in the aqueous phase of the emulsion or on the surface of the micro-

94

spheres when solvent evaporation approached completion. Free crystal formation was eliminated or greatly reduced for drug payloads of 25% or less if agitation was stopped well before solvent evaporation was complete and the emulsifier removed from the aqueous phase (Bissery et al., 1983). Solvent evaporation was then taken to completion in emulsifier-free water.

Microspheres containing up to 25% progesterone or CCNU were spherical and had very smooth surfaces (Fig. 1). There was no evidence of macroscopic pores. Formation of free progesterone crystals had no effect on the surface structure of (±)-PLA microspheres when the progesterone content was less than 31% (Fig. 1). This was not the case for CCNU/(±)-PLA microspheres, which showed rippled and rough surfaces when prepared under conditions that allowed free CCNU crystal formation (Benoît et al., 1983). When the progesterone payload was increased above 35%, drug crystals could be seen attached firmly to the surface of the microspheres. This effect was more pronounced with microspheres containing 68.3% progesterone (Fig. 2). Since these crystals did not wash off during the isolation step, microspheres with this type of structure had an actual payload that approached theoretical values. There was little loss of the drug during fabrication and isolation. However, a significant portion of the drug payload might not be effectively incorporated inside the microspheres, and this would have a pronounced effect on release and profile kinetics. It is also interesting to note that no more than 25% CCNU by weight could be incorporated within the microspheres, irrespective of the emulsifier used. No more than 35% progesterone could be introduced inside the microspheres in the presence of

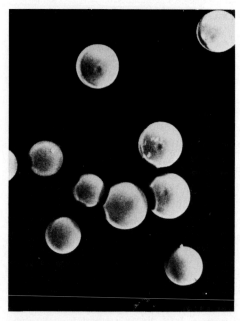

Figure 1. Scanning electron photomicrograph of (±)-PLA microspheres containing 23.2% progesterone (magnification, × 25).

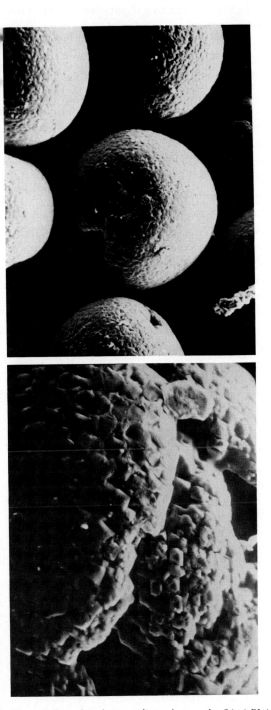

Figure 2. Scanning electron photomicrograph of ($\pm$)-PLA microspheres containing 68.3% progesterone (at two different magnifications: $\times$ 125 and $\times$ 500).

poly(vinyl alcohol), whereas up to 70% progesterone by weight were incorporated within the microspheres by using methylcellulose as the emulsifier.

3.1. Differential thermal analysis (DTA)

This technique was used to study the physical and chemical changes that the microspheres could undergo on a heating cycle (30–200°C). This temperature programme was applied on the different samples and inert reference material. In the case of the melting phase transition of progesterone, a sharp endotherm was observed at 133°C (Fig. 3), corresponding exactly to the melting point of progesterone. Figure 4 shows that poly((±)-lactide) had a thermal event at 57°C which is attributed to the glass transition temperature (T_G) of (±)-PLA. Progesterone-loaded microspheres, prepared by the standard procedure with a drug payload of 22.3%, had an inflection at 53°C, close to the T_G of poly((±)-lactide) alone (Fig. 5), but there was no sharp peak at 133°C, characteristic of crystalline progesterone melting point (Fig. 3). Hence, this was evidence that no crystalline progesterone domains were present in the microspheres. The progesterone was present either in a molecular dispersion or a solid solution state in the (±)-PLA polymer. The progesterone did not crystallize as the microspheres hardened because methylene chloride evaporation, and therefore (±)-PLA solidification, was carried out at 22°C, well below the T_G of (±)-PLA. Progesterone molecules were probably entrapped within the (±)-PLA molecules, without any ability to accumulate and produce solid aggregates in the microspheres.

Microspheres containing 31.7% progesterone behaved similarly to the microspheres previously described, whereas microspheres with 68.3% progesterone presented one phase transition at 132°C (Fig. 6). This sharp peak corresponded to the melting point of progesterone and provided evidence that at least some of this compound existed in the microspheres in a solid state. This evidence is consistent with

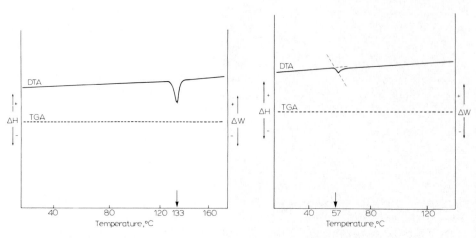

Figure 3. Differential thermal analysis of pure progesterone. TGA, thermal gravimetric analysis.

Figure 4. Differential thermal analysis of pure (±)-PLA polymer.

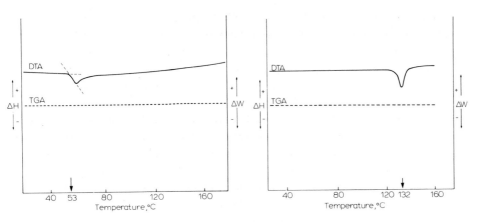

Figure 5. Differential thermal analysis of (±)-PLA microspheres containing 22.3% progesterone.

Figure 6. Differential thermal analysis of (±)-PLA microspheres containing 68.3% progesterone.

the SEM examinations, which indicated that drug crystals were embedded on the microsphere surfaces (Fig. 2). The disappearance of the T_G event between 53 and 57°C could be attributed to the small amount of polymer in these high-loaded progesterone microspheres. In all cases, the thermal gravimetric analysis (TGA) curves remained constant, indicating that no loss of weight occurred during the different DTA experiments.

3.2. CCNU release from the microspheres

Results on the stability of CCNU and progesterone in the microspheres were reported recently (Benita et al., 1984b). Shelf life stability of lomustine incorporated in the microspheres was decreased as compared with unencapsulated lomustine. Decomposition rate increased with increasing temperature, probably due to the molecular dispersion in the poly((±)-lactide). A similar but moderated effect was also observed with the progesterone microspheres. The CCNU results were particularly interesting, since this active ingredient is water- and pH-sensitive. CCNU, relatively stable at pH 1, had a half-life of 40 minutes in phosphate buffer, pH 7.4, and 208 minutes in Tris buffer, pH 7.2, at 37°C (Benoît, 1983). It appeared that decomposition rate was also dependent on the nature of the buffer used. Therefore, it was not possible to determine exactly the accumulated amount of CCNU released from the microspheres in the sink solution by the HPLC method.

To confirm that at least part of the CCNU remained intact in the sink solution, an organic extraction of the aqueous phase was made using hexane after 120 minutes of incubation in both buffers. CCNU can be extracted by hexane, whereas its main polar degradation products (2-chloroethanol or cyclohexylamine) remain in the aqueous phase (Reed et al., 1975). Small quantities of CCNU were found in the hexane phase in both buffers. This was evidence that intact CCNU was present in the microspheres after immersion in buffer sink solutions. Moreover, the microspheres were not altered, and kept their surface characteristics, even after 22 days of incubation in a phosphate buffer containing 5% polysorbate 20 at 37°C (Fig. 7). In view of these results, another approach was used. The amount of CCNU released (more exactly, its main degradation product in acidic medium, nitrous acid) was determined by the Griess method, and the amount of CCNU remaining in the microspheres was then calculated. No linear dependence between the logarithm of the percentage of CCNU remaining in the microspheres and the time was observed, indicating that the kinetic data did not follow the first-order equation (Fig. 8). However, the interpretation of these release data is very difficult as a result of the degradation processes probably occurring simultaneously inside the microspheres and in the sink solution. Therefore, no clear conclusion could be drawn.

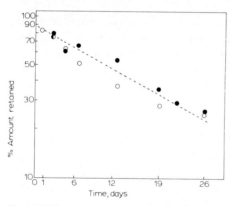

Figure 7. Scanning electron photomicrograph of (±)-PLA microspheres containing 17.1% CCNU after 22 days immersion in a phosphate buffer solution comprising 5% polysorbate 20.

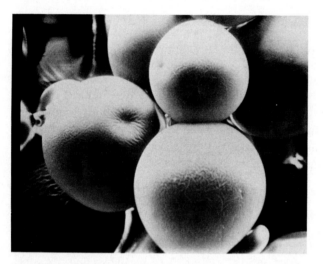

Figure 8. First-order release plots of CCNU from two similar batches of microspheres (22.3% payload) in a phosphate buffer sink solution containing 5% polysorbate 20.

3.3. Release kinetics of progesterone from the microspheres

DTA analysis and SEM observations (Figs. 1 and 5) indicated that progesterone was intimately mixed with the polymer in the (±)-PLA microspheres, as was also confirmed by transmission electron microscopy. No pores or channels could be detected, even at high magnification. All this evidence led to the conclusion that progesterone-loaded microspheres (up to 32%) consisted of a homogeneous matrix phase. Progesterone release from the (±)-PLA microspheres should, therefore, follow the equation which describes the desorption kinetics of a dissolved drug from a monolithic spherical device. Since the kinetic equation is too complex, it can be reduced to two approximations which are valid for different portions of the desorption curve and which are reliable to better than 1% (Baker and Lonsdale, 1974). The early time approximation which holds over the initial portion of the curve is expressed by the following equation:

$$\frac{Q'}{W_0} = \left(\frac{Dt}{r^2\pi}\right)^{\frac{1}{2}} - 3\frac{Dt}{r^2} \qquad \{1\}$$

where Q' is the amount released at time t, W_0 is the initial amount in the microspheres, D is the diffusion coefficient of the drug in the polymer, r is the radius of the microspheres. Equation 1 is valid for $Q'/W_0 < 0.4$. The late time approximation is given by:

$$\frac{Q'}{W_0} = 1 - \frac{6}{\pi^2}e^{-\frac{\pi^2 Dt}{r^2}} \qquad \{2\}$$

Equation 2 is in fact a first-order equation valid for $Q'/W_0 > 0.6$.

According to these equations, the overall progesterone release should not follow either a first-order equation or a square root of time equation. For the purpose of confirming this, the non-linear least-squares regression search procedure was used (Benita et al., 1984a). This statistical method, using the kinetic experimental results without any further transformation, was applied to identify the drug release mechanism from matrix tablets. Since two kinetic models are expected, the chi-square, χ^2, test should be used which is useful for comparison purposes. It is in fact a measure of the deviation of the expected curves from the experimental curve. The expected curves are calculated by a curvefit computer program which consists of a least-squares fit to a non-linear function with a linearization of the fitting function. Therefore, the resultant values of χ^2 for the first-order expected equation having the following expression:

$$Q' = W_0(1-e^{-k_1 t}) \qquad \{3\}$$

and for the square root of time expected equation represented by:

$$Q' = kt^{1/2} \qquad \{4\}$$

can be compared in order to determine which of the two models better describes the experimental kinetic data obtained. The expected amount released will be calculated by means of Equations 3 and 4, respectively, and compared with the observed amount released.

According to the definition, a value of χ^2 equal to 0 indicates that the observed kinetic data and the expected kinetic data are identical. The smallest χ^2 value obtained during the comparison will designate the correct release model. Therefore, χ^2 is an evaluation of the accuracy of fit to the experimental data. The computer program used is based on the method of non-linear least-squares, which is a technique for fitting the data with a function which is not linear in its parameters. According to this method, the optimal parameter values are obtained by minimizing χ^2 with respect to each of the parameters simultaneously. This search leads to the best-fit curve expressed by the appropriate minimum value of χ^2 for each of the two expected kinetic models, taking into consideration the experimental data obtained. The two expected curves as predicted by the first-order kinetic pattern and square root of time equation are shown in Figure 9 and compared with the observed kinetic data.

It can be seen from Figure 9 that none of the kinetic models fits the experimental release data of progesterone from microspheres (24.4% payload). This result is also confirmed by the χ^2 values of 10.1 and 33.5 for the first-order and square root of time equations, respectively. Similar kinetic behaviour was observed in various batches of microspheres containing less than 32% progesterone. Analysis of different portions of the release curve according to Equations 1 and 2 showed that no linear relationship was observed between the initial amount released and the square root

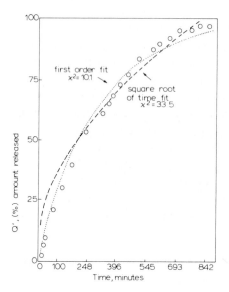

Figure 9. Fitting and comparison of predicted release curves as reported by the computer according to the square root of time (---) and first-order (···) equations to observed kinetic data (o) yielded by (±)-PLA microspheres containing 24.4% progesterone.

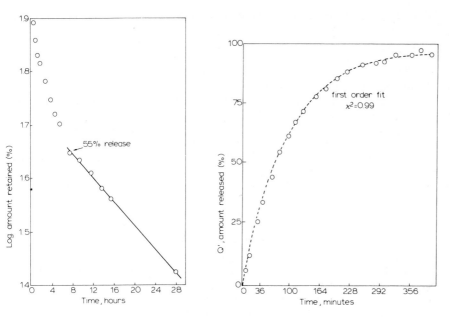

Figure 10. Apparent first-order progesterone release profile from ($\pm$)-PLA microspheres (24.4% payload) in the final portion of the release curve.

Figure 11. Fitting of first-order predicted release curve to observed kinetics data (o) yielded by ($\pm$)-PLA microspheres containing 68.3% progesterone.

of time. However, late release of progesterone from the microspheres was found to follow a first-order kinetic pattern according to Equation 2 (Fig. 10). In contrast, high progesterone payload microspheres exhibited a release profile which conformed with first-order kinetics (Fig. 11). The square root of time expected curve was so far from the kinetic data observed that it was totally rejected by the computer. These results were corroborated by the χ^2 values obtained, which were 0.99 and 67.00 for the first-order and square root of time kinetic models, respectively. The kinetic profile observed indicated that progesterone release from the high payload micro-spheres probably followed a dissolution process rather than a leaching process through a homogeneous matrix. Therefore, it was very interesting to note that increasing the progesterone content in the microspheres altered the morphology of the microspheres and led to different release kinetic patterns.

References

Baker, R.W. and Lonsdale, H.K. (1974) in Controlled Release of Biologically Active Agents (Tanquary, A.C. and Lacey, R.E., Eds.), Vol. 47, pp. 15–71, Plenum Press, New York.

Beck, L.R., Cowsar, D.R., Lewis, D.H., Gibson, J.W. and Flowers, C.E. (1979a) Am. J. Obstet. Gynecol. 135, 419–426.

Beck, L.R., Cowsar, D.R., Lewis, D.H., Cosgrove, R.J., Riddle, C.T., Lowry, S.L. and Epperly, T. (1979b) Fertil. Steril. 31, 545–551.

Benita, S., Shani, J., Abdulrazik, M. and Samuni, A. (1984a) J. Pharm. Pharmacol. 36, 222–228.

Benita, S., Benoît, J.P., Puisieux, F. and Thies, C. (1984b) J. Pharm. Sci., in press.

Benoît, J.P. (1983) Préparation et Caractérisation de Microsphères Biodégradables pour Chimioembolisation, Ph. D. Thesis, Université de Paris-Sud, Paris.

Benoît, J.P., Puisieux, F., Thies, C. and Benita, S. (1983) 3rd International Conference on Pharmaceutical Technology (APGI), Vol. III, pp. 240–249, Paris.

Bissery, M.C., Thies, C. and Puisieux, F. (1983) Communication, 10th International Symposium on Controlled Release of Bioactive Materials, San Francisco.

Friedman, M. and Groves, M.J. (1983) 3rd International Conference on Pharmaceutical Technology (APGI), Vol. III, pp. 179–184, Paris.

Gurny, R., Peppas, N.A., Harrington, D.D. and Banker, G.S. (1981) Drug Develop. Ind. Pharm. 7, 1–25.

Hashida, M., Yoshioka, T., Muranishi, S. and Sezaki, M. (1980) Chem. Pharm. Bull. 78, 1009–1016.

Loo, T.L. and Dion, R.L. (1965) J. Pharm. Sci. 54, 809–811.

Mason, N., Thies, C. and Cicero, T.J. (1976) J. Pharm. Sci. 65, 847–850.

Reed, D.J., May, H.E., Boose, R.B., Gregory, K.M. and Beilstein, M.A. (1975) Cancer Res. 35, 568–576.

Sabet, V.M., Zourab, S.M. and Said, W. (1982) J. Disper. Sci. Techn. 3, 419–433.

Sugibayashi, K., Morimoto, V., Nadai, T. and Kato, Y. (1977) Chem. Pharm. Bull. 25, 3433–3434.

Wakiyama, N., Juni, K. and Nakano, M. (1982) Chem. Pharm. Bull. 30, 2621–2628.

Widder, J.K., Seney, A.E. and Sears, B. (1982) J. Pharm. Sci. 71, 379–387.

Wise, D.L., Fellman, T.D., Sanderson, J.E. and Wensworth, R.L. (1979) in Drug Carriers in Biology and Medicine (Gregoriadis, G., Ed.), pp. 237–270, Academic Press, London.

Yoshioka, T., Hashida, M., Muranishi, S. and Sezaki, H. (1981) Int. J. Pharm. 8, 131–141.

Microspheres and Drug Therapy. Pharmaceutical, Immunological and Medical Aspects
edited by S.S. Davis, L. Illum, J.G. McVie and E. Tomlinson
© *1984, Elsevier Science Publishers B.V.*

103

CHAPTER 3

Design of biodegradable polyalkylcyanoacrylate nanoparticles as a drug carrier

P. Couvreur, V. Lenaerts, D. Leyh, P. Guiot and M. Roland

1. Introduction

The entrapment of cytotoxic drugs inside carriers that can be taken up by endocytosis, such as liposomes, improves drug specificity and reduces toxicity towards healthy cells (Rahman et al., 1974; Gregoriadis, 1974). Work in this field has resulted in the development of polyacrylamide nanocapsules (Speiser, 1976; Marty et al., 1978). These nanocapsules may also be helpful in promoting cellular uptake via endocytosis for compounds that normally do not gain access to lysosomes (Couvreur et al., 1977). Polyacrylamide capsules (diameter, approximately 200 nm) are more stable than liposomes in biological fluids and during storage due to their polymeric nature (Krupp, 1976; Kimelberg et al., 1975). Furthermore, they can entrap various molecules in a stable and reproducible way (Speiser, 1976; Couvreur et al., 1977). However, it is unlikely that these lysosomotropic colloidal carriers will be digested by lysosomal enzymes, and this may restrict their clinical use. With these considerations in mind we recently developed biodegradable nanoparticles prepared by polymerization of various alkylcyanoacrylate monomers (Couvreur et al., 1979a, 1982b). Similar polymers are used in surgery as sutures and adhesive agents (Collins et al., 1969; Heisterkamp et al., 1969).

This paper describes the preparation of polyalkylcyanoacrylate nanoparticles as well as the techniques used in attaching cytostatic drugs to the particles. Data concerning the degradability and the release of drugs from these nanoparticles are also presented.

2. Preparation of polyalkylcyanoacrylate nanoparticles

The most significant advantage of alkylcyanoacrylates over other acrylic derivates used previously for preparing nanoparticles is the polymerization process. In contrast to other acrylic derivates, which require an energy input for the polymerization process which can affect the stability of the adsorbed drug, the alkylcyanoacrylates can be polymerized easily without such a contribution.

Nanoparticles are prepared by adding the monomer to an aqueous solution of a

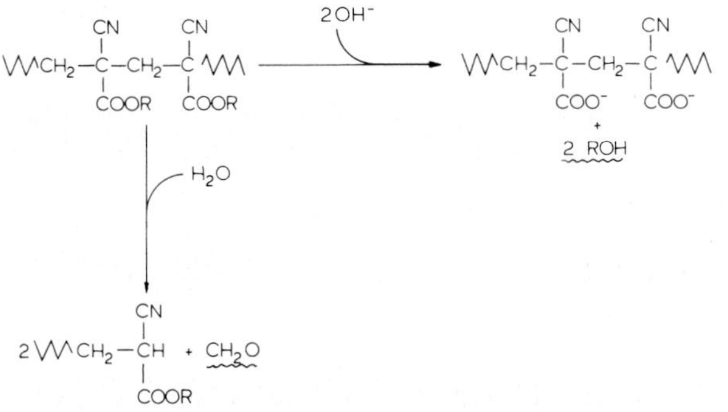

Figure 1. Polymerization mechanism for cyanoacrylic monomers (Donnelly et al., 1977).

surface-active agent under vigorous stirring. The pH value of the polymerization medium lies between 2 and 4. The alkylcyanoacrylate is polymerized at ambient temperature and the biologically active substance is introduced into the medium either before the addition of the monomer or after polymerization. The pH of the medium determines both the polymerization rate and the degree of adsorption of the drug when the latter is ionizable. The polymerization process is slowed down when the pH is reduced and the adsorption of the drug reaches a maximum when it is in a non-ionized form (Couvreur et al., 1979a).

More recently, it was discovered, surprisingly, that polyalkylcyanoacrylate nanoparticles can be prepared by polymerization of an alkylcyanoacrylate in an aqueous medium in the absence of surface-active agents. In some cases, it is also possible to avoid the use of an acid in the polymerization medium. This is sometimes desirable because the adsorbed drug could be adversely affected or decomposed. The surfactant-free media used for the preparation of nanoparticles generally contain poly(ethylene glycol) 200 (10%), glucose (5%), lactose (9.5%) or dextran 70 (1%) in an aqueous solution of citric acid (Couvreur et al., 1983). It is important to note that alkylcyanoacrylates are practically insoluble in water. Therefore, it was unexpected that a monomer of this type added to an aqueous medium free of surfactant could polymerize and form submicroscopic particles of a diameter smaller than 100 nm. Furthermore, it was also surprising that nanoparticles could be prepared by adding an alkyl cyanoacrylate to a non-acidic aqueous medium as these monomers are very reactive. The monomers polymerize very quickly, by an anionic polymerization mechanism (Fig. 1), as soon as they come into contact with alkaline substances or with non-acidified water (Donnelly et al., 1977).

3. Morphological characterization

Scanning electron microscopy of the nanoparticles shows generally spherical particles of a diameter of about 200 nm (Fig. 2). Furthermore, electron microscopic examination of the freeze-fracture replicas reveals the existence of an internal structure for

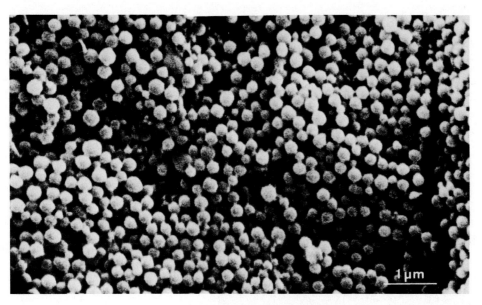

Figure 2. Morphological appearance of polymethylcyanoacrylate nanoparticles in the scanning electron microscope.

the polybutylcyanoacrylate nanoparticles (Couvreur et al., 1979a; Kante et al., 1980; Guiot and Couvreur, 1983). The particles are extremely porous and show a large surface available for drug adsorption. The internal structure is not homogeneous (Fig. 3), but consists of a granulous nucleus surrounded by a more homogeneous ring. This zone cannot be considered as an envelope since there is no clear discontinuity between it and the nucleus. From a total of 250 distribution profiles, the range in radius distribution was from 25 to 340 nm, and the average radius $\pm$ S.D. was 80.6 $\pm$ 73.2 nm. The average external surface of particles was 148,800 nm^2 and the average volume per particle was 11×10^6 nm^3. These results were confirmed by using a laser light-scattering technique (nanosizer).

4. Molecular weight measurements

Nanoparticles were prepared with and without the use of surfactants at various pH values ranging between 2.9 and 4.1. The molecular weights of these preparations were determined using a HPLC-GPC chromatograph with a μStyragel column. The molecular weight determinations were made using poly(ethylene glycol) as a standard. Figure 4 shows the chromatogram of polyisobutylcyanoacrylate nanoparticles prepared at pH 3.6 without surface-active agents. The presence of only one peak demonstrates that the analysed polymer was homogenous. Furthermore, the symmetry of the peak suggests a uniform distribution of the molecules with a calculated molecular weight ranging between 500 and 1000. Thus, the nanoparticles appear to be built by

106

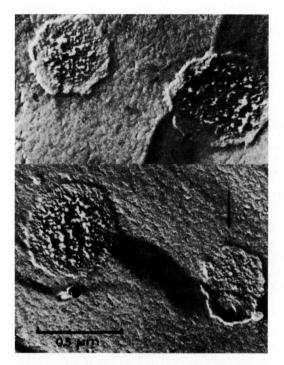

Figure 3. General appearance of a freeze-fracture replica from spray-frozen sample of a polybutylcyanoacrylate nanoparticle suspension (Kante et al., 1980).

an entanglement of numerous small oligomeric subunits rather than by the rolling up of one or a few long polymer chains. Figure 5 shows that the molecular weight of these oligomers is proportional to the pH of the preparation medium. However, when the nanoparticles were prepared by polymerization of the butyl cyanoacrylic monomer in an aqueous medium containing Pluronic F68 (1%) as a surfactant, the chromatogram appeared quite different (Fig. 6). Indeed, three different peaks were

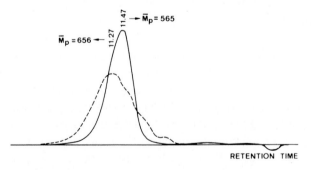

Figure 4. Chromatogram of polyisobutylcyanoacrylate nanoparticles prepared at pH 3.55 (—) and neutralized at pH 7 (---).

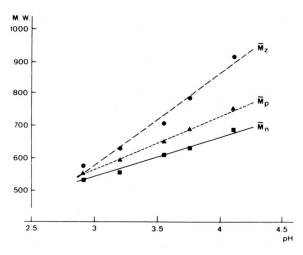

Figure 5. The effect of the pH of nanoparticle preparation on the molecular weight.

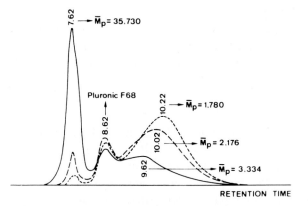

Figure 6. Gel permeation chromatogram for polyisobutylcyanoacrylate nanoparticles prepared with Pluronic F68 as stabilizer. pH of nanoparticle preparation: pH 4.5, —; pH 3.8, ---; pH 3.3, ⋯.

observed: the central one corresponded to the Pluronic, whereas the extreme ones corresponded to a bimodal distribution of polymer molecular weights. The mean molecular weight of the heaviest fraction was calculated to be greater than 35,000, while the molecular weight of the lightest one was about 2,000.

These data suggest that the procedure for the preparation of nanoparticles can greatly modify the molecular weight of the polymeric subunits forming the nanoparticles. These observations could be of significance in the later discussion of toxicological and pharmacological results.

5. Degradation of nanoparticles

The ability of the cyanoacrylate monomers to polymerize quickly and to adhere firmly to tissues has evoked considerable medical interest in their potential as haemostatic agents and tissue adhesives (Leonard et al., 1966; Matsumoto et al., 1967). A characteristic of these polymers is that their rate of degradation is dependent on the length of their alkyl chain. Moreover, histotoxicity seems to be dependent upon the half-life of biodegradation, which is prolonged with increasing alkyl chain length (Wilkinson and San Antonio, 1972). Likewise, the polymerization speed increases with the chain length of the monomer. It was found by many authors that the in vitro degradation of polyalkylcyanoacrylate follows a chemical pattern, leading to the production of formaldehyde and cyanoacetate (Leonard et al., 1966; Vezin and Florence, 1980). It was shown that degradation took place at the polymer surface and was independent of any esterase present (Vezin and Florence, 1978). Wade and Leonard (1972) have shown that the disappearance of an implanted polymeric block is only for a minor part due to degration via the formaldehyde-producing pathway. However, no other degradation mechanism was identified. Also, the in vivo behaviour of nanoparticles studied by autoradiography and by metabolization and toxicological experiments was difficult to explain by a degradation process forming only formaldehyde (Kante et al., 1982; Couvreur et al., 1982a; Grislain et al., 1983). For this reason, it was very important to identify and quantify the main degradation mechanism of polyisobutyl-cyanoacrylate nanoparticles under biological conditions.

5.1. Chemical degradation

Nanoparticles were suspended either in a 0.05 N phosphate buffer, pH 7.0, or a 0.01 N NaOH solution, pH 12.0. After 24 hours incubation, the degradation products (isobutanol and formaldehyde) were measured, after removal of the remaining polymer by ultracentrifugation at 21,000 rpm for 2 hours. The formaldehyde concentration was determined in 3 ml of the supernatant after reaction with chromotropic acid according to the method of Bricker and Johnson (1945). The isobutanol concentration was determined by a gas chromatography method. 1.25 mg of isopentanol were added as internal standard to a 5 ml sample of the supernatant. The chromatograms were interpreted by the ratio of sample peak height over internal standard peak height. Both alcohols were extracted by 2.5 ml diethyl ether and the extracts were injected into a column (6 feet × 1/8 inch) filled with Chromosorb (W-AW-DMCS, 80–100 mesh) containing 10% Carbowax 20M. The temperature of the injector and of the flame ionization detector was 200°C and the temperature of the oven was 120°C. The carrier-gas (N_2) flow was 30 ml/min. At the same time, the degradation of the nanoparticles due to ester hydrolysed was followed by an automatic titrimetric method. During the pH-stat work, the titrant was added as soon as the pH of the sample differed from a preselected value (pH 10.5). By proper choice of the speed for titrant addition, it was possible to keep the pH exactly at the desired value. Addition of 0.1 N NaOH was recorded as a function of time. This experiment was made on a 50 ml nanoparticle suspension containing 1.7 mg of polymer per ml.

The contribution of the formaldehyde pathway to the degradation of polyisobutyl-cyanoacrylate nanoparticles was surprisingly small for all pH values tested. Indeed, the amount of formaldehyde produced in 24 hours at pH 7.0 was 5% of the theoretical quantity that would have been produced if the polymer had been entirely degraded by this method. At pH 12, this value reached only 7%. Conversely, isobutanol production was 85% of the theoretical quantity in the alkaline medum. These results suggest the presence of an alternative degradation pathway to that of chain hydrolysis with production of formaldehyde. This new pathway, consisting of the hydrolysis of the ester function, is the main degradation route at basic pH values. Furthermore, this was confirmed by determination of the acid produced by the ester hydrolysis (Fig. 7). Indeed, consumption of NaOH corresponded to the hydrolysis of 94% of the ester functions present in the incubation medium.

5.2. Enzymatic degradation

The nanoparticles were suspended in a phosphate-buffered (0.05 N, pH 7) isoosmolar sucrose solution containing various concentrations of rat liver microsomes. The concentration of polymer was 2 mg/ml at the beginning of the degradation process. The isobutanol present was measured by the GLC method described above after centrifugation of the samples at 21,000 rpm for 2 hours. In the same way, the isobutanol was measured after different incubation times in the presence of a given concentration of rat liver microsomes (1.88 mg protein/ml). The effect of liver microsomes on the ester hydrolysis of polyisobutylcyanoacrylate nanoparticles was clearly demonstrated. Indeed, the relation between the amount of isobutanol produced in 30 minutes and the concentration of liver microsomes was linear up to 4 mg protein/ml, where the curve reached a plateau (Fig. 8), probably because of a relative lack of nanoparticles. Furthermore, the rate of production of isobutanol as a function of time was constant for at least 45 minutes (Fig. 9). After that time, a plateau was reached, which could be due to an enzymatic inhibition by one of the products. These results implied that, under physiological conditions, the polyisobutylcyanoacrylate

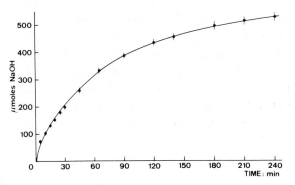

Figure 7. Plot of NaOH required to compensate the acidity resulting from polymer degradation at pH 10.5 as a function of time. Each point is the mean ± S.D. of three experiments (Lenaerts et al., 1983).

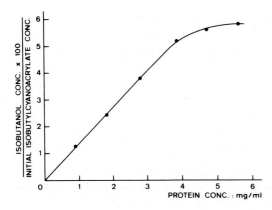

Figure 8. Isobutanol produced by ester hydrolysis of polyisobutylcyanoacrylate nanoparticles in 30 minutes in the presence of various concentrations of rat liver microsomes (Lenaerts et al., 1983).

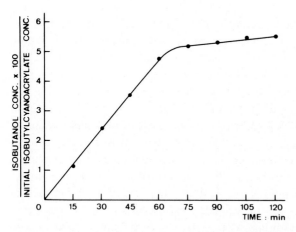

Figure 9. Isobutanol produced by ester hydrolysis of polyisobutylcyanoacrylate nanoparticles in the presence of rat liver microsomes (1.88 mg proteins/ml) as a function of time (Lenaerts et al., 1983).

nanoparticles were degraded mainly by an enzymatic process. By this process, the polymeric chain remains intact, but gradually becomes more and more hydrophilic, until it is water-soluble. The production of formaldehyde via chemical degradation seems to play a marginal role in the overall degradation of nanoparticles under physiological conditions. The suggestion of Vezin and Florence (1978), that esterases do not affect the degradation rate, is contested. Furthermore, our results show that the use of formaldehyde production as the only indicator for polymer degradation can lead to erroneous conclusions.

6. Drug adsorption and drug release

6.1. Drug adsorption on nanoparticles

Owing to their small size and porous nature, nanoparticles are able to adsorb efficiently a wide variety of drugs. Examples are listed in Table 1. The drugs to be associated to the carrier can be dissolved in the polymerization medium before addition
of the cyanoacrylic monomer or in the already prepared nanoparticle suspension.

6.2. Drug release from nanoparticles

It was important to test the hypothesis that the drug is released from the nanoparticles as a consequence of polymer degradation. For this reason, we compared the
kinetics of release of drug from the carrier and of polymer degradation.

^{14}C-labelled nanoparticles loaded with [^{3}H]actinomycin D (2 ml) were incubated
at 37°C in 50-ml portions of an isotonic medium buffered at various pH values (0.05
M acetate buffer, pH 4.9, 0.05 M phosphate buffer, pH 7, and 0.05 M borate buffer,
pH 9). Samples (5 ml) were taken out at various times and centrifuged (21,000 rpm;
2 hours). ^{14}C and ^{3}H activities were measured by liquid scintillation counting in the
supernatant and the sediment dissolved by dimethylformamide.

Figure 10 shows an excellent correlation between the release of [^{3}H]actinomycin
D from the particles and the degradation of the ^{14}C-labelled polymer into water-soluble compounds. An increase in the degradation rate at higher pH values was also
confirmed. However, the correlation between drug release and degradation rate was
observed at all pH values tested. This strict correlation is only possible if the drug
is distributed homogeneously in the polymeric mass of the particle. Since the biodegradability of polyalkylcyanoacrylates depends on the nature of the alkyl chain it is
possible to choose a polymer that has a biodegradability corresponding to the pro-

TABLE 1

Adsorption of different drugs on several polyalkylcyanoacrylate nanoparticle formulations

Drug	Concentration* (μg/ml)	Adsorption (%) on polyalkylcyanoacrylate nanoparticles			
		Methyl	Ethyl	Isobutyl	Hexyl
Adriamycin	1,000	—	—	94	61
Dactinomycin	55	92	86	70	—
Vinblastine	1,000	58	66	46	—
Vincristine	300	—	—	57	—
Penicillin V	1,000	50	37	—	—
Insulin	12 IU	40	44	40	93
Methotrexate	120	15	15	—	—

* Concentration of the drug in the polymerization medium.

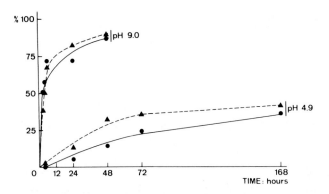

Figure 10. Quantities (%) of ^{3}H (▲) and ^{14}C (●) released from [^{3}H]actinomycin D-loaded ^{14}C-labelled polyisobutylcyanoacrylate nanoparticles as a function of time in different pH conditions (Lenaerts et al., 1983).

gramme established for the drug-release. Thus, the degradation kinetics of these nanoparticles as well as the release of the adsorbed drug can be perfectly controlled and programmed according to the desired therapeutic effect. This objective can also be achieved by using appropriate mixtures of nanoparticles (Couvreur et al., 1979b).

6.3. Application to the parenteral administration of insulin
The parenteral administration of insulin associated to degradable polyalkylcyano-acrylate nanoparticles is an interesting example of drug release in vivo (Couvreur et al., 1980b).

Nanoparticles were prepared by polymerization of different monomers (i.e., methyl, ethyl, isobutyl and butyl cyanoacrylates) according to the previously de-scribed method (Couvreur et al., 1979b, 1980a). Insulin (at a concentration of 10.5 IU/ml) was allowed to adsorb onto the particles obtained by polymerization of 13.5 mg monomer/ml final suspension. Different formulations were investigated using groups of six female Wistar rats made diabetic by intravenous injection of 60 mg streptozotocin/kg body weight. 52.5 IU/kg insulin were administered subcutaneously. Test groups receiving insulin adsorbed on polyalkylcyanoacrylate nanoparticles were compared for hypoglycaemic action with control groups receiving free insulin. Blood samples were collected from the tail vein at regular time intervals, and blood-glucose levels were determined enzymatically, using glucose oxidase. Results were expressed as a percentage of the initial blood-glucose levels. Figure 11 shows that nanoparticles were effective in prolonging the hypoglycaemic action after subcutaneous adminis-tration to diabetic rats. Indeed, the initial blood-glucose levels were retained after 8 hours for the control groups and after 20, 24 and 26 hours for the rats that had received insulin adsorbed onto polyethylcyanoacrylate nanoparticles, polyisobutyl-cyanoacrylate nanoparticles and polybutylcyanoacrylate nanoparticles, respectively. These results are in accordance with the degradation rates of the polymers and demonstrate that the drug was not altered by its linkage to nanoparticles. Therefore,

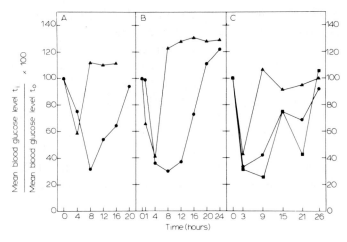

Figure 11. Comparison of blood-glucose levels between groups of six female Wistar rats receiving subcutaneously either 52.5 IU/kg free insulin (▲) or 52.5 IU/kg insulin adsorbed on nanoparticles (●) obtained by polymerization of ethyl cyanoacrylate (A), isobutyl cyanoacrylate (B) or butyl cyanoacrylate (C) monomers (Couvreur et al., 1980b).

longer alkyl chain lengths are thought to be able to provoke longer hyperglycaemic effects since their degradation rate is lower.

7. Conclusions

This paper describes the design of a biodegradable particulate drug carrier. Although favourable results have been obtained using experimental tumour models and the toxicity of doxorubicin has been reduced by linking it to nanoparticles (Brasseur et al., 1980; Couvreur et al., 1982a), an important problem remains, namely the excessive accumulation of the carrier by the reticuloendothelial system (Grislain et al., 1983), especially by the Kupffer cells of the liver (Lenaerts et al., 1983). In a few limited cases, such characteristics of the in vivo distribution of nanoparticles could be favourably exploited in the treatment of parasitic (leishmaniasis) or infectious diseases (cryptococcis, hystoplasmosis). However, in the field of anticancer chemotherapy, capture of nanoparticles by liver, spleen and bone marrow could hinder the availability of the associated drug to the tumoural tissue. Therefore, a second carrier generation with higher tissue specificity has been proposed, which can be guided in the body by an external intervention. Among the possibilities, we chose the production of nanoparticles possessing magnetic susceptibility. We demonstrated that such magnetized nanoparticles were able to reduce the accumulation of the carried drug in the reticuloendothelial system and that higher levels of drug were obtained at the desired target organ (Ibrahim et al., 1983). A third generation of drug carriers with a better cell specificity has also been considered following the discovery of a method

114

for the production of monoclonal antibodies (Köhler and Milstein, 1975). Indeed, specificity of interaction between antibodies and antigens has stimulated numerous researches in the field of drug-targeting, especially for application in cancer chemotherapy. The lack of success obtained in in vivo experiments with drug-antibody molecular complexes can be partly attributed to the poor loading capacity of immunoglobulins. Therefore, we have considered another strategy, consisting of the entrapment of a larger number of active molecules inside polycyanoacrylic nanoparticles coated with monoclonal antibodies (Couvreur and Aubry, 1983). The specific interaction between antibody-coated nanoparticles and antigenic tumour cells has also been confirmed. Using a spacer molecule, we showed that it was possible to build a system with both of the antibody-immunoreactive portions on the outside of the carrier (Couvreur and Aubry, 1983).

Acknowledgements

This work was supported by grants from the SOPAR company and the 'Institut pour l'Encouragement de la Recherche Scientifique dans l'Industrie et l'Agriculture'. We are also grateful to the 'Fonds National de la Recherche Scientifique' of Belgium. The excellent technical assistance of Mr. Bulckens and Mr. Van Diest is greatly appreciated.

References

Brasseur, F., Couvreur, P., Kante, B., Deckers-Passau, L., Roland, M., Deckers, C. and Speiser, P. (1980) Eur. J. Cancer 16, 1441–1445.

Bricker, C.E. and Johnson, H.R. (1945) Ind. Eng. Chem. 17, 400–402.

Collins, J.A., Pani, K.C., Seidenstein, M., Brandes, G. and Leonard, F. (1969) Surgery 65, 256–259.

Couvreur, P. and Aubry J. (1983) in Topics in Pharmaceutical Sciences (Breemer, D.D., Ed.), Elsevier, Amsterdam, pp. 305–316.

Couvreur, P., Tulkens, P., Roland, M., Trouet, A. and Speiser P. (1977) FEBS Lett. 84, 323–326.

Couvreur, P., Kante, B., Roland, M., Guiot, P., Baudhuin, P. and Speiser, P. (1979a) J. Pharm. Pharmacol. 31, 331–332.

Couvreur, P., Kante, B., Roland, M. and Speiser, P. (1979b) J. Pharm. Sci. 68, 1521–1524.

Couvreur, P., Kante, B., Lenaerts, V., Scailteur, V., Roland, M. and Speiser, P. (1980a) J. Pharm. Sci. 69, 199–202.

Couvreur, P., Lenaerts, V., Kante, B., Roland, M. and Speiser, P. (1980b) Acta Pharm. Technol. 26, 220–222.

Couvreur, P., Kante, B., Grislain, L., Roland, M. and Speiser, P. (1982a) J. Pharm. Sci. 71, 790–792.

Couvreur, P., Roland M. and Speiser P. (1982b) US Patent 4,329,332.

Couvreur, P., Roland, M. and Speiser P. (1983) U.S. Patent Request, 370,892.

Donnelly, E.F., Johnston, D.S., Pepper, D.C. and Dunn, D.J. (1977) Polym. Lett. Ed. 15, 399–405

Gregoriadis, G. (1974) Biochem. Soc. Trans. 2, 117–119.

Grislain, L., Couvreur, P., Lenaerts, V., Roland, M., Deprez-Decampeneere, D. and Speiser, P. (1983) Int. J. Pharmaceut. 15, 335–345.

Guiot, P. and Couvreur, P. (1983) J. Pharm. Belg. 38, 130–134.

Heisterkamp, C.H., Simmons, R.L., Vernick, J. and Matsumoto, T. (1969) J. Trauma 9, 587–593.

Ibrahim, A., Couvreur, P., Roland, M. and Speiser, P. (1983) J. Pharm. Pharmacol. 35, 59–61.

Kante, B., Couvreur, P., Lenaerts, V., Guiot, P., Roland, M., Baudhuin, P. and Speiser, P. (1980) Int. J. Pharmaceut. 7, 45–53.

Kante, B., Couvreur, P., Dubois-Krack, G., De Meester, C., Guiot, P., Roland, M., Mercier, M. and Speiser, P. (1982) J. Pharm. Sci. 71, 786–790.

Kimelberg, H.K., Mayhew, E. and Papahajopoulos, D. (1975) Life Sci. 17, 715–723.

Köhler, G. and Milstein, C. (1975) Nature 256, 495–497.

Krupp, L., Chobanian, A.V. and Brecher, P.I. (1976) Biochem. Biophys. Res. Commun. 72, 1251–1258.

Lenaerts, V., Nagelkerke, J.F., Van Berkel, T.J.C., Couvreur, P., Grislain, L., Roland, M. and Speiser, P. (1982) in Sinusoidal Liver Cells (Knook D.L. and Wisse E., Eds), pp. 343–352, Elsevier, Amsterdam.

Lenaerts, V., Couvreur, P., Christiaens-Leyh, D., Joiris, E., Roland, M., Rollman, B. and Speiser, P. (1983) Biomaterials 5, 65–68.

Leonard, F., Kulkarni, R.K., Brandes, G., Nelson, J. and Cameron, J.J. (1966) J. Appl. Polym. Sci. 10, 259–272.

Marty, J., Oppenheim, R.C. and Speiser, P. (1978) Pharm. Acta Helv. 53, 17–23.

Matsumoto, M.T., Pani, K.C., Hardaway, R.M. and Leonard, F. (1967) Arch. Surg. 94, 153–156.

Rahman, Y.E., Cerny, E.A., Tollaksen, S.L., Wright, B.J., Nance, S.L. and Tompson, J.F. (1974) Proc. Soc. Exp. Biol. Med. 146, 1173–1176.

Speiser, P. (1976) Prog. Colloid. Polym. Sci. 59, 48–54.

Vezin, N.R. and Florence, A.T. (1978) J. Pharm. Pharmacol. 27, 5P.

Vezin, N.R. and Florence, A.T. (1980) J. Biomed. Mat. Res. 14, 93–106.

Wade, W.R. and Leonard, F. (1972) J. Biomed. Mat. Res. 6, 215–221.

Wilkinson, T.S. and San Antionio, S. (1972) Arch. Derm. 106, 834–836.

Microspheres and Drug Therapy. Pharmaceutical, Immunological and Medical Aspects
edited by S.S. Davis, L. Illum, J.G. McVie and E. Tomlinson
© *1984, Elsevier Science Publishers B.V.*

CHAPTER 4

Development and testing of proteinaceous nanoparticles containing cytotoxics

Richard C. Oppenheim, Elizabeth M. Gipps, John F. Forbes and Robert H. Whitehead

1. Introduction

Traditional chemotherapy is sometimes inefficient and/or dangerous. Over the last few years, a number of ways have been devised to deliver the correct amount of the correct drug to the correct site at the correct time. Whilst drug solutions can be locally perfused into a diseased area, or drugs can be released from an embolized drug delivery system, such procedures presuppose a clear identification of an accessible diseased target area. This essentially external approach to targeting, whilst being clinically useful, does not address the main problem of modern pharmaceutics.

Before any drug delivery system can be designed to target effectively to diseased cells, we need to have a much better understanding of the properties and behaviour of the surfaces of such cells. Considerable work still remains to be done to determine how the circulatory system of the body interacts with variously administered delivery systems. Until such basic information is established, the development of modern drug delivery systems will be severely limited. Any drug delivery system which purports to target selectively to diseased cells must lead to a reduction in dose and/or increase in therapeutic index.

If we are to devise drug delivery systems which will target to individual diseased cells, it is appropriate to consider only those systems that have a size of the same order as the diseased cell. Hence, effective targeting will involve the development and testing (both in vitro and in vivo) of colloidal drug delivery systems. If we can achieve an association between the delivery system and the outside surface of the cell, the drug will be released to perfuse the cell locally, and hopefully sufficient will interact with and penetrate through the membrane to cause the desired therapeutic response.

Most cells become diseased by an intracellular derangement. Hence, it is sensible to concentrate the efforts in delivering the drug as close as possible to its site of action within the cell. Consequently, methods of delivering drugs into target cells, and nowhere else, have to be considered. One of the drug delivery systems that can do this is based on hardened desolvated macromolecules.

2. General method of making proteinaceous nanoparticles

The microencapsulation literature contains many references to the simple coacervation of macromolecules including proteins. In summary, an aqueous solution of the macromolecule is gradually desolvated by the addition of a strongly hydrophilic electrolyte or a water-miscible solvent in which the macromolecule is insoluble. When sufficient desolvating agent has been added, phase separation occurs (as represented by the phase boundary in Figure 1) and coacervate droplets appear. In traditional simple coacervation, these high-energy droplets deposit onto the dispersed insoluble or immiscible bulk core material and coalesce, thereby reducing the high interfacial free energy associated with the droplets. The coating on the core is then hardened by cooling and chemical cross-linking with aldehydes, such as formaldehyde or glutaraldehyde. The coacervation process can be thought of as the end result of the gradual removal of water from an extended flexible macromolecule which results in the macromolecule gradually 'rolling up' in the increasingly adverse environment.

Just on the isotropic side of the coacervate phase boundary, represented by the point × in Figure 1, the discrete macromolecules can be considered to be in an extensively desolvated state but still not sufficiently desolvated to associate with other macromolecules to form a coacervate. It was proposed that the macromolecules (or small aggregates of them) could be fixed in this state by adding glutaraldehyde, just as is done in simple coacervation procedures and in other analogous procedures. Following work initially in Zurich and subsequently at Parkville, we were able to show that discrete submicron solid particles could be made (Marty et al., 1978; The Pharmaceutical Society of Victoria and Speiser, 1974). These were styled nanoparticles (Marty and Oppenheim, 1977) to distinguish them from the larger and already well-established microparticles (Ekman and Sjöholm, 1975) and macro-aggregates (Rhodes et al., 1969).

This particular way of making solid, submicron drug delivery systems or nanoparticles was initially described in terms of a wide range of macromolecules including the proteins gelatin and albumin. All the work reported here on the incorporation

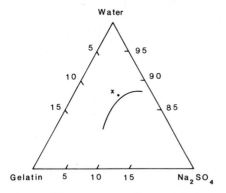

Figure 1. Three component diagram (gelatin, water, sodium sulphate).

of cytotoxics into nanoparticles and the in vitro and in vivo testing of the delivery systems has used human serum albumin as the macromolecule. This material was chosen because of the desire to use the delivery system eventually in humans and the excellent clinical record of other particulate systems based on human serum albumin.

The extent of desolvation and approach to the coacervation phase boundary can be monitored by nephelometry. As the boundary is approached, there is a sharp rise in the intensity of the scattered light just before the system becomes visibly turbid and coacervation has occurred. Resolvation of the macromolecule by the addition of solvents such as isopropanol or water reduces the intensity of the scattered light. The ideal points on the desolvation/resolvation profile for hardening are indicated in Figure 2.

Usually an excess of glutaraldehyde is added and, after the hardening reaction has proceeded for a defined time, the excess is removed by an addition reaction with sodium metabisulphite. The nanoparticles are separated from free unincorporated drug and the other low-molecular-weight impurities by passage through a gel permeation chromatography column. Sephadex G-50m is usually used as the packing.

Figure 3 is a scanning electron micrograph of a typical batch of nanoparticles. Even at the highest magnification routinely used (× 30,000), there has never been any suggestion that these nanoparticles have pores. This nonporous character of proteinaceous nanoparticles is different from other types of nanoparticles, such as those based on alkylcyanoacrylate, which appear to be quite porous (Couvreur et al., 1979). This lack of porosity means that if drugs are to be linked to preformed nanoparticles, only the outer surface is available and the payloads would be expected to be quite low. However, the drug would be quite accessible once the drug delivery system had been administered in vivo. On the other hand, a higher payload should result if the drug is added to the system before the macromolecule is desolvated and hardened. However the drug, molecularly dispersed throughout the solid nanoparticles, would only be available if the nanoparticle was degraded in vivo.

An extensive body of information is available concerning the extent and type of

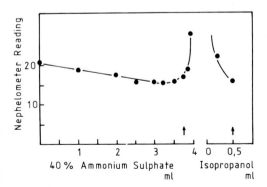

Figure 2. Light scattering profile for the desolvation and resolvation of human serum albumin. The ideal points for hardening are indicated by arrows.

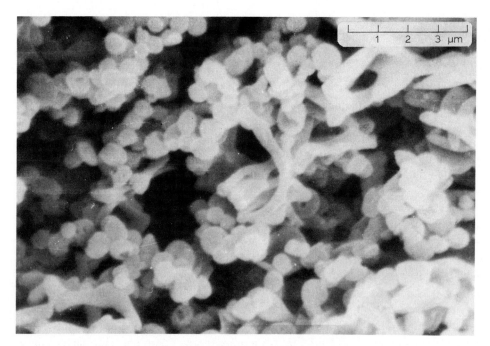

Figure 3. Scanning electron micrograph of a batch of albumin-based nanoparticles.

binding of drugs to albumin, particularly when the albumin is in a well-solvated state. There is very little data available on the binding when the albumin is not so well solvated, as will occur when proteinaceous nanoparticles are made. A detailed discussion of this problem and the related problem of how to maximise payloads is available elsewhere (Oppenheim, 1984).

As summarised in Table 1, we have found that the payload that is achievable ranges from less than 1% to more than 15%, depending on the drug and the macromolecule.

TABLE 1

Drug payloads achieved in a variety of proteinaceous nanoparticles

Drug	Nanoparticle base	Payload (%)
Melphalan	Human serum albumin	0.19
Sodium diatrizoate	Human serum albumin	0.5
Prednisolone	Human serum albumin	3.0
Sodium salicylate	Gelatin	6.0
Sodium stibogluconate	Bovine serum albumin	9.0
Sodium aurothiomalate	Gelatin	10.0
Potassium triamcinolone acetonide 21-phosphate	Rabbit serum albumin	15.7

Marty (1977) found that the inclusion of a surface-active agent in the starting system improved the dispersibility of the final product, even though most of the surfactant is separated from the nanoparticles in the size-exclusion chromotography purification step. Polysorbate 80 was originally used, but this was found to be unsuitable since its cloud point was lowered upon the addition of the desolvating agent to below the working temperature of 35°C. The resultant cloudiness interfered with the nephelometer monitoring of the desolvation of the albumin. Polysorbate 20 was found not to interfere with the monitoring and has been used subsequently to make various proteinaceous nanoparticle products.

Whilst it might be possible to make a solid nanoparticle containing a high payload of the desired drug, and that delivery system has all the desired in vitro properties, there is always the potential problem of administering to the body a protein which has been chemically modified. Kennedy (1983) has shown that when nanoparticles made from bovine serum albumin are injected into the knee joints of rabbits, there is an adverse temporary increase in joint diameter upon the second and subsequent administrations of the drug delivery system. However, nanoparticulate products based on gelatin did not cause any adverse response when injected into the joints.

Upon repeated intravenous administration of gelatin nanoparticles to rodents no gross antigenic response has been observed (Oppenheim, 1981). More recently, Gipps (1983) has repeatedly injected human serum albumin nanoparticles intravenously into mice and again no adverse response has been observed. Whilst this is encouraging and enables continuation of the development of proteinaceous nanoparticles, before such a system could be considered for human use, very careful screening of the delivery system will be required.

Having provided this background to the production of proteinaceous nanoparticles, the question of a delivery system for cytotoxic agents can be addressed.

3. Incorporation of cytotoxics into proteinaceous nanoparticles

In designing a drug delivery system for use in cancer chemotherapy four questions have to be answered: 1. Can the delivery system associate with or be taken up by the target cancer cells? 2. Can cytotoxic agents of choice be incorporated into nanoparticles? 3. Can sufficient of the agent be incorporated to be cytotoxic in vitro? 4. Is the drug delivery system effective in vivo?

These four questions have been considered in an attempt to devise a proteinaceous nanoparticle delivery system containing either 5-fluorouracil or doxorubicin. It was our objective to achieve one or both of the following: 1. Reduce the in vivo therapeutically effective dose. 2. Increase the therapeutic index.

Two cell lines were chosen for the study. The B16 mouse melanoma is a rapidly growing transplantable tumour which arose spontaneously in a C57 BL/6 mouse. When grown in fluid culture, the cells adhere to the plastic or glass of the culture flask in which they are grown and they are not inhibited by contact (Kolb and Mansfield, 1980). In soft agar assay, colony formation of the B16 line is decreased by a number of cytotoxic agents, including 5-fluorouracil (Stephens et al., 1977) and doxorubicin (Stephens and Peacock, 1978). The concentration of doxorubicin hydrochloride needed to inhibit the growth of this cell line by 50% has been reported by Tsuruo and Fidler (1981) as being between 7 and 13 ng/ml for 10^5 cells.

The other cell line chosen came from a breast adenocarcinoma in the mouse induced by a virus (MMTV). This normally develops a mouse mammary tumour in older (post-breeding age) female mice of the RIII strain (Schlomm et al., 1977). It is not inhibited by contact, and adheres to glass and plastic. In vitro, both cell lines can be grown in RPMI 1640 medium containing 15% foetal calf serum, 2 mM L-glutamine, 50 IU Penicillin and 100 μg/ml streptomycin. The cells were maintained in fluid medium in plastic culture flasks in an incubator at 37°C in a 5% carbon dioxide in air atmosphere with 100% humidity. The medium was changed weekly, or more frequently if required.

When B16 is grown in fluid culture, the cells take from 12 to 24 hours after seeding to enter the exponential growth phase and the doubling time has been reported by Kolb and Mansfield (1980) to be about 18 hours in RPMI 1640. Preliminary experiments in our laboratories gave similar results for the B16 line and analogous results for the MMTV line.

3.1. Association of nanoparticles with target cells

Since the proteinaceous nanoparticles can be considered as nonporous matrices with the drug molecularly dispersed throughout the matrix, drug release would depend on the degradation of the nanoparticle by lysosomal enzymes after the nanoparticle has been taken across the cell membrane by some form of vacuolation. To show that such a lysosomotropic drug delivery system can, in fact, cross the cell membrane rather than just associating with it, the surface of the nanoparticles can be conjugated with fluorescein isothiocyanate (FITC) (Oppenheim and Stewart, 1979). Upon incubation with both the B16 and the MMTV cell lines and then upon examination under a fluorescence microscope, it was found that for FITC-conjugated human serum albumin-based nanoparticles, there was a concentrated fluorescence in the cytoplasm with a dark nuclear shadow (Gipps, 1983). The background contained a very diffuse fluorescence. If the nanoparticles were only adsorbing or adhering to the cell membrane surface, the whole of the cells would show as fluorescent. Hence, for these cell lines, the proteinaceous nanoparticles appear to be endocytosed by the cells, as Oppenheim and Stewart (1979) found earlier for other tumour lines.

3.2. Obtaining a usable payload

FITC can be surface-conjugated to proteinaceous nanoparticles and such nanoparticles can also be tagged with ^{99m}Tc (Oppenheim et al., 1978). This indicates that there are amino and oxygen based moieties on the surface which could act as anchor points for drug conjugation. However, in order to maximise the payload, these potential sites were not pursued, rather attempts were made to incorporate separately 5-fluorouracil and doxorubicin into the nanoparticles.

5-Fluorouracil is appreciably soluble and stable in water and does not bind strongly to proteins. It is not vulnerable to attack by glutaraldehyde but can undergo covalent addition with bisulphite (Rork and Pitman, 1975). Doxorubicin as the hydrochloride has fair stability in water but the amino group is a potential site for reaction with glutaraldehyde. It was known (Oppenheim, 1981) that methotrexate had severe problems in linkage since masses of yellow flocculant conjugate were formed when attempts were made to make proteinaceous nanoparticles containing methotrexate.

Nanoparticles containing separately 5-fluorouracil and doxorubicin were made following the general method outlined earlier. Ammonium sulphate (40% aqueous solution) was used to desolvate the 2.5% human serum albumin, 1.0% 5-fluorouracil and 2% polysorbate 20 solution. After hardening with glutaraldehyde, the system was passed through a 45 × 800 mm Sephadex G-50m column. The void volume containing the desalted nanoparticles was freeze-dried. The resultant cake can be stored for at least 4 years before reconstitution to produce a colloidal dispersion suitable for parenteral administration.

The salt peak was read at 266 nm, a maximum absorbance wavelength for 5-fluorouracil. The maximum possible interaction between the unincorporated 5-fluorouracil and the residual bisulphite produces an insignificant contribution to the absorbance over the time span taken to make the measurement. After contributions by other possible contaminants, a payload of around 8% (i.e., 100 mg of nanoparticles contained 8 mg 5-fluorouracil) was found. This compares favourably with the 0.25% payload found by Hashida et al. (1977) for their emulsion type system and 2.3% payload found by Morimoto et al. (1980) for their heat-stabilised albumin microspheres.

In a similar way, proteinaceous-based nanoparticles containing doxorubicin were made. No problems were encountered with the addition of the glutaraldehyde. The salt peak was first cleaned up by high-pressure liquid chromatography using a C18 reverse-phase column and then the amount of doxorubicin analysed by fluorescence spectroscopy. Payloads of 2.5% were achieved. This is an unoptimised result and further work is in progress to increase the payload. It is comparable to the 1% obtained by Forssen and Tökés (1979) and the 4% obtained by Widder et al. (1979), but lower than the 14% reported by Couvreur et al. (1982) for their methylcyanoacrylate nanoparticles.

Determining the payload of drug in the nanoparticle by calculating the difference between that added initially and the amount that is unincorporated in the salt peak can be subject to criticism. However, careful evaluation (Gipps, 1983) of potential losses of the drug have shown that these are insignificantly small and that the drugs are either in the nanoparticles or in the salt peak. If the payloads have been overstated, then the nanoparticles used in the in vitro and in vivo experiments described below are more potent than has been assumed. Thus, this type of payload calculation gives the worst case situation.

Storage of the purified drug-containing nanoparticles in water or saline for up to

7 days at room temperature, followed by analysis of the aqueous phase, showed that no drug could be detected in the supernatant, so confirming the nonporous drug-imbedded-in-matrix picture of proteinaceous nanoparticles.

Full details of the manufacture and physical testing of these nanoparticles containing cytotoxics is available elsewhere (Oppenheim et al., 1984).

3.3. In vitro testing

Despite the recent work of Tritton et al. (1983) showing that free unbound doxorubicin may have some toxicity at the membrane surface, the assumption has been made in this work that the desired site of action is intracellular. The FITC-conjugated nanoparticles showed that it is possible to obtain intracellular delivery, and it appears possible to incorporate 5-fluorouracil and doxorubicin into separate lots of human serum albumin-based nanoparticles. Whilst these are necessary prerequisites for effective intracellular therapy, it must also be shown that the payload of drug can be released from the delivery system at the site of action. Whilst incubation with lysosomal enzymes may provide nanoparticle degradation and drug release, there may be complicating factors when whole cells are used. Accordingly, two types of in vitro experiments were undertaken with B16 and MMTV-cell lines growing in RPMI 1640 medium.

As described by Gipps et al. (1984), initially a dose response relationship was established. From this, not only can the absolute weight of drug containing nanoparticles required to kill tumour cells be established but also an estimate can be made of the possible dose needed in animal studies. By choosing two mid-range doses, a growth kinetic profile of the tumour lines can be determined.

3.3.1. Dose response

1×10^5 cells of the B16 and MMTV lines were separately incubated with nanoparticles containing 5-fluorouracil or doxorubicin. After 4 days, the number of viable cells was determined. In untreated cultures, the number of viable cells was almost four times that at the beginning of the dose response experiments. The results for each drug with each cell line were similar, in that at the highest concentration of the nanoparticles containing the cytotoxics, the tumour cells were killed. However, at the lower concentrations, there is only inhibition of the growth. Table 2 gives typical results for 5-fluorouracil with the MMTV cell line.

The activity of the cytotoxic nanoparticles ranges from half the activity of the free drug at relatively high drug concentrations to less than 10% at the lower concentrations. This change in responsiveness, whilst disappointing, may be an artefact of the in vitro experiment and final judgement needs to be reserved for the in vivo experiments.

3.3.2. Growth kinetics

Again using 1×10^5 cells of the individual lines, the growth kinetics over 4 days were studied. When untreated cells were grown, approximately 24 hours elapsed after the cells had been seeded before the cells adhered to the plastic plates and started to divide. Thereafter, both cell lines had a doubling time of approximately 24 hours. Since

TABLE 2

Average number of cells ($\times 10^5$), present after 4 days incubation of 1×10^5 MMTV cells

Dose of 5-fluorouracil ($\mu g/ml$)	Free drug	Nanoparticles containing 5-fluorouracil
50	0.05 ±0.05	0.11±0.025
15	0.094±0.07	1.92±0.16
5	0.13 ±0.02	2.17±1.04
1.5	0.09 ±0.07	2.26±0.05
0.5	0.36 ±0.12	1.69±0.1

Eight replicates of untreated cells grew to $(2.88 \pm 0.98) \times 10^5$.

the medium was not replaced during the experiment, the supply of nutrients is limited and growth of the cells is slowed after about 3–4 days. The results of both lines with both drugs are similar and Figure 4 shows the typical results obtained for 5-fluorouracil and the B16 melanoma.

Free 5-fluorouracil at either concentration severely inhibits the growth of the cells whilst not killing them completely. Incubation with the larger amount of 5-fluorouracil incorporated in nanoparticles also inhibited the cell growth. However, the smaller amount of drug in nanoparticles, whilst inhibitory, did not stop the development of the cells. The doubling time was extended to about 120 hours.

Low doses of drug-free nanoparticles do not significantly affect the growth of the cells. Using an amount of drug-free nanoparticles equivalent to that used to deliver the highest doses of drug, there was a slowing of the onset of division of the cells, although growth, when started, was normal.

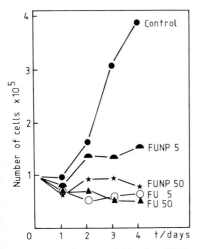

Figure 4. In vitro growth kinetics of B16 melanoma in the presence of 5-fluorouracil (FU) and 5-fluorouracil in nanoparticles (FUNP). Doses of 5 or 50 $\mu g/ml$ 5-fluorouracil as indicated.

These two types of in vitro testing of proteinaceous nanoparticles show that the drug is present in sufficient concentration in an available form to exert a cytotoxic and cytostatic effect. Since high doses of the drugs incorporated into nanoparticles do kill the cells, the nanoparticles are being degraded and the cytotoxic agent being released. The potency of these cytotoxic nanoparticles is lower than the free drug, which may be due to less of the drug reaching the interior of the cell because of incorporation into nanoparticles, or incomplete degradation of the nanoparticles.

3.4. In vivo testing

In the in vitro test systems there are no anatomical barriers between the administered nanoparticles and the target cells, and only the target cells are contained within this system. Since the in vitro experiments had shown that incorporation of the drug into the nanoparticles did not destroy all the activity of the drug, the problems of anatomical barriers and the effect of non-target cells can be examined in appropriate in vivo experiments.

Two types of animal experiments were performed. As Gipps et al. (1984) show, it is important to consider both survival time and acute toxicity following administration of a novel drug delivery system. If the in vivo targeting to the tumour cells is efficient, it is expected that there should be a reduction in dose and an increase in therapeutic index.

Subcutaneous injection of 0.2 ml containing 1×10^5 viable cells into the left groin of 9–12-week-old female C57 BL mice, enabled the in vivo dose response of the nanoparticles containing 5-fluorouracil to be assessed. Six mice were assigned randomly to the treatment group and also to the control group receiving free 5-fluorouracil. The chemotherapeutic agent was administered intravenously on days 2, 4 and 7 after implantation. Table 3 combines the results of two parallel experiments.

The free drug results in an increase in survival time at around 200 mg/kg. At higher doses it is clear that there is drug toxicity as the survival times fall below the control

TABLE 3

Mean and standard deviation of survival times in days of C57 BL/6 mice ($n = 6$) with SC B16 melanoma treated intravenously

Total dose, mg/kg, 5-fluorouracil equivalence	Free drug	Nanoparticle form
50	27.0±10.6	29.2±12.4
100	28.7± 8.9	26.0± 9.1
200	*33.5± 7.7	28.2± 8.4
Drug control ($n = 8$):		24.2± 4.8 days
300	**10.0± 0.9	26.0± 5.7
400	**9.7± 2.1	*37.7± 9.7
Drug control ($n = 12$);		26.7± 4.8 days

By Student's t-test: * $P \leqslant 0.05$; ** $P \leqslant 0.01$.

of drug-free treatment. The highest dose of fluorouracil in nanoparticles shows a significant increase in survival time.

The treatment of an intraperitoneally implanted fluid MMTV tumour cell suspension by intraperitoneal administration of free doxorubicin and doxorubicin in nanoparticles also shows an initial increase followed by a decrease in survival time for the free drug and an increase (but not statistically significant increase) for the nanoparticle system. Hence, the dose of cytotoxic required for an increase in survival is increased by incorporating the drug into nanoparticles.

Acute toxicity studies would give an estimate of the change in therapeutic index. The LD_{50} for free fluorouracil was found to be 658 mg/kg following four 0.5-ml intravenous injections over 2 hours. For the nanoparticle form it was more than 1000 mg (5-fluorouracil)/kg. No upper limit could be established since the volume injected was large and the mice showed signs of fluid overload. The analogous figures for doxorubicin were 25 mg/kg for free drug and more than 125 mg/kg for the nanoparticle product.

So combining the dose response data with the acute toxicity data, we find that the therapeutic index (measured as the ratio of the toxic dose to the therapeutic dose) for free 5-fluorouracil seems to be around 1.5 whilst for the nanoparticle-delivered 5-fluorouracil it is about 2.5. For doxorubicin, the free drug has a therapeutic index of about 1.6 whilst for the nanoparticle form it is around 3. The delivery of doxorubicin by nanoparticles would also be likely to decrease the cardiotoxicity of the drug, which is one of the major problems in chronic toxicity studies.

4. Conclusions

Solid, nonporous, submicron particles can be made by desolvating and hardening proteins. These proteinaceous nanoparticles are internalized into tumour cells. When either 5-fluorouracil or doxorubicin are incorporated into human serum albumin-based nanoparticles, cytotoxicity is retained both in vitro and in vivo, but diminished as compared to the free drug. However, for both drugs the therapeutic index is increased. Provided payloads, particularly of the doxorubicin product, can be increased, the nanoparticle drug delivery system may be a means of improving chemotherapy with these drugs.

Acknowledgements

The financial support (C76/15138) of the Australian Research Grants Committee is gratefully acknowledged. We thank Hoffman LaRoche and Pharmitalia for donation of 5-fluorouracil and doxorubicin, respectively. The support received from E.R. Squibb & Sons for the general nanoparticle program is gratefully acknowledged.

128

References

Couvreur, P., Kante, B., Roland, M., Guiot, P., Baudwin, P. and Speiser, P. (1979) J. Pharm. Pharmacol. 31, 331–332.

Couvreur, P., Roland, M. and Speiser, P. (1982) U.S. Patent, 4,329,332.

Ekman, B. and Sjöholm, I. (1975) Nature 257, 825–826.

Forssen, E.A. and Tökés, Z. (1979) Biochem. Biophys. Res. Commun. 91, 1295–1301.

Gipps, E.M. (1983) The Incorporation of Cytotoxics into Nanoparticles, M. Pharm. thesis, Victorian College of Pharmacy.

Gipps, E.M., Oppenheim, R.C., Forbes J. and Whitehead, R. (1984), submitted.

Hashida, M., Muranishi, S. and Sezaki, H. (1977) Chem. Pharm. Bull. 25, 2410–2418.

Kennedy, K.T. (1983) Preparation and Testing of Nanoparticles containing Triamcinolone Acetonide, M. Pharm. thesis, Victorian College of Pharmacy.

Kolb, C.A. and Mansfield, J.M. (1980) Oncology 37, 343–352.

Marty, J.J. (1977) The Preparation, Purification and Properties of Nanoparticles, D. Pharm. thesis, Pharmaceutical Society of Victoria.

Marty, J.J. and Oppenheim, R.C. (1977) Aust. J. Pharm. Sci. 6, 65–76.

Marty, J.J., Oppenheim, R.C. and Speiser, P. (1978) Pharm. Acta. Helv. 53, 17–23.

Morimoto, Y., Akimoto, M., Sugibayashi, K., Nadai, T. and Kato, Y. (1980) Chem. Pharm. Bull. 28, 3087–3092.

Oppenheim, R.C. (1981) Int. J. Pharmaceut. 8, 217–234.

Oppenheim, R.C. (1984) in Polymeric Microparticles (Guiot, P. and Couvreur, P., Eds.), CRC Press, Boca Raton, in press.

Oppenheim, R.C. and Stewart, N.F. (1979) Drug. Dev. Ind. Pharm. 5, 563–571.

Oppenheim, R.C., Marty, J.J. and Stewart, N.F. (1978) Aust. J. Pharm. Sci. 7, 113–117.

Oppenheim, R.C., Gipps, E.M., Forbes, J. and Whitehead, R. (1984), submitted.

Rhodes, B.A., Zolle, I., Buchanan, J.W. and Wagner, H.N. (1969) Radiology 92, 1453–1460.

Rork, G.S. and Pitman, I.H. (1975) J. Pharm. Sci. 64, 216–220.

Schlomm, J., Colcher, D., Drohan, W., Kettman, R., Michalides, R., Vlahakis, G. and Young, J. (1977) Cancer 39, 2727–2733.

Stephens, T.C. and Peacock, J.H. (1978) Br. J. Cancer 38, 591–598.

Stephens, T.C., Peacock, J.H. and Steel, G.G. (1977) Br. J. Cancer 36, 84–93.

The Pharmaceutical Society of Victoria and Speiser, P. (1974) Australian Provisional Patent PB 8951/74 and, e.g., U.S. Patent 4,107,288.

Tritton, T.R., Yee, G. and Wingard, L.B. Jr. (1983) Fed. Proc. 42, 284–287.

Tsuruo, T. and Fidler, I.J. (1981) Cancer Res. 41, 3058–3064.

Widder, K.J., Senyei, A.E. and Ranney, D.F. (1979) Adv. Pharmacol. Chemotherap. 16, 213–271.

Microspheres and Drug Therapy. Pharmaceutical, Immunological and Medical Aspects
edited by S.S. Davis, L. Illum, J.G. McVie and E. Tomlinson
© *1984, Elsevier Science Publishers B.V.*

CHAPTER 5

Targeting anticancer drugs to the cell surface by preparation of immobilized derivatives

Thomas R. Tritton and Lemuel B. Wingard, Jr.

1. Introduction

Adriamycin is the most prominent member of the anthracycline class of antineoplastic antibiotics. This drug as well as several of its congeneric relatives play an important role in the treatment of cancer in humans. Since the anthracyclines have a wide spectrum of clinical activity against several kinds of neoplasms, including both the leukemias and solid tumors, much interest has developed concerning the mechanism of action of these agents. Adding to the urgency is the fact that most anthracycline drugs have a serious cardiotoxic side effect, and it has been assumed by workers in the field that a better understanding of the molecular mechanism of the drug might lead to the design of both more active and less toxic new agents.

Proposals seeking to explain the cytotoxic anticancer action of adriamycin have been in three general areas. First, the original ideas in this field derived from the fact that the structure of adriamycin confers upon the molecule a high affinity for binding to DNA by intercalation (DiMarco, 1975). Thus, non-covalent interaction with DNA causing physical blockade of the template for replication and/or transcription could lead to derangement of cell growth. Of course, it is well known that many kinds of molecules have the property of being effective intercalating agents without also having any antineoplastic or pharmacologic properties. In addition, there are adriamycin derivatives (for example, *N*-acetyladriamycin-14-valerate (Sengupta et al., 1977)) which have little or no affinity for DNA but which are still effective agents. Consequently, the direct DNA binding hypothesis suffers both from a lack of explanation for the specific antineoplastic effect of the drug and from the apparent fact that DNA binding is not necessary and sufficient for drug action.

The second type of hypothesis for analyzing the mechanism of action of the anthracyclines again stems from the fact that quinone containing molecules of this type can be reduced by one-electron or two-electron processes (Bachur et al., 1979; Moore, 1977). In the one-electron case, pathways can be postulated that would lead to the formation of reactive anthracycline alkylating agents. Such a reactive agent could then, analogously to other anticancer drugs such as the nitrogen mustards, alkylate sensitive cellular sites, including the genome or other critical intracellular molecules. Although this is an attractive hypothesis on chemical grounds, little evidence exists which supports this mechanism in vivo (Kennedy et al., 1983, Fisher et al., 1983). Reduction of an anthracycline can also potentially lead to the formation of reactive oxygen species, such as superoxide, peroxide or hydroxyl radicals, which could in turn be dangerous to essential cellular sites. Certainly, these kinds of reactions occur in cells exposed to adriamycin and other anthracyclines, but the importance of such oxidative reactions in the cellular toxicity of the drugs has not been firmly established. Evidence exists both for and against this hypothesis (Tannoch and Guttman, 1981; Kennedy et al., 1983).

The third major explanation for the anticancer action of adriamycin is that it acts at the level of the plasma membrane (Tritton et al., 1978). This argument, just as with direct DNA binding, originally came from structural considerations. Most of the anthracyclines, including adriamycin, are amphipathic molecules with both polar and non-polar character. Thus, inherent in their molecular structure is the ability to interact with and thereby disrupt membrane organization. The original experimental evidence supporting this notion is of two basic types: (1) Adriamycin has been shown to interact with both lipid and protein components of membranes with reasonable affinity (Tritton et al., 1978; Mikkelson, et al., 1977; Sinha and Chignell, 1979) and (2) binding to membranes elicits a number of specific changes in their biological properties; in fact, a long record of publications of cell surface membrane activities of anthracyclines exists in the literature (Tritton and Hickman, 1984). This list, however, cannot be taken as proof that the cell surface is the target for drug action or that any of the affected properties of the cell surface are the critical lesion in the mechanism of drug action. Rather, we have undertaken a direct way to show that adriamycin could be an active agent under conditions where it only interacts with the cell surface, and consequently has no access to DNA or other intracellular targets.

2. Preparation of immobilized adriamycin

One of the most useful and straightforward ways to separate cell surface from intracellular actions of a molecule is to immobilize it on insoluble supports (Venter, 1982; Wingard, 1983). Thus, covalent attachment of a ligand to a polymeric material should yield a reagent useful in testing a membrane target hypothesis. We proposed three criteria which were necessary to validate this idea for adriamycin: (1) the dimensions of the polymer used for immobilization should be larger than cells so as to prevent internalization of the drug by endocytotic processes, (2) the attachment of the drug to support should be covalent so as to provide a permanent and irreversible linkage and (3) a method for detecting leakage of free adriamycin from the polymer has to be available. This latter point is especially critical since the presence of low-molecular-weight native drug, which will be taken inside cells by normal uptake mechanisms, would prevent the formation of any decisive conclusions on the role of intracellular versus extracellular sites of action.

Our strategy has been to use both agarose and cross-linked poly(vinyl alcohol) as the polymeric support and to attach the drug molecule by several different chemistries and in different orientations (Tritton and Yee, 1982; Tritton et al., 1983; Wingard and Tritton, 1983; Wingard et al., 1984). Three of the more useful products we have prepared are shown in Figure 1. Structure A is obtained by reaction of the free amino group on the sugar portion of the adriamycin molecule with imidazolyl carbamate groups on agarose polymer of average size about 100 μm. The covalent linkage is then a carbamate. Structure B also uses the amino functionality of the drug for covalent attachment, but the linking chemistry differs from A. In addition, B employs a poly(vinyl alcohol) support. Structure C, also using poly(vinyl alcohol), joins the anthracycline to the polymer through the drug ring system, using a diazonium ion intermediate. In this case carminomycin was used in place of adriamycin since the presence of the strongly activating -OH group should better promote electrophilic substitution than the $-OCH_3$ of adriamycin. The product shown is the *ortho* deriva-

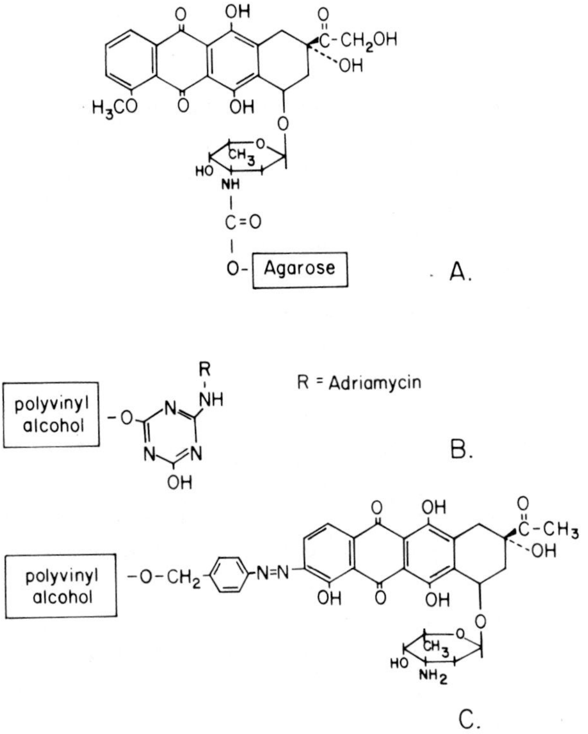

Figure 1. Structures of the various forms of immobilized adriamycin and carminomycin discussed in the text. Synthetic details may be found in Tritton and Yee (1982), Wingard and Tritton (1983) and Wingard et al. (1984). A, Adriamycin immobilized to agarose via reaction of the drug amino group with imidazolyl carbamate linked to the polymer. B, Adriamycin immobilized to cross-linked poly(vinyl alcohol) via reaction of the drug amino group with cyanuric chloride-activated polymer. C, Carminomycin immobilized to cross-linked poly(vinyl alcohol) via reaction of the drug ring system with a diazotized coupling.

tive but the *para* derivative is also possible; we have not analyzed the distribution between the two potential classes of substitution.

Following the synthesis of the immobilized anthracyclines it becomes necessary to remove all traces of non-covalently attached drug. This is accomplished by extensive and continuous washing of the polymers with large volumes of buffer (generally 0.1 M borate, pH 8.0), water and organic solvents (acetonitrile, methanol). This washing phase can take several weeks before acceptably low levels of drug release are obtained. Release is monitored by evaporating a large volume of solvent wash (usually methanol) and then analyzing the residue by high-pressure liquid chromatography. The washing is continued until either no detectable drug is released or the release rate is so low that it can be considered negligible.

The Tökés group has tackled this same problem with somewhat different approaches to the methodology (Tökés et al., 1982; Rogers et al., 1983). Their work is described in the following chapter.

3. Results with agarose immobilization

Our original work in this area used the agarose immobilization chemistry of Figure 1A (Tritton and Yee, 1982). The experimental protocol was to expose a culture of tumor cells (generally the murine cell lines Leukemia 1210 or Sarcoma 180) to immobilized drug and other test conditions for a period of time, and then separate the culture into two aliquots. One aliquot is analyzed for cytotoxicity by cloning the cells in soft agar (Chu and Fisher, 1968). This assay is a measure of cell survival following exposure to a drug; in all cases similar results have been obtained by measuring the cell growth rate in the continuous presence of drug. The second aliquot of cells is extracted and analyzed by high-pressure liquid chromatography for the presence of free adriamycin. Our HPLC system (a reversed-phase μBondapak phenyl system) is capable of recording and quantitating all known adriamycin metabolites, although metabolism is not generally seen in the type of experiments reported here. The sensitivity of the HPLC system is such that we detect intracellular drug at concentrations below that causing cytotoxicity. Thus, we have a good working operational definition of the amount of intracellular drug which is necessary to cause cell death when the anthracycline is given as free, native agent.

Table 1 shows some typical experimental results. Agarose beads without attached adriamycin are not cytotoxic and, as expected, do not reveal any intracellular drug by HPLC analysis. Native, free adriamycin causes the expected dose-dependent cell kill and the accumulated cellular content of drug correlates with cytotoxicity. A notable point here is that even though 10^{-9} M adriamycin is not active, we can still detect cellular accumulation. When the polymer-immobilized adriamycin is used for the first time, cell kill is observed but an amount of free drug is detected in the extracted cells. This occurs despite the fact that extensive washing had reduced the spontaneous release rate to less than detectable levels. The amount of drug found inside the cells

TABLE 1

Survival of L1210 clones in soft agar following exposure to free and immobilized adriamycin

Treatment	% Survival	Cell-associated adriamycin
Control cells	100	0
+ Agarose	100	0
+ 10^{-9} M adriamycin	99	8
+ 5×10^{-8} M adriamycin	60	60
+ 1×10^{-7} M adriamycin	41	110
+ 50 mg freshly prepared agarose-/adriamycin	58	29
+ 50 mg recycled agarose-adriamycin	63	0
+ 100 mg recycled agarose-adriamycin	32	0

The polymeric support in these experiments is agarose and the chemical linkage is an N-alkyl carbamate (Fig. 1). 50 ml of cells (1 × 10^5/ml) were exposed to the indicated treatment for 2 hours. 1 ml was then cloned and 49 ml extracted for HPLC analysis of intracellular adriamycin as previously described (Tritton and Yee, 1982). The cell-associated adriamycin is given in arbitrary fluorescence units; a value of 0 means that none could be detected.

exposed to immobilized adriamycin is less than that found in cells exposed to 5 × 10^{-8} M free adriamycin, which caused similar cytotoxicity. However, a convincing argument could not be made from these results and we could not at this point make any conclusions about the relative importance of cell surface versus intracellular effects of the drug. However, if the once-used immobilized drug preparation is recycled, the material is still cytotoxic but no free drug is found associated with the cells by HPLC. We have also confirmed the absence of drug by radioimmunoassay. Consequently, we conclude that an agent that was heretofore postulated to have intracellular DNA as the major target may still be active even when restricted solely to interaction at the cell surface.

We are not certain why the agarose-immobilized adriamycin needs to be recycled once before no detectable free drug is released upon exposure to cells. One explanation is that small fragments of the polymer exist in the preparation and that these particles can be taken up by endocytosis and dismantled by lysosomal or other cellular degradative processes. In this case, the first exposure to cells causes removal of this small amount of material so that in subsequent exposure to immobilized drug, cytotoxic activity is maintained but no drug is available to be taken inside the cells. In support of this explanation is the indication that with poly(vinyl alcohol) polymers (see below) prior exposure to cells is not generally required before activity without drug uptake is observed.

In the experiments described so far, we do not know the effective concentration of drug when using agarose-immobilized adriamycin. The ambiguity arises because, although we can determine the total concentration of drug attached to the polymer, we do not a priori know how much of the covalently attached drug is on the surface of the beads, and thus available to interact with cells, compared to how much is on the inside of the beads and inaccessible to cellular contact. Our approach to this problem has been to embed the agarose complex in Epon, cut serial sections with a microtome, and observe the cross-sections in a fluorescence microscope. All sections examined show a perfectly uniform distribution of drug fluorescence. Thus, during the coupling reaction, which lasts several hours, the drug can attach to the polymer equally well at all exterior and interior sites. This is a fortunate circumstance because it greatly simplifies the calculation of available drug at the surface of the polymer. We know the total concentration of attached adriamycin and that the drug molecules are uniformly distributed throughout the polymer; since we also know the surface-to-volume ratio, it is a straightforward matter to calculate the available concentration of drug when exposed to cells. In the experiments of Table 1, we came to the surprising conclusion that immobilized adriamycin is at least two to three orders of magnitude more potent than free adriamycin. Because of this finding, we believe that the cell surface represents a very attractive target for anticancer drug action, both because of its apparent high level of sensitivity and because toxic side effects (e.g., cardiotoxicity) may be mediated by intracellular events which would not be triggered by non-penetrating adriamycin derivatives.

The extraordinary sensitivity of tumor cells to cell surface attack by adriamycin may also explain another phenomenon associated with the drug. It has been known for several years that many cell types accumulate adriamycin by facilitated diffusion (reviewed in Skovsgaard and Nissen, 1982). Thus, uptake of free drug is by a carrier molecule, most likely a protein. A question that could be asked is — why have cells evolved a mechanism for internalizing a substance which is toxic? One explanation is that the uptake mechanism occurs via a route which is normally present for concentrating needed nutrients, for example, sugars. An alternative explanation based on our results is that the uptake mechanism does not exist fundamentally to take the drug inside the cells, but rather to get rid of the offending molecule from the site where it is doing the most harm, i.e., at the cell surface. By this hypothesis, the cells take in membrane toxic agents where they can be degraded, metabolized or sequestered by normal routes and consequently removed from dangerous locations on the cell-surface membrane.

4. Results with poly(vinyl alcohol) immobilization

The results described so far allow us to draw certain conclusions, but also raise a number of additional questions. We would like to know, for example, if the nature of the immobilization support is important for maintaining cytotoxic activity and whether the exact chemistry and orientation of drug attachment are critical for drug action. To address these questions we synthesized the two additional types of immobilized anthracyclines (Wingard and Tritton 1983; Wingard et al., 1984) whose structures are shown in Figure 1. The experimental procedures used to analyze these prep-

TABLE 2

Survival of S180 clones in soft agar following exposure to adriamycin immobilized on poly(vinyl alcohol) via attachment through cyanuric chloride

Treatment	% Survival	Cell-associated adriamycin
Control cells	100	0
+ 10^{-7} M adriamycin	52	49
+ 100 mg immobilized adriamycin		
2 hours exposure	81	0
20 hours exposure	41	0

See Figure 1. The experiment was conducted as described in the legend to Table 1.

arations were identical to those used in the agarose-adriamycin experiments described above.

Table 2 shows the combined cell survival and HPLC analysis for adriamycin-poly-(vinyl alcohol) polymers. It is clear that this polymer is also capable of supporting adriamycin in an actively cytotoxic mode and we can tentatively conclude that the nature of the support is probably not a major factor in the design of this general reagent. Comparing the results of Tables 1 and 2, it is also evident that both forms of amino group attachment of adriamycin to the support maintain productive cytotoxic activity. This is somewhat fortunate since reactions at the animo group are often capable of inactivating native, free adriamycin (Arcamone, 1981). Lastly, again comparing Tables 1 and 2, we have shown that immobilized adriamycin is cytotoxic towards both S180 and L1210 cell lines. Therefore, the action at the cell surface does not appear to be limited to a single cell type.

Table 3 shows an experiment designed to test the orientational specificity of the drug-attachment site on the polymer. In the results of both Tables 1 and 2 the adriamycin molecule is attached through the amino sugar moiety, and thus presents approximately the same view of the molecule when approached by a cell. The reverse view, i.e., attachment through the ring system (aglycone) portion of the molecule was

TABLE 3

Survival of S180 clones in soft agar following exposure to carminomycin immobilized on poly(vinyl alcohol) via attachment through diazonium coupling

Treatment	% Survival	Cell-associated carminomycin
Control	100	0
+ 180 mg immobilized carminomycin	19	0

The experiment was conducted as described in the legend to Table 1.

obtained by preparing the carminomycin-poly(vinyl alcohol) conjugate shown in Figure 1C. Carminomycin was used instead of adriamycin for technical reasons, as explained above, but we expect the primary mechanism of action of both agents to be the same. The results described in Table 3 show that carminomycin immobilized in this way is also actively cytotoxic without entering the cell. This result suggests that a precise orientation of the drug at its site of cell-surface attachment is not required for biological activity. Rather, the mere presence of the drug is sufficient to cause derangement of cell growth. One possible implication of this conclusion is that a formal drug receptor, which by ordinary definitions would require a precise ligand orientation, is not present at the cell surface. In a certain sense this is reassuring, since there is no reason to expect cells to have a receptor for a toxic agent and no literature exists supporting such a postulate. On the contrary, our own previous work using photoaffinity labeling (Yee et al., 1984) did not reveal the presence of a cell-surface anthracycline receptor. Furthermore, we have shown a strong connection between the cytotoxic action of adriamycin and cell-surface membrane fluidity (Murphree et al., 1981; Siegfried et al., 1983). Thus, if a global property of membranes, such as fluidity, is the target property whose modulation mediates drug cytotoxicity, then a specific identifiable receptor should not necessarily be expected to be present in the membrane.

5. Conclusion

The results described here suggest strongly that the anthracycline anticancer drugs can mediate their cytotoxic action through cell surface interaction. It cannot be concluded that adriamycin itself works solely at the plasma membrane level because the immobilized drug is a different entity and, in effect, is forced by virtue of its structure to interact with a more limited subset of potential cellular targets than is the native drug, which distributes throughout the cell. The importance of this work lies not so much with adriamycin then, but with the demonstration that the cell surface can be a worthy target for antineoplastic drug action as a general principle. Emphasizing this conclusion is the fact that astonishingly small amounts of immobilized drug need to interact with the cell surface in order to initiate the cytotoxic response. This suggests that a fruitful approach to a new class of anticancer drugs would be to design non-penetrating low-molecular-weight agents which take advantage of the cell surface-mediated mechanism of cell kill. Two major problems must be faced in order to accomplish this: (1) a definition and understanding of the molecular mechanisms by which a cell-surface event can lead to the shutdown of cellular function and eventual cell death and (2) the application of these principles into practical clinical protocols. Such are the goals of future efforts in this area.

Acknowledgements

We thank the NIH (CA 28852 and RR 05416) and American Cancer Society (CH-212 and In-58 S) for financial support. T.R. Tritton is the recipient of a Research Career Development Award (CA 00684).

References

Arcamone, F. (1981) Doxorubicin: Anticancer Antibiotics, Academic Press, New York.

Bachur, N.R., Gordon, S.L., Gee, M.V. and Kon, H. (1979) Proc. Natl. Acad. Sci. U.S.A. 76, 954–957.

Chu, M.-Y. and Fischer, G.A. (1968) Biochem. Pharm. 17, 753–767.

DiMarco, A. (1975) Cancer Chemo. Therap. Rep. 6, 91–106.

Fisher, J., Ramakrishnon, K. and Reevar, J.F. (1983) Biochemistry 22, 1347–1355.

Kennedy, K.A., Siegfried, J.A., Sartorelli, A.C. and Tritton, T.R. (1983) Cancer Res. 43, 54–59.

Mikkelson, R.B., Lin, P.-S. and Wallach, D.F.H. (1977) J. Mol. Med. 2, 33–40.

Moore, H.W. (1977) Science 197, 527–532.

Murphree, S.A., Tritton, T.R., Smith, P.L. and Sartorelli, A.C. (1981) Biochim. Biophys. Acta 649, 317–324.

Rogers, K.E., Carr, B.I. and Tökés, Z.A. (1983) Cancer Res. 43, 2741–2748.

Sengupta, S.K., Seshadri, R., Modest, E.J. and Israel, M. (1977) Proc. Am. Assoc. Cancer Res. 17, 109.

Siegfried, J.A., Kennedy, K.A., Sartorelli, A.C. and Tritton, T.R. (1983) J. Biol. Chem. 258, 339–343.

Sinha, B. and Chignell, C.F. (1979) Biochem. Biophys. Res. Commun. 86, 1051–1057.

Skovsgaard, T. and Nissen, N.I. (1982) Pharmac. Ther. 18, 293–311.

Tannoch, I. and Gutman, P. (1981) Br. J. Cancer 43, 245–248.

Tökés, Z.A., Rogers, K.E. and Rembaum, A. (1982) Proc. Natl. Acad. Sci. U.S.A. 79, 2026–2030.

Tritton, T.R., Murphree, S.A. and Sartorelli, A.C. (1978) Biochim. Biophys. Res. Commun. 84, 802–808.

Tritton, T.R. and Hickman, J.A. (1983) in Oncology Series: Cancer Chemotherapy II (McGuire, W.L. and Muggia, F., Eds.), Martinus Nijhoff, Boston, in press.

Tritton, T.R., Wingard, L.B. and Yee, G. (1983) Fed. Proc. 42, 284–287.

Tritton, T.R. and Yee, G. (1982) Science 217, 248–250.

Venter, J.C. (1982) Pharm. Rev. 34, 153–187.

Wingard, L.B. (1983) Biochem. Pharm. 32, 2647–2652.

Wingard, L.B. and Tritton, T.R. (1983) in Affinity Chromatography and Biological Recognition (Chaiken, I.M., Wilchek, M. and Parikh, I., (Eds.), Academic Press, New York, in press.

Wingard, L.B., Tritton, T.R. and Egler, K.A. (1984), submitted.

Yee, G., Carey, M. and Tritton, T.R. (1984) Cancer Res. 44, 1898–1903.

Microspheres and Drug Therapy. Pharmaceutical, Immunological and Medical Aspects
edited by S.S. Davis, L. Illum, J.G. McVie and E. Tomlinson
© 1984, Elsevier Science Publishers B.V.

Use of microspheres to direct the cytotoxic action of adriamycin to the cell surface

Zoltán A. Tökès, Kevin L. Ross and Kathryn E. Rogers

1. Prologue

1.1. Experience with liposome-entrapped adriamycin

The aminoglycosidic anthracycline, adriamycin (Adr), is widely used in the treatment of various human neoplasms. Chronic cardiotoxicity, immune-suppressive activity, significant dermatologic toxicity after accidental extravasation, and the eventual development of highly resistant tumor clones severely limit the clinical use of this drug. In order to overcome these limitations, efforts were directed toward the development of alternative modes of drug delivery. Our laboratory elected an approach to camouflage Adr by entrapment into anionic liposomes. The rationale for these experiments was to exploit the elevated endocytotic activities of tumor cells and to save the myocardial cells which are deficient in such activities. The drug was bound to phosphatidylcholine in a molar ratio of 1:2 and entrapped in a mixture of lipids composed of a 7:3:1 molar ratio of phosphatidylcholine, cholesterol and phosphatidylserine (Forssen and Tökès, 1979). The resulting vesicles, having an average diameter of 0.09 μm, retained the full anti-tumor activity of Adr as determined in the murine Sarcoma 180 tumor model. Significantly increased cytotoxic activity was observed against Lewis lung carcinoma and murine leukemias L1210 and P388 (Forssen and Tökès, 1981, 1983a). In all of these studies a marked reduction of host toxicity was also achieved. Young mice, after two courses of treatments with liposome-entrapped Adr at a dose of 10 mg/kg, gained the same weight in 10 weeks as the untreated controls, indicating an overall reduction of host toxicity by entrapment (Forssen and Tökès, 1981). At treatment levels of either 20 or 40 mg/kg total dose, mice receiving the liposome-entrapped drug failed to develop significant acute or chronic cardiotoxicity. Using the same experimental conditions with free drug or with empty liposomes combined with free drug, severe chronic cardiotoxicity could be demonstrated (Forssen and Tökès, 1981). The marked immune-suppressive activity of the free drug as measured by hemagglutinin titers against xenogenic erythrocyte antigens and by peripheral leukocyte counts was also eliminated by entrapment (Forssen and Tökès, 1983a). Moreover, the severe tissue damage which occurs when Adr is extravasated during infusion has also been attenuated by encapsulation (Forssen and Tökès,

1983b). Similar findings have been made in other laboratories (Mayhew and Papahadjopoulos, 1983).

Two interesting observations have emerged from these studies. The first was the lack of correlation between the amount of drug associated with a given tissue and the accumulated toxicity. The reduction in myocardial and dermal toxicity by the entrapped Adr was not directly related to the drug exposure in the tissue. This suggests that the mode of drug disposition into subcellular compartments may be more crucial than the absolute amount of drug (Forssen and Tökès, 1983a,b). The second set of observations was the rarity of complete cures and the relative ineffectiveness of liposomes against drug-resistant tumor types. For example, Lewis lung carcinoma treated with Adr-liposomes showed significant reduction in tumor volume. However, after 4 weeks of treatment, an apparently resistant population of tumor cells emerged and grew aggressively. These observations prompted us to search for additional modes of drug delivery.

2. Microspheres

2.1. The rationale for designing microsphere carriers for chemotherapeutic agents

In order to overcome resistance, different approaches for drug presentation were considered. The objectives were to direct a large number of drug molecules predominantly to one cellular domain, the cell surface, and to deliver them simultaneously so that the cell would receive an accentuated effect of the drug-binding all at once. The rationale for this approach comes from two sets of past experiences, namely, lectin-mediated and polymer-hapten-mediated cytotoxicity.

Lectins are well-recognized macromolecules due to their noncovalent binding to carbohydrate groups without modifying them chemically. They usually have two or four binding sites which can attach to glycosylated cell surface components (Andersson and Melchers, 1977). Examples are Concanavalin A (Con A) and wheat germ agglutinin (WGA), both of which are known to bind to lymphocyte cell surfaces. Within a well-defined concentration range, they are known to stimulate lymphoblastogenesis. For example, Con A at a concentration of $1-5$ $\mu g/ml$ per 10^5 lymphocytes will bind to the cell surface and provide a signal for cell division. It is believed that cross-linking of cell surface glycoproteins, acting as Con A receptors, significantly contributes to this signaling process. Lower concentrations of lectins are not effective to stimulate the cells, and higher concentrations result in lectin-mediated cytotoxicity. There appears to be a critical concentration of lectin bound to the cell surface, above which the cell cannot escape from the overwhelming consequences of cross-linked receptors. Subunits of lectins with a single binding site are not effective in producing toxicity, even at higher concentrations.

Similar cross-linking of lymphocyte surface components is observed with haptens covalently attached to carriers and their corresponding immunoglobulin membrane receptors (Melchers, 1979). For successful stimulation of lymphocytes by antigen, simultaneous binding to at least two receptors is necessary. A solution of low-molecular-weight haptens is not sufficient for lymphoblastogenesis. However, if several hapten molecules are covalently attached to a carrier macromolecule and allowed to interact with specific lymphocytes possessing cell surface receptors for the hapten, a successful stimulation of cell division occurs. Furthermore, if the concentration of hapten-carrier complexes increases, or if the hapten is covalently linked to polymers providing a highly repetitious structure, the specific lymphocytes can be killed selectively. These observations suggest again that beyond a critical concentration of hapten-carrier complexes, the excessive cross-linking of immunoglobulin receptors may lead to cytotoxicity.

These two sets of observations prompted us to attach Adr covalently to polymeric carriers with the hope to accomplish an overwhelming perturbation of cell-surface components, leading to cytotoxicity. Although we had no evidence for the existence of specific cell-surface receptors, ample observations of the membrane-perturbing activities of free Adr have been reported (Tritton and Hickman, 1983). In addition, Taylor and coworkers (1982) have already isolated two distinct macromolecular lipids with high affinity of binding to Adr, suggesting the existence of molecules in the membrane for selective drug binding. For the carrier polymers we have chosen polyglutaraldehyde microspheres, because of their available aldehyde groups for the covalent coupling of aminoglycosidic anthracyclines.

A summary of our experience with Adr coupled to polyglutaraldehyde microspheres is provided below. This is not intended as a review of all polymer-bound forms of Adr. In the preceding chapter, Drs. Tritton and Wingard summarize a similar approach using agarose beads or cross-linked poly(vinyl alcohol) as support for Adr and carminomycin.

2.2. Preparation of polymer-bound adriamycin, Adr-PGL

Polyglutaraldehyde microspheres (PGL) were prepared according to the previously published procedures of Margel et al. (1979). The resulting polymers were washed and sized (Tökès et al., 1982). The average diameter of the microspheres used for drug coupling was 4500 Å, as determined by small-angle light scattering with laser flow cytometry and confirmed by scanning electron microscopy (Tökès et al., 1982). Coupling of Adr was accomplished by continuous shaking of a 100 mg/ml suspension of PGL with 5–10 mg/ml of drug in a medium adjusted to pH 6.5 with dilute hydrochloric acid. The resultant drug-polymer complexes (Adr-PGL) were extensively washed in order to ensure that only the covalently coupled drug molecules remained in the suspension. Three observations suggested the formation of stable imino complexes by Schiff base condensation between the Adr amino groups and the aldehyde groups of PGL. First, the reduction of aldehyde groups by LiBH$_4$ eliminated the reaction, second, the analog N-acetyldaunorubicin with blocked amino groups failed to couple to PGL. Finally, the stability of attachment was demonstrated in the presence of fetal calf serum, liposomes, leukemia cells, rat hepatocytes and sarcoma cells.

After 72 hours of incubation with these cells, the Adr-PGL microspheres can be re-covered and repeatedly retested for cytotoxicity. No decrease in activity was observed after repeated use of the complexes.

The amount of drug coupled to PGL can be varied. Adr-PGL preparations have been made to contain 2.5–45 nmol of drug per mg of PGL. Since these microspheres have low porosity, an assumption is made that Adr is primarily coupled to the sur-face of polymers. The surface-density of drug can be varied from approximately one to 20 molecules per 1000 Å^2. However, not every molecule may have equal access to interact with plasma membrane components.

2.3. In vitro interaction with sensitive and drug-resistant murine leukemia cells, L1210. The toxicity of free Adr and Adr-PGL was evaluated using a cytostatic assay, inhibi-tion of colony formation in soft agar and radiochromium release (Tökès et al., 1982; Rogers and Tökès, 1984). In the cytostatic assay, L1210 cells were incubated for 72 hours (four to six doubling times of untreated cells) with various concentrations of the two forms of the drug. The concentration which results in 50% inhibition of growth, IC$_{50}$, was 28 nM for free Adr and 15 nM for Adr-PGL. The actual drug con-centration available in Adr-PGL may be significantly lower due to topologic restric-tions on the coupled molecules. Consequently, the inhibitory activity of the polymer-bound drug may be considerably higher.

The results of clonogenic assays using the sensitive and resistant L1210 cells are summarized in Table 1. As judged by the D_q values, representing the lowest concen-tration of drug that cells can tolerate without loss of viability, Adr-PGL is signifi-cantly more toxic. The polymer-bound drug was approximately five times more toxic with the sensitive cells and 15 times more toxic with the resistant cells at D_q concen-tration. Similarly, Adr-PGL incubated with the resistant cells was approximately 12

TABLE 1

Sensitivity of murine leukemic cell lines to free or polymer-coupled adriamycin

Cell line	Form of Adr	Adr concentration (nM)	
		D_q	50% survival
L1210$_S$	Free	4.3	3.5
	Polymer-bound	0.9	2.5
L1210$_R$	Free	62.0	100.0
	Polymer-bound	3.9	8.0

Sensitivity was measured by the colony-forming ability of individual cells assayed in soft agarose. D_q repre-sents the quasi-threshold values, indicating the lowest concentration for drug-induced damage that cells can sustain without a loss of viability (Rogers and Tökès, 1984). L1210$_S$ are sensitive and L1210$_R$ are re-sistant cells.

times more active than the free drug, reducing survival by 50% (Rogers and Tökès, 1983).

Scanning electron microscopy revealed extensive cell surface modification by Adr-PGL. As illustrated in Figure 1, L1210 cells developed blebs, which eventually led to cytolysis. Only the drug-covered microspheres formed patches on the cell surface. Plain PGL microspheres failed to bind to the cell. The representative transmission electron micrograph in Figure 2 illustrates the positions of a large number of plain microspheres adjacent to an L1210 cell. Only four of the 200 microspheres appear to be in contact with the cell surface. In the same study, based on the position of 3000 Adr-PGLs, 20% of the microspheres were in direct contact with the plasma membrane (Rogers and Tökès, 1983). Less than 0.5% of Adr-PGLs were found in the cytoplasm and none were inside or in contact with the nucleus. Higher magnification of Adr-PGLs in contact with the cell surface of L1210 reveals the extent of microsphere-cell interactions (Fig. 3). Using similar electron micrographs, an estimation can be made of the surface area involved in these interactions. When Adr-PGL containing 40 nmol of Adr per mg of PGL was used for incubation, the surface area for contact between one microsphere and a cell was approximately $6.2 \times 10^6 \, \text{Å}^2$. More

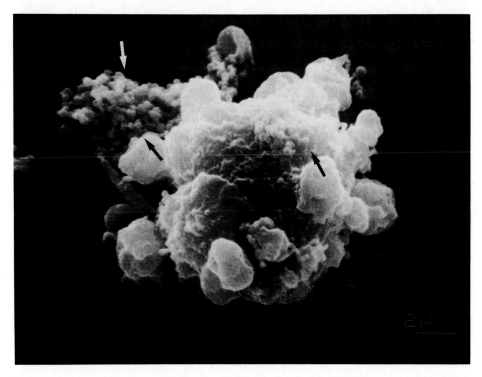

Figure 1. Scanning electron micrograph of an L1210 cell treated with Adr-PGL containing 10 μM Adr. The drug-covered microspheres are clumped together in patches (see arrows). The cell surface shows extensive blebbing (Tökès et al., 1982). (Reproduced from the Proceedings of the National Academy of Sciences, U.S.A.)

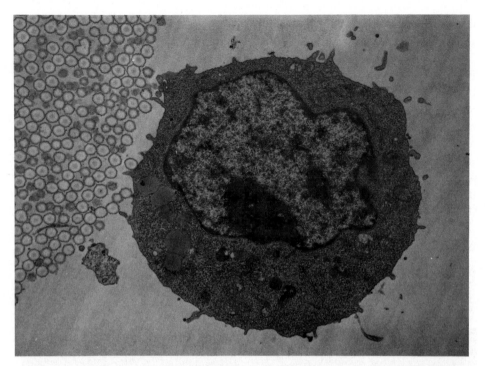

Figure 2. Transmission electron micrograph of an L1210 cell treated with plain PGL. Only four of the 200 microspheres appear at the vicinity of the plasma membrane. (Magnification, × 7,110.) (Reproduced from the Journal of the National Cancer Institute.)

than 50,000 Adr molecules could participate in such an area of cellular interaction.

These observations demonstrate that covalent attachment of Adr to a polymer results in microspheres which have a high affinity for the cell surface. After 72 hours incubation of microspheres containing 10 μM Adr with 6 × 10^4 cells in a complete cell culture medium supplemented with 10% fetal bovine serum, less than 0.08% of the drug was released from the polymers (Tökès et al., 1982). This amount of free drug is not sufficient to exert detectable cytotoxic activity. The observation that Adr-resistant cells are rendered sensitive suggests that a novel mode of cytotoxicity was created, and that this toxic interaction cannot be overcome by the cellular mechanisms which are responsible for drug resistance.

2.4. In vitro experiments with sensitive and resistant rat hepatocytes

Three types of rat liver hepatocytes were evaluated for their sensitivity to free Adr and Adr-PGL (Rogers et al., 1983). The established rat liver carcinoma cell line, RLC, can grow in a medium containing 10^{-7} M Adr without any inhibition. However, 33% inhibition of growth is observed when the equivalent amount of drug is present as Adr-PGL. Significant inhibition of growth is retained even at 10^{-9} M Adr concentration when the drug is coupled to microspheres. When carcinogen-altered,

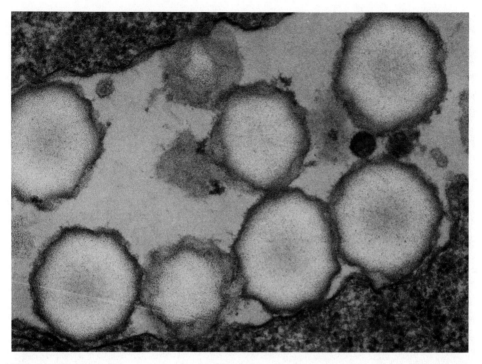

Figure 3. Transmission electron micrograph of Adr-PGL microspheres in contact with the cell surface of L1210 cell. The average diameter of a microsphere is 4500 Å.

drug-resistant rat hepatocytes were tested at an Adr concentration of 10^{-6} M, after a 24-hour exposure, the polymer-bound drug killed 32% of the cells, while the free drug had no detectable cytotoxic effect. When using the same conditions with normal rat hepatocytes, the Adr-PGLs were less toxic than the free drug. In all of these experiments greater than 99.5% of the drug remains covalently coupled to microspheres. Incubation of the resistant hepatocytes with polymer-bound Adr results in the loss of microvilli and extensive blebbing of the cell surface (Fig. 4). Continued incubation leads to cytolysis. Transmission electron microscopy demonstrates that less than 1% of the microspheres is internalized by either cell type. A representative transmission electron micrograph demonstrating the cell surface-bound Adr-PGLs on drug-resistant hepatocytes is shown in Figure 5. A survey of 25 cells and 2,000 microspheres was completed. Approximately 22% of the Adr-PGLs were found to be in close contact with the cell surfaces. None of the microspheres were observed in contact with the nuclear membrane or inside the nucleus (Rogers et al., 1983).

These findings are consistent with the observations obtained with L1210 cells and support further the validity of the objectives for the polymer-bound Adr as stated earlier.

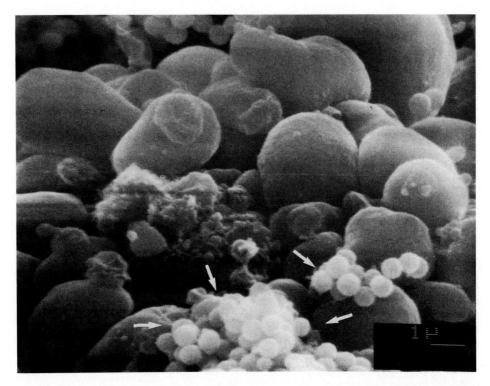

Figure 4. Scanning electron micrograph of the cell surface of a resistant rat liver hepatocyte treated with Adr-PGL microspheres, containing 10 μM Adr. Arrows indicate the position of aggregated microspheres. The extensive blebbing subsequently leads to cytolysis.

2.5. In vitro studies with human cancer cells

The human leukemia cell line, CCRF-CEM, and its resistant subclones were tested with Adr-PGL in cytostatic assays. The IC_{50} values were identical (11–12 nM) with the free and bound drug, using the sensitive clone. Since only a portion of the bound Adr is accessible to the cell, this form of drug appears to be even more active than the free form (Tökès et al., 1982). The two resistant clones (IC_{50} of 320 and 390 nM with the free drug) became highly sensitive to the polymer-bound Adr (IC_{50} of 20 nM for each clone).

The study was further extended to 50 freshly obtained human cancer specimens. These studies were performed using the clonogenic assay at two drug concentrations: 0.1 and 10 μg/ml. Again, the effects of free Adr and Adr-PGL were compared. A marked increase in cytotoxicity was observed in 35% of the specimens at 0.1 μg/ml and in 55% of the specimens at 10 μg/ml due to the covalent attachment of Adr to PGL. Indistinguishable results were obtained with Adr-PGL in 45 and 25% of the specimens at 0.1 and 10 μg drug/ml, respectively. Decreased activity was observed in 20% of the samples. The most striking increase was obtained with lung and ovarian cancer specimens, where more than half the tumor specimens demonstrated an increased sensitivity to the polymer-bound form of Adr (Tökès et al., 1983).

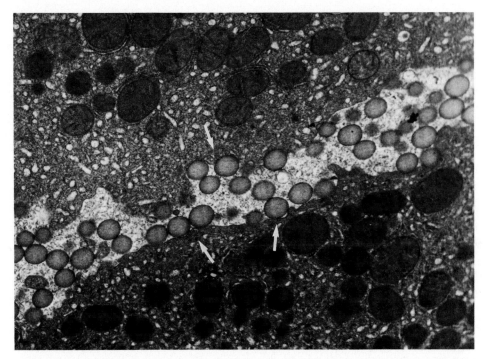

Figure 5. Transmission electron micrograph of carcinogen-altered drug-resistant rat hepatocytes reacted with Adr-PGL microspheres. The space between the two cells is filled with microspheres, many of which are tightly bound to the cell surface (arrows indicate the position of typical surface-bound microspheres).

2.6. *In vivo studies with polymer-bound adriamycin*

Only preliminary results are available from in vivo experiments conducted with Adr-PGL in mice. Most of the relevant experiments are currently in progress. Plain microspheres injected intraperitoneally or intravenously are well tolerated; however, no results are available on long-term toxicity. Radioiodinated microspheres were used for in vivo tissue-distribution studies. The plasma clearance curves were biphasic and nearly identical for both the plain and drug-coupled PGLs. Coupling of Adr to microspheres caused a marked elevation of Adr-PGL in the lung. 8 hours after injection, the amount of ^{125}I-labelled Adr-PGL was approximately six times greater in the lung than the ^{125}I-labelled plain PGL (Rogers, Neri and Tökès, unpublished observation). This observation suggests that Adr bound to microspheres may be useful for the treatment of lung metastases.

3. *Summary and future directions*

The synthesis of Adr-PGL was undertaken in order to test the validity of forcing the drug action to the cell surface and to obtain a desired cytotoxicity. The development of a therapeutic agent was not the immediate objective. The experiments summarized above clearly demonstrate the validity of the concept that overwhelming membrane perturbations can be accomplished by polymer-bound anthracyclines. These perturbations lead to a mechanism of cytotoxicity which is effective in overcoming resistant cells. The challenge now is to define the ideal carrier for the drug which will provide the optimal therapeutic benefit. The variety of available polymers which can serve as drug carriers is immense, which is an attractive feature of this approach. Some of these carriers may accumulate in the lung, and may therefore help to treat those types of metastatic tumors which frequently colonize this organ.

The drug-polymer complexes are also useful in identifying those plasma membrane components which have a selective affinity for the drug. These components may serve as a port of entry into the cell and may transport the free drug across the plasma membrane. Preliminary experiments indicate that two membrane proteins from L1210 cells bind selectively to Adr-PGL but not to the plain PGL (Rogers and Tökès, unpublished observations). If these membrane proteins indeed act as receptors for the sensitive cells, the question is raised as to whether they become modified in the resistant clones. The availability of drug-microsphere complexes for the affinity purification of these membrane entities will help significantly to answer this question.

The mechanism by which the Adr-PGL-induced membrane perturbation is translated into cytotoxicity is of considerable interest. The plasma membrane as a potential target site for cancer chemotherapy has been overlooked for decades, yet this is the target site that appears to be exploited by both the activated macrophages and natural killer cells of the host's immune system. Neither of these cells recognizes specific molecules on the tumor cells, instead they appear to exploit the malignant cell's increased sensitivity to cytolysis.

Acknowledgements

During the early phases of this research, we benefited significantly from collaboration with Dr. Alan Rembaum of Jet Propulsion Laboratories, whose contributions are gratefully acknowledged. Experiments using normal and carcinogen-treated drug-resistant hepatocytes from rats were performed in collaboration with Dr. Brian I. Carr, City of Hope, Duarte, CA, whose help is appreciated. The authors wish to thank Ms. Ruth Olivo for her expert technical assistance. In addition, we wish to thank Mary Kirchen and Dr. Grace J. Marshall for the use of the electron microscopes and for their interest and assistance with this project. We also thank Dr. Anthony Neri for useful comments. The experiments that have been outlined were supported in part by National Institutes of Health, Grant CA-21271 and by the Weingart Foundation.

References

Andersson, J. and Melchers, F. (1977). In Cell Surface Reviews. (Poste, G. and Nicolson, G.L., Eds.), Vol. 3, 601–618.

Forssen, E.A. and Tökès, Z.A. (1979) Biochem. Biophys. Res. Commun. 91, 1295–1301.

Forssen, E.A. and Tökès, Z.A. (1981) Proc. Natl. Acad. Sci. U.S.A. 78, 1873–1877.

Forssen, E.A. and Tökès, Z.A. (1983a) Cancer Res. 43, 546–550.

Forssen, E.A. and Tökès, Z.A. (1983b) Cancer Treatment Rep. 67, 481–484.

Margel, S., Zisblatt, S. and Rembaum, A. (1979) J. Immunol. Methods 28, 341–353.

Mayhew, E. and Papahadjopoulos, D. (1983) In Liposomes, (Ostro, M.J., Ed.), pp. 289–341, Marcel Dekker, Inc., New York.

Melchers, F. (1979) In B Lymphocytes in the Immune Response (Cooper, M., Mosier, D.E., Scher, I. and Vitetta, E.S., Eds.), pp. 271–274, Elsevier/North Holland Inc., New York.

Rogers, K.E. and Tökès, Z.A. (1984) J. Natl. Canc. Inst., in press.

Rogers, K.E., Carr, B.I. and Tökès, Z.A. (1983) Cancer Res. 43, 2741–2748.

Taylor, R.F., Teague, L.A. and Yesair, D.W. (1982) Cancer Res. 41, 4316–4323.

Tökès, Z.A., Rogers, K.E. and Rembaum, A. (1982) Proc. Natl. Acad. Sci. U.S.A. 79, 2026–2030.

Tökès, Z.A., Rogers, K.E., Daniels, A.M. and Daniels, J.R. (1983) Proc. Am. Assoc. Cancer Res. 24, 255 (1006).

Tritton, T.R. and Hickman, J.A. (1983) In Cancer Chemotherapy (Muggia, F., Ed.), Martinus Nijhoff, The Hague, in press.

Microspheres and Drug Therapy. Pharmaceutical, Immunological and Medical Aspects
edited by S.S. Davis, L. Illum, J.G. McVie and E. Tomlinson
© *1984, Elsevier Science Publishers B.V.*

The manufacture, particle size analysis and release characteristics of three-ply walled microcapsules

B. Warburton

Initial work (Warburton, 1981; Morris and Warburton, 1982) has explored the properties of novel n-ply walled microcapsules. These are produced by a multiple emulsion process. If n is an even number the cores of the microcapsules will be oleophilic in nature and if n is odd the cores will be hydrophilic in nature.

The walls of these microcapsules are constructed from two dissimilar polymers which need to be pharmaceutically acceptable. One polymer needs to be hydrophilic, examples being gum acacia, gelatin and some cellulose ethers. The other polymer is more critical in specification, and examples are certain grades of ethyl cellulose and cellulose acetate phthalate. Manufacturing conditions and recipe variations can control the number of cores produced from a few to one and information about this core structure can be obtained from the analysis of the particle size distribution.

Microcapsules are normally formed as an aqueous suspension and, in favourable cases, they can be obtained as a fine running powder.

The kinetics of release of simple model drugs is discussed.

References

Morris, N.J. and Warburton, B. (1982) J. Pharm. Pharmacol. 34, 475–479.
Warburton, B. (1981) U.K. Patent, 2,009,698.

Passive targeting — Occlusion, cellular uptake and local injection

Microspheres and Drug Therapy. Pharmaceutical, Immunological and Medical Aspects
edited by S.S. Davis, L. Illum, J.G. McVie and E. Tomlinson
© *1984, Elsevier Science Publishers B.V.*

153

CHAPTER 1

Biodegradable starch microspheres – A new medical tool

Bernt Lindberg, Knut Lote and Heitti Teder

1. General introduction

Embolization by means of injection of foreign materials into the circulation seems to have been known for a long time (Dawbarn, 1904), but not until the last decade has this possibility become the subject of extensive research and application (Young, 1981).

Various materials have been used (Kunstlinger et al., 1981), and embolization has been performed for various diagnostic and therapeutic purposes. An important goal has been to occlude tumors either by permanent occlusion in order to achieve necrosis or by transient occlusion in combination with drug therapy, where the occluding materials also may serve as drug carriers (Chuang and Wallace, 1981).

In 1974 the technique of microembolization with degradable cross-linked starch microspheres was introduced by Dr. Ulf Rothman at the Department of Experimental Research, Malmö General Hospital. Further development of the microsphere was carried out by Pharmacia, Uppsala.

Degradable starch microspheres (DSM) were first used experimentally for scintigraphic imaging in the diagnosis of lung emboli. During the development of starch microspheres for scintigraphy, it was found that the microspheres were extremely well tolerated when given intravenously. The lungs of dogs could be loaded with large amounts (0.1 g/kg body weight) without adverse effects (Wulff, 1975). This finding led to the idea of injecting DSM intraarterially, to produce a transient reduction of arterial blood flow (Rothman et al., 1976).

There are many potential applications for transient occlusion of the blood flow by means of DSM. The most important feature of DSM is that the degradation time can be regulated by means of the degree of cross-linking to suit various organs and applications. DSM have been applied to the liver, kidney and mesenterium without any harm.

When injected intraarterially into the target organ, microspheres of a suitable size become trapped in its arterioles (Fig. 1). If a drug is dissolved in the microsphere suspension, it will be retained in the blood vessels of the target organ as long as the blood flow is blocked or considerably reduced. If the drug can cross the capillary walls and enter the cells of the target organ within the time of circulatory arrest, an

154

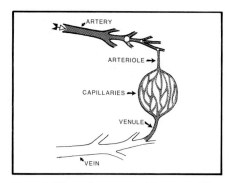

Figure 1. Microspheres trapped in an arteriole.

effective targeting would be achieved, and the systemic concentration of the drug could be reduced. This would be expected to reduce undesirable systemic drug effects.

Transient ischemia causes hypoxia. This renders the organ less susceptible to low linear energy-transfer ionising radiation damage, and thus DSM-induced ischemia offers a means of protecting healthy tissues from harmful effects of radiotherapy.

Temporary arrest of blood flow would inhibit the dissipation of heat by the circulation. The cooling effect of the blood flow is a problem in therapeutic applications of hyperthermia. Administration of DSM would, by a purely hydrodynamic effect, help facilitate local hyperthermia.

In the following sections the general physical and chemical properties of DSM are described, and their effect on the pharmacokinetics of anticancer drugs delivered together with DSM via the hepatic artery, as well as their effect and safety for radioprotection, will be illustrated.

The concept of DSM for the targeting of drugs is summarized in Box 1.

2. Physical and chemical properties of degradable starch microspheres

2.1. General properties

Our cross-linked starch microspheres are made by emulsion polymerization of a soluble potato starch hydrolysate, specially produced for a polymerization process designed to yield particulate material for parenteral use.

The microspheres swell in water and exhibit gel characteristics. They are not fully rigid but are slightly deformable. Thus, they can adapt their shape to the vascular environment. During enzymatic degradation they maintain their integrity for a considerable time before they finally collapse and disappear.

By using microspheres of defined size distributions the circulation can be arrested at desired levels of the vascular tree of the target organ. Thus, the microspheres may be custom made to suit each potential application. Microsphere fractions in the range of 1–500 μm in diameter and with degradation times from minutes to hours can be

THE DSM CONCEPT

Degradable Starch Microspheres (DSM)

consisting of crosslinked starch.

Properties

- Completely degradable by endogenous amylase.
- Mean diameter can be varied, $1-500$ μm.
- SPHEREX®, mean diameter ~ 45 μm.

Mode of action

- Temporary reduction or arrest of blood flow by intrarterial administration.
- The size is chosen so that the DSM are entrapped in the arterioles of the target organ.
- The rate of degradation is regulated by the degree of cross-linking.

Effects of blood flow arrest

- Drugs added to the injection medium are localised to the area of DSM entrapment.
- Hypoxia is induced in the target organ.
- Dissipation of heat by the blood circulation is reduced.

prepared. Currently, DSM with a mean diameter of about 40–45 μm are used for most of the intraarterial applications (proprietary name, Spherex®), and Figure 2 shows their size distribution.

The pharmaceutical form of Spherex® is a stable suspension in saline. The pharmaceutical properties have been discussed elsewhere (Russell, 1983).

2.2. Degradation kinetics

The degradation properties of starch microspheres are characterized in vitro by agitation of DSM with hog pancreas amylase at pH 7.0 (phosphate buffer) at 37°C. 10 mg of DSM are agitated in 20 ml of calcium-containing amylase at a concentration

156

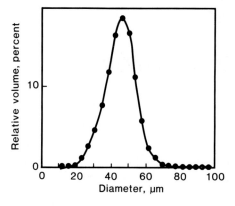

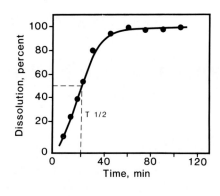

Figure 2. Volume size distribution of DSM (Spherex).

Figure 3. In vitro amylase degradation of DSM (Spherex). Dissolution vs. time, 4.0 μkat/l hog pancreas amylase (20 ml/10 mg microspheres, pH 7.0 (phosphate buffer), 37°C).

of 4.0 μkat/l. α-Amylase has an activity optimum between pH 6 and 7 (Fischer and Stein, 1960) and its activity is effectively stopped by raising the pH above 11.

The amount of material dissolved by amylase action is measured as glucose equivalents in the supernatant by the anthrone method (Jenner, 1967). A typical dissolution curve is shown in Figure 3. The half-life, $T_{1/2}$, is defined as the time it takes for the microspheres to lose half of their mass by the action of amylase. Spherex has an in vitro half-life of 20–30 minutes under the conditions specified here.

The dissolved fragments, although measured as glucose equivalents, are not glucose, but consist of glucose units, cross-linked glucose units or substituted glucose units. These oligomers have a wide distribution of molecular weights, with a maximum at about 1,000 daltons.

Investigations on microspheres with sharp size distributions have shown that $T_{1/2}$ is proportional to the mean diameter (Fig. 4). The dissolution rate thus seems to be somehow related to the ratio between volume and surface of the microsphere. This would be in accordance with some rate-controlling surface barrier affecting the diffusion of enzyme or degradation products. $T_{1/2}$ is also proportional to the degree of cross-linking (Fig. 5).

Lindberg et al. (1983) investigated the amylase degradation of DSM by means of microcalorimetry. It was found that $T_{1/2}$ correlates with calorimetric rate parameters (Fig 6). This indicates that the dissolution rate is proportional to the enzymatic bond-breaking rate. The heat of reaction is inversely proportional to the amount of cross-linker used (Fig. 7), indicating that a smaller number of bonds are broken when the degree of cross-linking is increased. Microscopic examination shows that below a certain amylase level the microspheres decrease in optical density but retain their diameter and integrity for a considerable time, after which they disappear rather

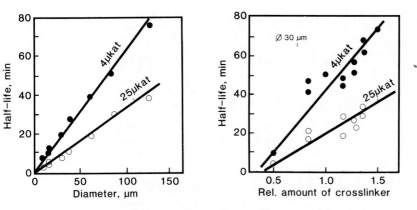

Figure 4. In vitro amylase degradation of DSM. Half-life, $T_{1/2}$, vs. mean diameter.

Figure 5. In vitro amylase degradation of DSM (mean diameter, 30 μm). Half-life, $T_{1/2}$, vs. relative amount of cross-linker used in the synthesis of the DSM.

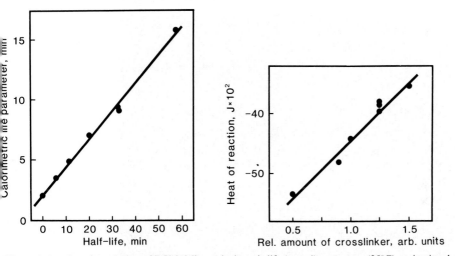

Figure 6. Amylase degradation of DSM. Microcalorimetric life (rate^{-1}) parameter (25°C) vs. in vitro half-life, $T_{1/2}$ (mean diameter, 30 μm). From Lindberg et al. (1983).

Figure 7. Amylase degradation of DSM. Heat of reaction (25°C) vs. the relative amount of cross-linker used in the synthesis of the DSM (mean diameter, 30 μm). From Lindberg et al. (1983).

abruptly without breaking up into smaller fragments (Fig. 8). However, when agitated with a large amount of amylase, (as is the case during the determination of $T_{1/2}$), the microspheres are degraded from the periphery, with a continuous decrease in the diameter and number of microspheres, as shown in Figure 9.

Although there exists a certain correlation between the in vitro parameter, $T_{1/2}$, and the return of DSM-arrested blood flow, restoration of the blood flow is to a large extent determined by parameters related to the particulate nature of the micro-

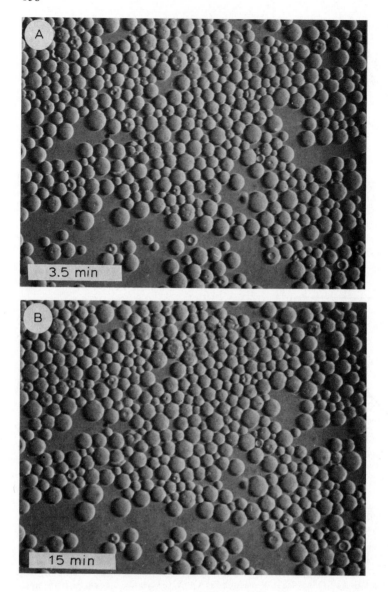

spheres, which are not well characterized by $T_{1/2}$. Thus, $T_{1/2}$ provides a suitable reproducible parameter for the analytical specifications, but, as a measure of the effect of the microspheres in the circulation, $T_{1/2}$ is insufficient.

In an investigation by Tuma et al. (1982) on the dog kidney, the arrest of blood flow was studied with microspheres of two different sizes, 36 and 58 μm mean diameter. The results are described by Dr. Tuma in the following chapter. Figure 2 of that chapter shows the kinetics of the arrest. The product of the diameter and the dose of microspheres (mg) correlates with the half-life for the arrest of blood flow (Lindberg, 1983), as shown in Figure 3 of the same chapter. The weight of microspheres

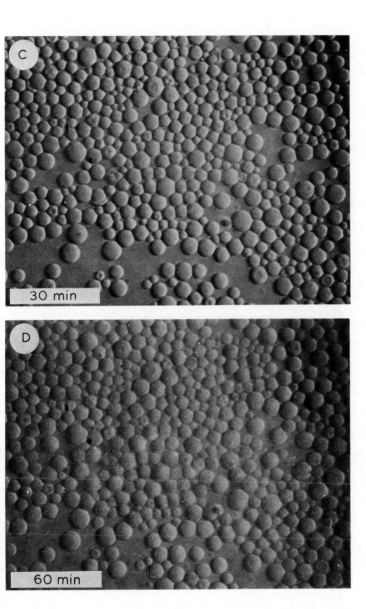

would reflect their number, and the product of size (represented by the diameter) and number would thus be a measure of their ability to arrest the blood flow.

2.3. Mechanism of degradation

Malmquist (1982) performed an in vitro morphometric kinetic study with various ratios of amylase to a defined amount of Spherex. Since amylase levels vary extensively between different species (Table 1), sera from various animals were used in this investigation. The general result is shown in Figure 10, in which the total amount of amylase is plotted logarithmically against degradation time. The degradation time, t, is

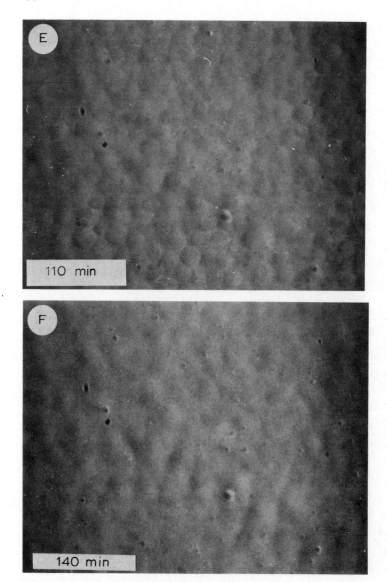

Figure 8. Photographs of amylase degradation of DSM (mean diameter, 40 μm). Amylase concentration 25 μkat/l at ambient temperature. The optical density of the microspheres decreases with time. They retain their integrity and diameter until they become invisible ($\times$ 100). A, 3.5; B, 15; C, 30; D, 60; E, 110; F, 140 minutes.

defined as the time for about 90% of the original number of microspheres to disappear. The shape of the curve indicates a transition from one exponential mode of kinetics to another at an amylase level of about 0.1 μkat/60 mg of microspheres. (The microspheres were supplied as a suspension of 60 mg/ml). This behaviour suggests that the mechanism of degradation is governed by a Michaelis-Menten type of enzymatic hydrolysis in a diffusion controlled system (Ceska et al., 1969).

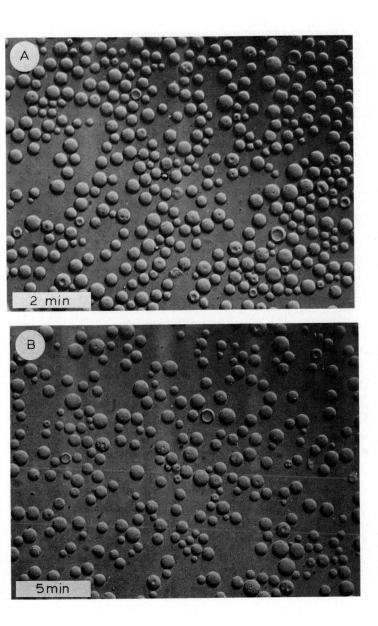

Figures 11 and 12 show the change of diameter and number of microspheres, respectively, with time during the observation time which ends at *t* (as defined above),
with various ratios of amylase to Spherex. The ratios refer to 1 ml of a Spherex suspension containing 60 mg microspheres, mixed with 5, 10, 20 or 40 ml of human serum.
Table 2 shows examples of data used for the construction of the figures. These figures
show clearly that a transition from a mode with unchanged diameter and number (amylase level, 1:5) to a mode with diminishing diameter and number takes place as the avail-

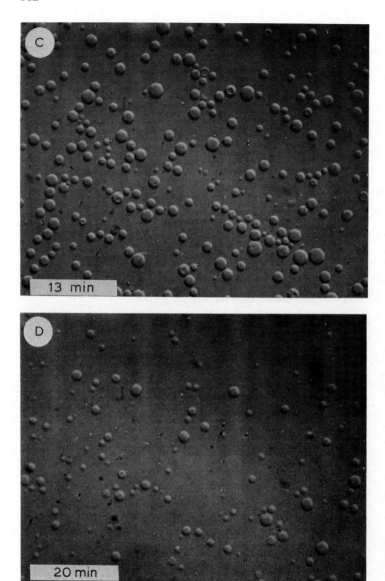

able quantity of amylase per weight of DSM increases. In addition, the product of the mean diameter and number of microspheres was found to represent the ability of DSM to arrest blood flow, as illustrated in Figure 13. This figure seems to suggest that the two modes of degradation shown in Figures 8 and 9 may perhaps be regarded as very simplified models for the two extreme situations in the circulation, i.e., (1) Complete arrest of the blood flow by a sudden entrapment of microspheres in the arterioles would lead to a local depletion of amylase, which would be expected to correspond to the mode of degradation depicted in Figure 8. (2) A steady-state,

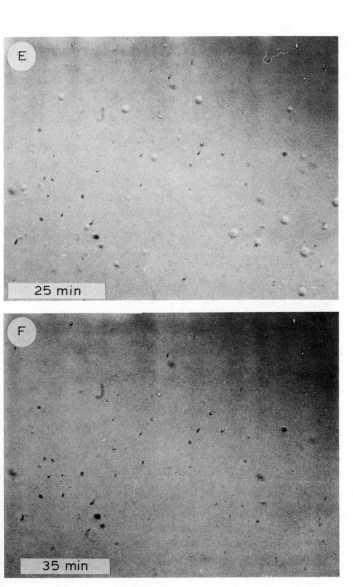

Figure 9. Photographs of amylase degradation of DSM (mean diameter, 40 μm). Amylase concentration 310 μkat/l at ambient temperature. The diameter of the microspheres decreases with time and the smallest microspheres disappear first ($\times$ 100). A, 2; B, 5; C, 13; D, 20; E, 25; F, 35 minutes.

whereby a continuous supply of new microspheres balances the losses by dissolution. This leakage of blood serum continuously supplies the microspheres with fresh amylase, resulting in the mode of degradation shown in Figure 9.

Our tentative interpretation of these observations is as follows. Starch has a high affinity for amylase, and DSM rapidly absorb it from the environment. The amylase seems to be able to penetrate the microsphere surface without difficulty. As soon as the hydrolysis has produced fragments small enough to escape from the matrix, or the matrix has become sufficiently degraded to allow the fragments to escape, the microsphere begins to lose mass. At amylase levels below saturation of the microsphere, the amylase concentration at the surface will be small, and since the degree of cross-linking may be highest at the surface, the surface could now be rather resistant to hydrolysis. The sphere thus retains its shape during a large part of the process.

Above the saturation limit, the amylase levels near the surface may be sufficient simultaneously to degrade the surface and to dissolve the sphere from the outside. In this case, the diameter would diminish gradually from the beginning.

The behaviour of the microspheres in the circulation is dependent on the dynamics of the exposure to endogenous amylase and cannot be characterized by a single analytical parameter, such as the half-life, $T_{1/2}$. The duration of the transient arrest of

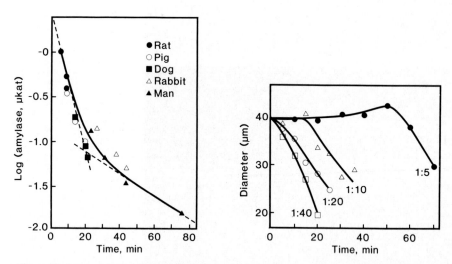

Figure 10. Amylase degradation of DSM (Spherex) in sera from various animals at 37°C. 1 ml of microspheres containing 60 mg/ml was mixed with various volumes of serum (5, 10, 20, 40 ml). The logarithm of the total amount of amylase available in the system has been plotted vs. the time it takes for about 90% of the original number of microspheres to disappear. Measured serum levels: rat, 109; pig, 34; dog, 20; rabbit, 15; man, 3.3 μkat/l. From Malmquist (1982).

Figure 11. The change in the mean diameter of DSM (Spherex) vs. time in human serum (3.3 μkat/l). Conditions as in Figure 10. From Malmquist (1982).

TABLE 1

Approximate α-amylase activity in various species

Species:	Rat	Pig	Dog	Cat	Rabbit	Man	Goat	Sheep
	100	50	40	40	10	3	1	0.7

Values are the mean from various literature sources, and are given in μkat/l.

blood flow would thus be dependent on the mode of administration (dose, speed of injection, etc.), and the possibilities for achieving optimal conditions of administration are currently under investigation.

2.4. Chemical structure

Our DSM are cross-linked by means of epichlorohydrin. For a long time epichlorohydrin cross-linking of polysaccharides was believed to give rise to single glycerol ether cross-links. A recent extensive study (Holmberg and Lindquist, 1984) has

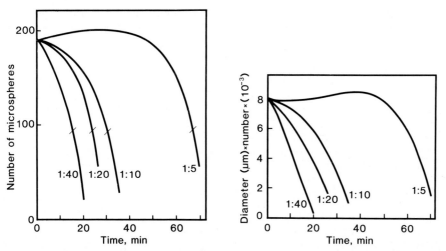

Figure 12. The change in the number of DSM (Spherex) in human serum (3.3 μkat/l). Conditions as in Figure 10. From Malmquist (1982).

Figure 13. The product of mean diameter and number vs. time from Figures 12 and 13. From Malmquist (1982).

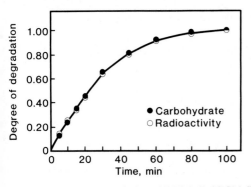

Figure 14. Amylase degradation of ^{14}C-labelled DSM. Dissolution measured as glucose (anthrone method) and as ^{14}C radioactivity vs. time.

TABLE 2

Amylase degradation of DSM in human serum (ml serum per 60 mg Spherex) showing the change of number and diameter of the DSM with time

Time (minutes)	5 ml serum		40 ml serum	
	Number	Mean diameter (μm)	Number	Mean diameter (μm)
0	200	40.0	200	40.0
5			167	39.8
10	193	39.3	138	32.4
15			95	27.0
20	200	40.5	20	19.5
30	202	40.8		
40	197	40.3		
50	181	42.6		
60	150	37.5		
70	60	29.4		

Data from Malmquist (1982).

shown that this is not so. In the case of dextran, about 80% of the cross-links are oligomeric. There is also a large proportion of oligomeric glycerol ether substituents present. In the case of starch, the content of oligomeric cross-links or substituents is less pronounced (Holmberg, 1984). In Spherex, 67% of the glucose units are unsubstituted.

Using ^{14}C-labelled epichlorohydrin, we have shown that the radioactivity levels in the dissolved material parallel those for carbohydrate (Fig. 14).

This shows that unsubstituted glucose is not preferentially attacked first by the enzyme, indicating that the epichlorohydrin-derived structural elements are randomly distributed.

A summary of the physical, chemical and degradation properties is given in Box 2.

3. Application of degradable starch microspheres

3.1. Introduction

Several investigations examining the feasibility and utility of our microsphere concept have been performed and published.

The primary action of DSM is the ability to produce a transient ischemia on

PROPERTIES OF DSM

Physical and chemical properties

- Manufactured by emulsion polymerisation of hydrolysed potato starch.
- Swell in water to gel particles.
- Can be fractionated into defined size distributions.
- Are dissolved by amylase without breaking up into visible fragments, and disappear gradually when viewed under the microscope.

Degradation kinetics

In vitro The half-life, $T^{1/2}$, is defined as the time it takes for half of the mass of the DMS to dissolve in an amylase solution.

- $T^{1/2}$ is proportional to the diameter.
- $T^{1/2}$ is proportional to the degree of crosslinking.

At lower levels of enzyme, degradation takes place from within with retention of apparent diameter.

At higher levels of amylase the diameter is gradually reduced, and the smallest spheres disappear first.

Diameter × number of microspheres is a measure of the blood flow stopping ability.

selected organ tissues after appropriate intraarterial infusion. This has been demonstrated in a series of studies on the liver, intestines and some other organs in animal models.

The results of these studies show that transient ischemia can be achieved by intraarterial injection of DSM, and that the transient ischemia produced by the microspheres is harmless.

The secondary action of DSM is the modification of drug distribution, when drugs are administered intraarterially together with DSM. This was investigated in a series of studies on the liver and kidney in various animal models. As examples of drugs and model compounds, inulin, 5-fluorouracil (5-FU), actinomycin D, ethacrynic acid, doxorubicin and ^{99}Tc-diethylenetriamine pentaacetic acid were used.

The main target organ for the therapeutic application of the present DSM product is the liver. The main therapeutic application is thus primary and secondary liver tumours. The liver has been chosen as the first target organ for several reasons:
Many types of tumours, and especially those with the primary site in the gastro-intestinal tract, often develop metastatic liver tumours;
Treatment of inoperable primary and secondary liver tumours is at present unsatisfactory;
The liver has a blood supply accessible for arterial infusion.

Other organs suitable for arterial infusion of drugs and DSM are the kidneys and the intestines.

In radiotherapy and hyperthermia, a reduction of blood flow may be of therapeutic value. Temporary ischemia and hypoxia of normal tissues at the time of irradiation can protect vital organs from radiation damage, and may thus reduce the risk of unacceptable radiation damage to healthy tissues. The use of DSM for hypoxic radioprotection has been established in animal models.

In tumours treated with hyperthermia, temporary blocking of tumour blood supply will deprive the heated tumour of the cooling effect of circulating blood and render the tumour more vulnerable to thermal necrosis.

A summary of current applications is given in Box 3 (see p. 169).

3.2. Transient ischemia

3.2.1. Experimental summary

The ability of DSM to cause transient ischemia has been demonstrated in a series of experimental studies.

A. Arfors et al. (1976) were the first to demonstrate that the intra-arterial injection of DSM produced a transient reduction of blood flow to an organ, pig intestine. The reduced tissue oxygen tension that followed the injection of the microspheres returned to control values after degradation of the spheres.

B. Lindell et al. (1977a) demonstrated in rats that the arterial blood flow to the liver was temporarily reduced following hepatic artery injection of the microspheres. In a later study, Lindell et al. (1977b) also demonstrated that the injection of DSM into the hepatic artery was followed by a proportionally greater reduction in the blood flow to liver tumours than to the healthy liver tissue. No adverse effects on hepatic cells were found after repeated administration of starch microspheres (Lindell et al., 1977a).

C. Forsberg et al. (1978a, b) studied the intestines and feet of the rat. Using flow measurements with tracer microsphere techniques, they showed that the injection of a suitable amount of DSM induced deep, but fully reversible ischemia in the organ. The period of occlusion was long enough to irradiate the ischemic organs under conditions of extreme hypoxia.

D. Tuma et al. (1982) found that injection of DSM into the renal arteries of dogs was followed by a reversible ischemia in the kidney, the duration of which was depen-

APPLICATIONS OF DSM

Modification of drug distribution

Prerequisites.
● Arterial supply suitable for selective catheterisation.
● Tolerance to transient circulatory arrest.

Pharmacokinetic effect. Lower concentration in peripheral blood with concomitant reduction of systemic toxicity. Higher concentration in the organ supplied by the injected artery.

Results. The pharmacokinetic effect has been established in animal models for kidney and liver.
The administration of cytostatic drugs to the liver has been evaluated in patients.

Radioprotection

Severe hypoxia at the time of irradiation reduces low-LET radiation damage.
Thus transient ischemia can protect radiosensitive normal tissues and permit increased tumor radiation doses at less cost in damage to normal tissues.
This effect has been established for skin, intestine, and kidneys in animals. With DSM-induced transient ischemia the radiation dose can be doubled.

Hyperthermia

Transient ischemia will reduce heat dissipation in heated tumors and is useful as an aid for localised hyperthermia.

dent on the number and size of the microspheres utilized (see the following chapter).

E. By in vivo microscopic observation of the DSM in the hamster cheek pouch, Tuma (the following chapter) showed that the microspheres are trapped at the arteriolar level and block blood flow in these microvessels. After degradation and reduction in size, they can pass along capillaries approximately 5 μm in diameter. The injection of DSM into the hamster cheek pouch failed to induce platelet aggregation or vasospasm.

F. Lote (1981a, b), Lote and Myking (1982) and Lote et al. (1980) investigated transient ischemia produced by DSM in the intestine of the cat. Special attention was paid to any possible immediate thrombogenic or later adverse effects. No evidence of any thrombotic hazards or harmful sequelae as a result of transient intestinal ischemia could be found. Also, DSM induced a more severe degree of small intestinal transient ischemia than ischemia produced by other methods.

G. In a flow study in the dog using a ^{133}Xe-wash-out method, Malmqvist et al. (1982) showed that a DSM dose level of 30 mg/kg Spherex injected into the hepatic artery caused a blood flow reduction of 15 minutes or more (Fig. 15).

H. In five patients Dakhil et al. (1982) studied the effect of DSM (Spherex) on hepatic arterial flow with angiography. It was possible with 900 mg of microspheres (Spherex) injected into the hepatic artery to transiently (for 15–30 minutes) reduce hepatic arterial flow by 80–100%.

3.2.2. Comparison of methods for production of transient mesenteric ischemia

It is possible to produce transient ischemia by proximal arterial occlusion, by arterial injection of vasoconstrictors, or by arterial injection of DSM. Few experiments compare the efficacy of available ischemia-inducing methods. Arfors et al. (1976) have shown that DSM injection is at least as effective as mesenteric arterial clamping for achieving intestinal hypoxia in the pig (Fig. 16). Lote et al. (1980) have compared the degree of temporary feline intestinal ischemia obtainable by arterial injection of DSM to intestinal ischemia, either produced by vasopressin injection (Lote et al., 1981) or induced by proximal mesenteric arterial occlusion (Lote and Lekven, 1982).

Mesenteric embolisation of DSM produced a more intense and more short-lived intestinal ischemia than arterial high-dose vasopressin injection (Fig. 17).

When feline small intestinal ischemia was induced by proximal clamping of the superior mesenteric artery and mucosal blood flow along the small intestine was determined by carbonized microsphere distribution, mucosal blood flow only de-

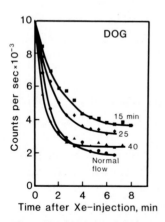
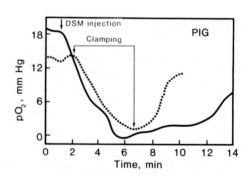

Figure 15. The effect of hepatic artery administration of DSM (Spherex) (30 mg/kg body weight) on liver artery blood flow in the dog. [133]Xenon-washout method with ^{133}Xe injections into the hepatic artery at normal flow and at various intervals after DSM injection (15, 25, 40 min). The initial slope of the ^{133}Xe decay curves reflects the blood flow. From Malmquist et al. (1982).

Figure 16. Reduction of oxygen tension after injection of DSM into the superior mesenteric artery in the pig, compared to oxygen tension after clamping of the artery. From Arfors et al. (1976).

creased to about 40% of control (Fig. 18, middle panel). In contrast, mesenteric arterial injection of DSM (bolus injection over 75–100 seconds) effectively blocked collateral blood flow, and consequently induced a more severe ischemia in all segments of the small intestine (Fig. 18, upper panel). High-dose mesenteric arterial vasopressin injection (0.15 IU followed by 0.075 IU/kg body weight/min) also reduced the mucosal blood flow considerably, but did not produce such intense ischemia as DSM injection (Fig. 18, lower panel).

In conclusion, mesenteric arterial embolisation by DSM is clearly a more efficient method for the induction of severe and transient feline small intestinal ischemia than either mesenteric arterial vasopressin infusion or proximal mesenteric arterial clamping.

A DSM-induced transient ischemia can be produced by a single bolus injection of DSM, but in animal experiments blood flow tends to rise 4–10 minutes after a single injection in rats (Fig. 19) or cats (Fig. 20). When an initial bolus injection of DSM was followed by a slow DSM infusion, blood flow in the superior mesenteric artery could be maintained at a much lower level for 10 minutes without risk for

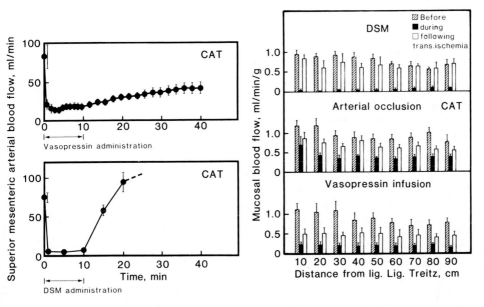

Figure 17. Upper panel: superior mesenteric arterial flow in cat (electromagnetic) before, during, and after injection of 0.15 IU/kg vasopressin followed by infusion of 0.075 IU/kg/min into the artery for 10 minutes (mean ± S.E., $n=9$). Lower panel: superior mesenteric arterial flow (electromagnetic) before, during, and following administration of DSM into the artery for 10 minutes (mean ± S.E., $n=41$). From Lote et al. (1981).

Figure 18. Mucosal blood flow (carbonized microsphere distribution) at 10-cm intervals along the feline small intestine before, during, and following transient ischemia induced by DSM (Spherex) (upper panel, $n=7$), proximal superior mesenteric artery occlusion (middle panel, $n=7$), or superior mesenteric vasopressin infusion (0.15 IU/kg followed by 0.075 IU/kg/min) (lower panel, $n=9$). Values are mean ± S.E.

mesenteric thrombosis (Fig. 21). A group of 15 animals treated in this way did not show any adverse effects when killed 14 days after severe transient intestinal ischemia.

3.2.3. *Clinical application of transient hepatic arterial ischemia*

The treatment of unresectable liver malignancies by temporary dearterialization using strangulating polyethylene slings around the hepatic artery has been tried (Bengmark et al., 1974). Rothman et al. (1976) suggested hepatic artery injection of DSM as an alternative method for temporarily interrupting hepatic arterial flow. In the first clinical investigation, Aronsen et al. (1979) combined continuous hepatic artery infusion of 5-fluorouracil with injections of DSM (mean diameter, 92 μm) three times daily for 14 days. 12 patients with secondary liver neoplasms of different origin were treated. The clinical effects and overall median survival time was 7 months, which is comparable to that obtained with hepatic artery ligation. However, any assessment of tumour response and survival should take into account the small

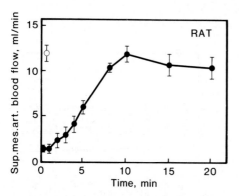

Figure 19. Electromagnetic blood flow registration by a flow probe on the superior mesenteric artery in eight rats after blockage with 1.4 × 10 DSM; mean diameter, 40 μm. Open circle = control flow. Values are mean ± S.E. From Forsberg (1978).

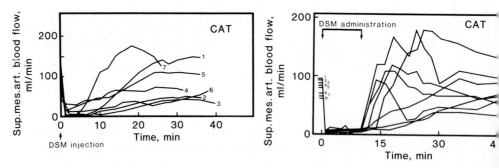

Figure 20. Superior mesenteric arterial blood flow in seven cats (electromagnetic) before and after bolus injection of DSM into the artery. From Lote et al. (1980).

Figure 21. Superior mesenteric arterial blood flow in eight cats (electromagnetic) before, during, and after an intraarterial bolus injection of DSM followed by a slow infusion for 10 minutes. From Lote (1981a).

number of patients studied and the fact that the primary tumours were of different origin and the secondary tumours in the liver varied greatly in size.

3.3. Modification of drug distribution and response

3.3.1. Experimental summary

The ability of DSM to modify drug distribution and drug response has been shown in the following experimental studies on animals:

A. Lindell et al. (1978) injected [14C]inulin together with DSM into the rat liver artery. Hepatic artery injection of inulin together with the microspheres resulted in

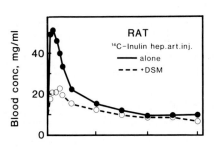
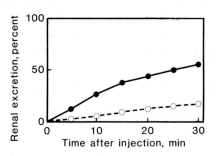

Figure 22. Administration into the rat liver artery of [14C]inulin or [14C]inulin plus DSM. Left panel: mean [14C]inulin concentrations in peripheral blood. Right panel: renal inulin excretion in percentage of administered inulin dose.

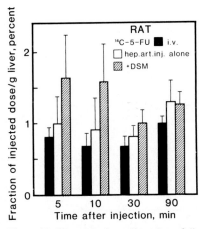
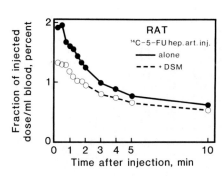

Figure 23. 14C activity in rat liver tissue following peripheral venous injection of 14C-labelled 5-fluorouracil ($\bar{n}=8$), hepatic artery injection of 14C-labelled 5-fluorouracil, alone ($\bar{n}=8$) or hepatic artery injection of 14C-labelled 5-fluorouracil mixed with DSM (Spherex) ($\bar{n}=8$). Mean values, percentage of injected 14C-labelled 5-fluorouracil dose/g liver tissue ($\pm$S.D.). From Teder et al. (1978).

Figure 24. 14C activity in peripheral blood after injection into the hepatic artery of 14C-labelled 5-fluorouracil alone, or mixed with DSM. Mean values, percent of injected 14C-labelled 5-fluorouracil dose/ml blood ($n=8$). From Teder et al. (1978).

increased inulin concentrations in the liver, compared to values found with inulin alone. The concentration of inulin in peripheral blood (Fig. 22, upper panel) was reduced in the presence of microspheres and the urinary excretion (Fig. 22, lower panel) of inulin was delayed. Injection of ^{14}C-labeled 5-fluorouracil together with DSM into the liver artery in rats (Teder et al., 1978) resulted in increased total ^{14}C activities in the liver compared to activities found with 5-fluorouracil injected alone into the hepatic artery or intravenously (Fig. 23). With microspheres there was also a reduction in the initial ^{14}C activities found in peripheral blood (Fig. 24).

In another experiment with rats, increased doxorubicin concentrations were found in the liver when injected into the hepatic artery together with DSM. (Fig. 25) (Teder, H., Nilsson, B., Ljungberg, J. and Aronsen K.F., unpublished results).

B. In another rat experiment Lindell et al. (1978) studied the tolerance of 5-fluorouracil (300 mg/kg body weight) injected into the hepatic artery with and without DSM. The experiments with microspheres resulted in increased survival when compared to injection of 5-fluorouracil (5-FU) alone (Fig. 26). This suggests that with microspheres there is an increased liver metabolism of 5-FU, and correspondingly a decreased systemic toxicity.

C. Tuma et al. (1982) investigated the effect of DSM on intraarterial injection of actinomycin D into the kidneys of dogs. The microspheres retarded wash-out of drug from the renal microcirculation. Blood flow recovered within 1 hour after injection. 23% of the total amount of the drug was retained in the kidney 1 hour after injection of the drug-microsphere combination. When the same amount of drug was selectively injected alone into a renal artery or given intravenously, 9% and 1.3% of the dose injected was found in kidney tissue 1 hour later (Table 3).

D. Arfors et al. (1979) investigated the effect of DSM on the injection of a diuretic,

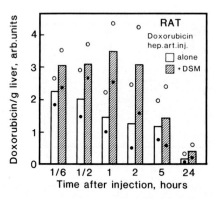
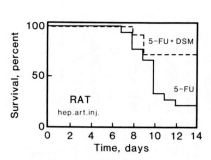

Figure 25. Doxorubicin (Adriamycin®) concentration in rat liver parenchyma (arbitrary units/g liver tissue) after injection into the liver artery of doxorubicin or a mixture of doxorubicin and DSM (Spherex). Median values, with maximum and minimum values indicated. From Teder et al. (1983).

Figure 26. Survival after injection into the rat liver artery of 5-fluorouracil (5-FU) (300 mg/kg body weight). Injection of 5-fluorouracil alone or 5-fluorouracil mixed with DSM ($\bar{n} = 2 \times 17$). From Lindell et al. (1978).

ethacrynic acid, into the renal artery of the dog. In these experiments, one kidney was injected with the drug, or drug plus DSM, while the other kidney served as control (Fig. 27). It was found that when ethacrynic acid and microspheres were injected together, diuresis was greater in the injected organ than that in the control, which displayed normal diuresis (Fig. 27, right panel). When ethacrynic acid was injected alone into one kidney, both kidneys were affected (Fig. 27, left panel). A comparison of the figures shows that microspheres prolong, as well as localize, the effect of the diuretic drug.

E. Lorelius et al. (1984) investigated the retention of ^{99}Tc-diethylenetriamine pentaacetic acid in rabbits with VX_2 tumours in the hind leg when injected into the external iliac artery together with DSM. When microspheres (Spherex) mixed with ^{99}Tc-diethylenetriamine pentaacetic acid were injected and followed by a slow injection

TABLE 3

Percent of the total amount of injected actinomycin D remaining in the dog kidney 60 minutes after injection

	Percent actinomycin D			
	Intravenously	Renal artery		
		Alone	With DSM	
			36 μm	58 μm
Cortex	1.0	8	18	20
Medulla	0.3	1	4	4
Total	1.3	9	22	24

Actinomycin D was injected either intravenously or into the renal artery, either alone or together with DSM with a mean diameter of 36 or 58 μm. Data from Tuma et al. (1982).

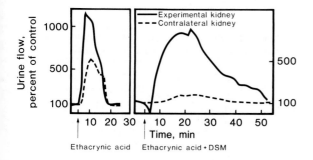

Figure 27. Diuretic effect of renal intraarterial injection of ethacrynic acid into the dog without (left panel) and with DSM (right panel). With DSM (60 mg) there is a prolonged effect. Without DSM there is a spillover effect on the contralateral kidney. From Arfors et al. (1979).

of microspheres alone, ^{99}Tc-diethylenetriamine pentaacetic acid was retained in the tumour at concentrations up to 11 times those obtained when ^{99}Tc-diethylenetri-amine pentaacetic acid alone was injected.

3.3.2. The effect of degradable starch microspheres on plasma pharmacokinetics of anticancer drugs injected into the hepatic artery of man

Modification of drug distribution by means of DSM has been applied clinically for the administration of anticancer drugs to patients with primary and secondary liver cancer in the following studies:

A. Dakhil et al. (1982) studied the effect of DSM on systemic carmustine exposure in five patients with liver malignancies. Carmustine was injected into the hepatic artery alone or mixed with microspheres (Spherex, 900 mg, mean diameter, 41 μm). When carmustine was injected together with the microspheres there was a consider-able reduction (34–92%) in systemic carmustine exposures and also a reduction (37–92%) of the systemic carmustine peak concentrations (Table 4).

B. In another study DSM were injected together with doxorubicin (Adriamycin) into the hepatic artery (Teder et al., 1983). Five patients with primary or secondary liver cancer were studied. In each patient two pharmacokinetic studies were made. Firstly, the patients were given doxorubicin alone (10 mg/m^2 body surface). 1 week later, the patients were given the same doxorubicin dose mixed with 900 mg of the microspheres (Spherex, mean diameter, 41 μm). The injection time was 10 seconds and the injected volume was 20 ml. Doxorubicin in plasma was analyzed by HPLC. Figure 28 shows the hepatic venous and systemic concentrations versus time in one typical patient (patient No. 2) after injection of doxorubicin alone or doxorubicin mixed with DSM.

In Table 5 the effect of the microspheres on the peak plasma concentration in all five patients is shown. In four of the patients, the hepatic venous peak was considera-bly reduced (75–92%) when microspheres were added. In peripheral blood the maxi-mum values were also reduced (41–69%). In case number five, the reduction of the hepatic venous peak was less pronounced and the maximum concentration in peri-pheral blood was higher with microspheres.

TABLE 4

Effect of DSM on the area under plasma concentration curve (AUC) ratio (carmustine concentration in peripheral blood × time) and peak ratio, following hepatic artery injection into six patients

Patient	AUC ratio	Peak ratio
1	0.08	0.08
2	0.1	0.14
3	0.4	0.32
4	0.55	0.44
5	0.66	0.62
6	0.66	0.3

From Dakhil et al. (1982). Ratios are value with DSM:value without DSM.

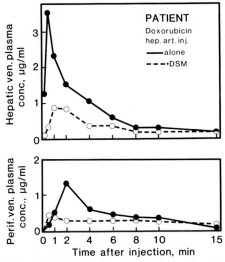

Figure 28. Injection of doxorubicin (Adriamycin®) into the hepatic artery of one patient. Doxorubicin alone or mixed with DSM (Spherex). Upper panel: hepatic venous plasma concentrations of doxorubicin. Lower panel: peripheral venous plasma concentrations of doxorubicin. From Teder et al. (1983).

TABLE 5

Reduction in initial peak values of doxorubicin (Adriamycin®) blood plasma concentration in hepatic and peripheral veins with DSM (Spherex) following hepatic artery injection into five patients

Patient	Percent reduction in initial peak value	
	Hepatic vein	Peripheral vein
1	−76	−46
2	−76	−69
3	−92	−42
4	−75	−41
5	−46	+1

From Teder et al. (1983).

Table 6 shows the effect of the microspheres on the areas under plasma concentration curves during the observation period in all patients. When doxorubicin and DSM were injected together the first four patients showed a 31–72% reduction in hepatic venous doxorubicin exposure (area under plasma concentration curve) and a 21–42% reduction in systemic doxorubicin exposure (area under plasma concentration curve). Patient number five had a large hepatic tumour with marked arteriovenous shunting, which may explain the unexpected result.

C. Gyves et al. (1983) studied the effect of two DSM doses on systemic mitomycin C exposure. When mitomycin C (10 mg/m^2) was injected together with 900 mg DSM (Spherex) over 1 minute into the hepatic artery, there was a 17–70% reduction in sys-

TABLE 6

Reduction in the area under curve (AUC) of doxorubicin (Adriamycin®), peripheral blood plasma concentration × time, with DSM (Spherex) following hepatic artery injection into five patients

Patient	Percent reduction in AUC	
	Hepatic vein	Peripheral vein
1	−60	−38
2	−56	−40
3	−72	−42
4	−31	−21
5	−14	+42

From Teder et al. (1983).

temic mitomycin C exposure (ten patients). Injection of 360 mg DSM together with the same mitomycin C dose (six patients) effected a 15–60% reduction in systemic mitomycin C exposure.

Conclusion: The results from the studies summarized in this section (3.3) show that drugs injected into an artery together with DSM remain longer in the target organ. This might increase the extraction ratio for the drug in the target organ, resulting in an increased local pharmacological effect and/or an increased metabolism of the drug.

3.4. Radioprotection

3.4.1. Introduction

Radiotherapy is an important tool for the treatment of malignant disease. Since both healthy and malignant cells are injured and killed by ionising radiation, the classical dilemma in radiotherapy is to select a radiation dose which will ensure tumour eradication without causing unacceptable damage to vital organs within the irradiated volume. The probability of lethal radiation damage to normal or malignant cells by increasing radiation doses is generally described by two sigmoid curves where the biological effect is a function of radiation dose (Fig. 29). Any means of enhancing tumour radiosensitivity or reducing normal tissue radiation damage will increase the separation of the response curves shown in Figure 29 and thereby increase the probability of tumour eradication at a given dose with less damage to normal tissue.

Injury caused by low linear energy-transfer ionising radiation is largely mediated by the interaction of highly reactive free radicals with molecular oxygen dissolved in irradiated tissues (Gray, 1961). Thus, severe ischemia and hypoxia at the time of irradiation can protect against radiation damage. Tissue oxygen tensions in excess of 30–40 mmHg (4–5 kPa) increase radiosensitivity only marginally, while complete anoxia is necessary to induce maximal radiation protection (Fig. 30).

Transient ischemia and hypoxia of normal tissues at the time of irradiation can

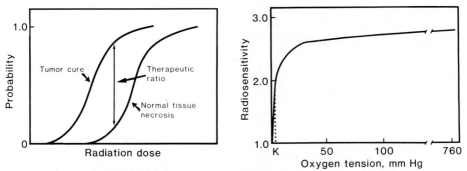

Figure 29. Theoretical curves describing the probabilities of tumour cure and development of normal tissue necrosis as a function of the radiation dose (redrawn from Bloomer and Hellman, 1975).

Figure 30. Experimental curve showing the influence of oxygen on radiosensitivity. From Gray (1961).

thus increase the radiation tolerance of hypoxic organs. This could substantially increase the therapeutic ratio in the radiotherapy of tumours at sites adjacent to dose-limiting organs, providing these organs tolerate transient hypoxia. An ideal ischemia-producing agent must induce intense temporary ischemia confined to and tolerated by normal tissues. Concurrent tumour ischemia and tumour radioprotection must be avoided. Therefore, normal tissues to be protected should have an accessible arterial supply separate from vessels supplying tumour tissue.

Ischemia induced by DSM has been demonstrated to be both intense and selective, and has been used for hypoxic radioprotection in experimental animal studies.

3.4.2. Experimental summary

Forsberg (1978), Forsberg and Jung (1978) and Forsberg et al. (1978a, b, 1979, 1981) investigated the effect of transient ischemia produced by DSM on the response to X-irradiation of the intestines, skin of the feet, and kidneys in rats. Lote (1981b) investigated whether the combination of DSM-induced ischemia and X-irradiation would induce thrombotic complications in cats. In this subsection, we summarize these studies:

A. Rats that had received an intraarterial injection of DSM (protected animals) and a subsequent in situ X-irradiation of the intestines (Forsberg and Jung, 1978) showed a smaller decrease in total body weight, and developed a much lower frequency of diarrhoea than animals which had not received microspheres (unprotected animals).

Histological evaluation of mucosal damage after irradiation of protected and non-protected ileal segments (Forsberg et al., 1978b) revealed that the effect of radiation was significantly less in protected segments (Fig. 31).

Fibrosis in the wall of the gut, determined 4 weeks after irradiation (Forsberg et al., 1979), was found to be significantly less frequent in protected than in nonprotected segments (Fig. 32).

Intestines protected by DSM-induced transient ischemia tolerated from 1.4 to 2.3 times higher radiation doses compared to unprotected bowel (Fig. 33).

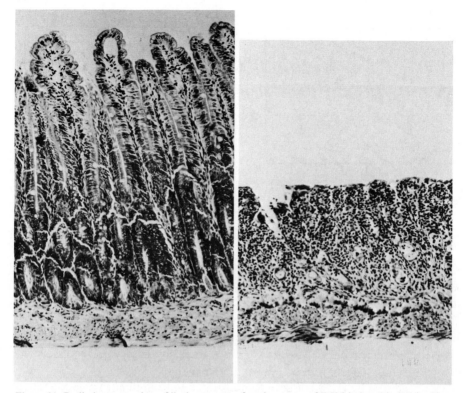

Figure 31. Radiation protection of ileal segments of rat by means of DSM-induced ischemia. Short-term effect 4 days after irradiation. Left: protected segment after a dose of 20 Gy. The villi heights are normal and the epithelial cells only slightly damaged (× 120). Right: non-protected segment after a dose of 10 Gy, showing maximum denudation of the epithelial structures. There is a marked inflammatory reaction (× 120).

B. When the hind foot of the rat (Forsberg et al., 1978a) was rendered temporarily ischemic by injection of degradable starch microspheres into the femoral artery, the skin-damaging effect of X-irradiation was 50% less in feet protected by ischemia than in unprotected feet.

C. In studies on rat kidneys, impairment of renal function as a result of radiation damage occurred in all nonprotected animals (Forsberg et al., 1981). Kidneys protected by DSM-induced transient ischemia tolerated 1.6 times higher doses compared to nonprotected controls.

D. Lote (1981b) found no evidence of thrombotic complications when cat intestine was irradiated during intense DSM-induced ischemia (Fig. 34, upper panel). Exposure to preceding irradiation did not increase the risk of thrombosis, and anticoagulant treatment was not required (Fig. 34, lower panel).

3.4.3. Clinical prospects

The radioprotective effect of transient DSM-induced ischemia has been demonstrated at single high-dose low linear energy-transfer radiation fractions in animal

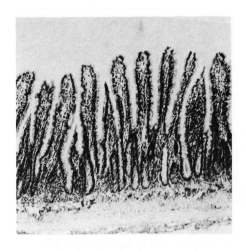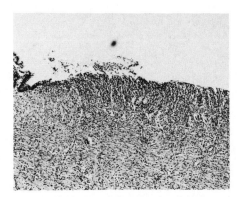

Figure 32. Radiation protection of ileal segments of rat by means of DSM-induced ischemia. Late effect 4 weeks after irradiation. Left: protected segment, after a dose of 20 Gy. No fibrosis can be seen, and the architecture of villi and crypts is almost entirely normal (× 65). Right: non-protected segment after a dose of 17.5 Gy. Heavy fibrosis and no mucosal regeneration (× 60).

studies. In clinical radiotherapy the total radiation dose is divided into smaller fractions, and usually delivered over a period of 3–6 weeks. Thus, the use of DSM for hypoxic radioprotective purposes in clinical radiotherapy demands either repeated arterial catheterizations or an indwelling intraarterial catheter, since the DSM must be administered with each treatment. For practical reasons this may only be possible for a relatively limited number of high-dose radiation fractions, i.e., an unconventional fractionation regime. Still, modest increments of the total tumour dose delivered may substantially increase the chances of cure, given the steep dose-response curves shown in Figure 30.

Important dose-limiting organs in clinical radiotherapy are the small intestine and the kidney. Both have well-defined arterial blood supply usually separate from vessels supplying many common abdominal tumours. Both tolerate transient ischemia.

3.5. Hyperthermia

The rationale for the use of DSM for the enhancement of local hyperthermia was advanced by Erichsen et al. (1984) as follows:

"The different vascular pattern of neoplastic tissue compared to normal tissue may play an important role in the tumour response to hyperthermia. A sluggish blood flow will minimize thermal dissipation in the tumour during heating. Occlusion of the hepatic artery during hyperthermia could further increase the effect on tumour cells by a decreased oxygenation and pH and deprivation of nutrients".

These authors designed a study to evaluate the effect of such a combination therapy. They inoculated the liver of 32 rats with tumour cells obtained from N-methyl-N-nitrosoguanidine-induced adenocarcinoma of the colon.

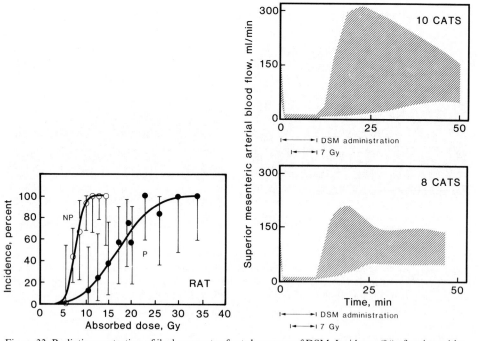

Figure 33. Radiation protection of ileal segments of rats by means of DSM. Incidence (%) of major epithelial damage in protected (P) and non-protected (NP) segments versus absorbed dose. Error bars represent 95% confidence limit. Curve obtained from probit analysis. For protected animals about a double dose of irradiation is required for the same incidence of damage as in the non-protected case. From Forsberg et al. (1978b).

Figure 34. Superior mesenteric arterial blood flow (electromagnetic) in cats. Upper panel: ten cats exposed to the combined trauma of DSM-induced ischemia and a surface radiation dose of 7 Gy delivered to the small intestine during ischemia. Lower panel: eight cats exposed to a surface radiation dose of 7 Gy to the intact abdomen followed after 72 hours by a second dose of 7 Gy delivered during severe DSM-induced ischemia. From Lote (1981b).

This study indicated that an occlusion of the hepatic artery during local microwave hyperthermia of the liver increased tumour destruction. The tumour volume was reduced about 70% 2 weeks after treatment compared with the control.

Further evaluation of the beneficial effect of DSM in hyperthermia is under investigation.

4. Toxicology and safety

4.1. Introduction

In this section we summarize the toxicological investigations carried out so far, and assess the tolerance to DSM by man from the aforementioned investigations in patients.

In assessing the toxicology of DSM, due consideration must be given to the nature of the substance. Most of the traditional models used for assessing the toxicity of pharmaceuticals were not relevant, since possible adverse effects were considered as a consequence of the occlusion.

Since the treatment of inoperable liver tumours has been proposed as one of the first clinical applications of DSM, a test model was set up in which DSM were repeatedly injected into the hepatic artery of the dog (section 4.2.1).

The effect of severe intestinal ischemia produced by injection of DSM into the mesenteric artery of the cat (section 4.2.2) was also investigated.

Acute intravenous toxicity studies with DSM were performed in the rabbit and the rat (section 4.2.3).

Acute intravenous toxicity studies of amylase degraded microspheres were performed in the mouse and rabbit (section 4.2.4).

Finally a mutagenicity test (Ames test) was performed on DSM following digestion with amylase simulating that occurring in human serum. The results revealed no mutagenicity.

4.2. Experimental summary

Intraarterial and acute intravenous toxicity of DSM has been investigated in the following studies on animals:

4.2.1 Prolonged intraarterial toxicity study — dog (Malmquist and Bodin, 1982a)

Permanent catheters were introduced in a retrograde direction into the gastroduodenal artery of six dogs. The catheters were placed near the bifurcation to the hepatic artery proper. Four of the dogs were treated with DSM, 30 mg/kg (Spherex, mean diameter, 41 μm), daily for 14 days. Two dogs served as controls. The first and last administrations were observed by fluoroscopy and the rate of injection was controlled in order to avoid back-flow via the common hepatic artery to the aorta. The animals were observed every day, and possible clinical symptoms were recorded. No adverse effects related to the repeated injection of DSM were observed.

At the termination, a complete autopsy and histopathological examination was performed on all animals. Lipid droplets were found in the Kupffer cells of the liver. This was attributed to the chronic catheterization rather than the substance, as the controls showed the same alterations. No adverse reactions related to the DSM injections were observed.

4.2.2. Intraarterial toxicity study – cat (Lote and Myking, 1982)

Severe intestinal ischemia lasting for 10 minutes was induced with DSM (Spherex) after laparotomy in 15 cats. At the end of the 14-day observation period, intestinal mucosal blood flow was determined by carbonized microsphere distribution, and the small intestine was examined histologically. No clinical signs of small intestinal injury were observed. The mean body weight increased from 2.4 to 2.5 kg during the observation period. Small intestinal mucosal blood flow was not significantly changed 14 days after DSM-induced transient ischemia. Histological evidence of intestinal injury was not seen, although PAS-positive starch fragments persisted within macrophages in ileal Peyer's patches (Fig. 35). It is well known that foreign particulate matter is rapidly removed from the circulation by macrophages located in the reticulo-endothelial system. The data from this study indicate that partly degraded starch particles taken up by macrophages may persist intracellularly for at least 14 days. Such starch persistence did not cause intestinal injury or inflammation.

4.2.3. Acute intravenous toxicity study — rat and rabbit (Malmquist and Waller, 1983; Malmquist et al., 1983)

DSM (Spherex) were injected intravenously into 30 rats and 12 rabbits at a dose level of 210 and 60 mg/kg, respectively. Clinical symptoms were recorded and blood gas analysis was performed in the rabbit.

The animals showed a transient tachypnea and a transient moderate disturbance of the ventilation/perfusion ratio as recorded by a decreased arterial PO_2. No lasting adverse effects could be demonstrated.

4.2.4. Acute intravenous toxicity study with degraded DSM — mouse and rabbit (Malmquist and Bodin, 1982b)

An intravenous toxicity study was performed using completely serum amylase-

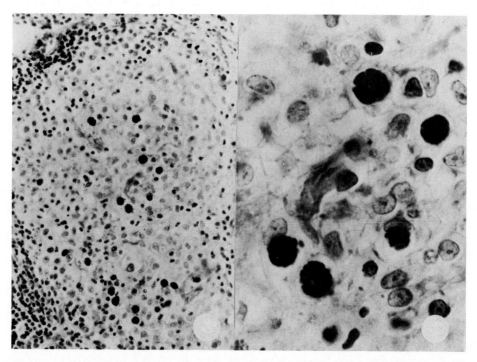

Figure 35. Left: germinal center of ileal Peyer's patch showing engulfed starch particles within macrophages 14 days after intense transient DSM-induced intestinal ischemia in the cat (Spherex). PAS stain, × 200. Right: same section at higher magnification. Several large starch-containing macrophages. PAS stain, × 810.

degraded DSM (Spherex). 50 ml/kg body weight, corresponding to 1500 mg of DSM/ kg, was injected intravenously into 20 mice and ten rabbits. The animals were observed for 1 week, after which they were killed and examined macroscopically.

Immediately after the administration, the rabbits showed a pronounced dyspnea. The symptoms disappeared rapidly, and after 1–2 hours there were no signs of abnormality. All animals survived the observation period. The post-mortem examination showed no signs of toxicity.

Conclusion: From the results of the studies in sections 4.2.1–3, it is concluded that DSM are well tolerated by the animals. No adverse effects associated with DSM injection were observed.

4.3. Tolerance to degradable starch microspheres in clinical studies

A. In the first clinical investigation (Aronsen et al., 1979 — section 3.2.3), where patients were treated with a dose of 150 mg DSM (mean diameter, 92 μm) three times daily for 14 days, all patients suffered more or less from nausea and tension in the liver region. Liver function tests fluctuated considerably and inconsistently in the individual patient as well as between the patients. The liver function tests did not indicate any damage to the liver parenchyma by the treatment. At autopsy there was no trace of foreign bodies or foreign body reaction in the liver or the lungs.

B. In a study where DSM (Spherex) were injected as a bolus together with doxorubicin (Teder et al., 1983 — section 3.3.2,B), the patients reported nausea and retrosternal/epigastric pain. These symptoms receded within 30 minutes after injection and had completely disappeared within 60 minutes. As no patient felt any discomfort during or after the injection with doxorubicin alone, the symptoms were thought to be caused by transient ischemia in the coeliac vascular region. When a dose of 360 mg microspheres was injected over a 4-minute period these symptoms were not observed.

Conclusion: From these results it may be concluded that the DSM levels proposed for clinical use would appear safe.

5. Conclusion and future prospects

In conclusion, we summarize the investigations in animals and man in Tables 7 and 8, respectively.

We would like to emphasize that in intraarterial administration of DSM mixed with drugs, the drug remains essentially free and may diffuse normally into the tissues or cells in the ischemic region. The pharmacokinetic studies in animals and man show that this leads to an increased drug concentration in the embolized region and to decreased systemic exposure. By this means the adverse effects of toxic drugs may be minimized and these drugs may also be administered more effectively.

We have also drawn attention to the fact that DSM-induced transient ischemia of normal tissues protects against damage by low linear energy-transfer ionizing

TABLE 7

Experimental animal models for investigation of the effect of intraarterially administered DSM

Species	Organ	Effect studied	Reference
Hamster	Cheek pouch	Behaviour in the microcirculation	Tuma (following chapter)
Rat	Liver	Transient ischemia	Lindell (1977) Lindell et al. (1977a,b)
		Drug pharmacokinetics	Teder et al. (1978) This chapter
		Drug pharmacokinetics and tolerance	Lindell et al. (1978)
		Hyperthermia	Erichsen et al. (1984)
	Foot	Transient ischemia	Forsberg (1978)
		Radiation protection	Forsberg et al. (1978a)
	Intestine	Transient ischemia	Forsberg and Jung (1978)
		Radiation protection	Forsberg et al. (1978b, 1979)
	Kidney	Radiation protection	Forsberg et al. (1981)
Rabbit	Leg	Pharmacokinetics	Lorelius et al. (1984)
Cat	Intestine	Transient ischemia	Lote et al. (1980)
		Possible thrombogenicity	Lote (1981a) Lote and Myking (1982)
		Possible thrombogenicity in combination with radiation	Lote (1981b)
Dog	Liver	Transient ischemia	Tuma et al. (1982) Malmquist et al. (1982)
		Toxicology	Malmquist and Bodin (1982a,b)
	Kidney	Transient ischemia and drug pharmacokinetics	Arfors et al. (1979) Tuma et al. (1982)
	Lung	Tolerance	Wulff (1975)
Pig	Intestine	Transient ischemia and tissue oxygen tension	Arfors et al. (1976)

TABLE 8

Published investigations in patients for pharmacokinetics and tolerance to drugs injected into the liver together with DSM

No. of patients	DSM	Drug	Reference
12	92 μm	5-Fluorouracil	Aronsen et al. (1979)
5	Spherex	Carmustine	Dakhil et al. (1982)
16	Spherex	Mitomycin C	Gyves et al. (1983)
5	Spherex	Doxorubicin	Teder et al. (1983)

radiation. This would permit the irradiation of tumours with higher doses leading to a better therapeutic ratio.

With the introduction of improved catheterization techniques and implantable injection/infusion devices, DSM-induced embolization will be facilitated. Thus, DSM-induced ischemia could become clinically attractive in the near future.

Although in this review we have only discussed the possibilities offered by unmodified DSM, the coupling of drugs or other active substances of therapeutic or diagnostic interest to DSM could provide alternative future applications.

Acknowledgements

We are indebted to Pharmacia AB for permission to use unpublished material and to R. Lindblom, Pharmacia Infusion, Uppsala, for coordination, suggestions and valuable discussions.

B. Lindberg is indebted to A. Nygren, G. Mälson, E. Dagérus, E.-L. Hartman and K. Granath, all of the Department of Chemical Research, Pharmacia Pharmaceuticals, Uppsala, for collaboration and assistance in the preparation and characterization of DSM, and to M. Malmqvist (Pharmacia Pharmaceuticals) for valuable discussions and providing of data, to H. Jenner and N.O. Bodin (both of Pharmacia Pharmaceuticals) for the measurements for Figure 14, and to J.O. Forsberg for providing Figures 31 and 32.

K. Lote is indebted to B. Rosengren, Department of Oncology, and J. Lekven at the Surgical Research Laboratory, University of Bergen, for support.

H. Teder is indebted to K.-F. Aronsen and U. Rothman, Department of Surgery, Malmö General Hospital, for support, and to J. Ljungberg, Department of Surgery, Malmö General Hospital, for collaboration and assistance.

We thank E. Johansson (Department of Biological Research, Pharmacia Pharmaceuticals, Uppsala) for redrawing the figures and G. Fahlström (Pharmacia Infusion, Uppsala) for skillful typing.

References

Arfors, K.-E., Forsberg, J.O., Larsson, B., Lewis, D.H., Rosengren, B. and Ödman (1976) Nature 262, 500–501.

Arfors, K.-E., Tuma, R.F. and Ågerup, B. (1979) Bibl. Anat. 18, 204–206.

Aronsen, K.F., Hellekant, C., Holmberg, J., Rothman, U. and Teder, H. (1979) Eur. Surg. Res. 11, 99–106.

Bengmark, S., Fredlund, P., Hafström, L.D. and Vang, J. (1974) in Progress in Surgery (Allgöwer, M., Bergentz, S.-E., Calne, R.Y. and Gruber, U.F., Eds.), Vol. 13, pp. 141–166, Karger, Basel.

Bloomer, W.D. and Hellman, S. (1975) N. Engl. J. Med. 293, 80–83.

Ceska, M., Birath, K. and Brown, B. (1969) Clin. Chir. Acta 26, 437–444.

Chuang, V.P. and Wallace, S. (1981) J. Am. Med. Assoc. 20, 1151–1152.

188

Dakhil, S., Ensminger, W., Cho, K., Niederhuber, J., Doan, K. and Wheeler, R. (1982) Cancer 50, 631–635.

Dawbarn, R.H.H. (1904) J. Am. Med. Assoc. 43, 292–795.

Erichsen, C., Bolmsjö, M., Hugander, A. and Jönsson, P.-E., et al. (1984), in press.

Fischer, E.M. and Stein, E.A. (1960) in The Enzymes (Doyer, D.D., Ed), Vol. 4, p. 338, Academic Press, New York.

Forsberg, J.O. (1978) Acta Chir. Scand. 144, 275–281.

Forsberg, J.O. and Jung, B (1978) Acta Radiol. 17, 353–361.

Forsberg, J.O., Jung, B. and Larsson, B. (1978a) Acta Radiol. 17, 199–208.

Forsberg, J.O., Jung, B. and Larsson, B. (1978b) Acta Radiol. 17, 485–486.

Forsberg, J.O., Jiborn, H. and Jung, B (1979) Acta Radiol. 18, 65–75.

Forsberg, J.O., Hillered, L., Graffman, S., Jung, B., Persson, E. and Selén, G. (1981) Scand. J. Urol. Nephrol. 15, 147–152.

Gray, L.H. (1961) Am. J. Roentgenol. 85, 803–815.

Gyves, J.W., Ensminger, W.D., Vanharken, D., Niederhuber, J., Stetson, P. and Walker, S. (1983) Clin. Pharm. Ther. 34, 259–265.

Holmberg, L. (1984) Thesis, University of Uppsala, Ch. 5.

Holmberg, L. and Lindquist, B. (1984) Carbohydr. Res., in press.

Jenner, H. (1967) Technicon Symposia 2, 203–207.

Kunstlinger, F., Prunelle, F., Chaumont, P. and Doyon, D. (1981) Am. J. Roentgenol. 136, 151–156.

Lindberg, B. (1983) in Proceedings of the International Conference of Commercial Applications and Implications of Biotechnology, pp. 863–876, Online Publications Ltd, Northwood.

Lindberg, B., Engdahl, K.-Å. and Ahlberg, P. (1983) Starch/Stärke 35, 313–315.

Lindell, B. (1977) Thesis, University of Lund.

Lindell, B., Aronsen, K.F. and Rothman, U. (1977a) Eur. Surg. Res. 9, 347–356.

Lindell, B., Aronsen, K.F., Rothman, U. and Sjögren, H.O. (1977b) Res. Exp. Med. 171, 63–70.

Lindell, B., Aronsen, K.F., Nosslin, B. and Rothman, U. (1978) Ann. Surg., 187, 95–99.

Lorelius, L.E., Benedetto, A.R., Blumhardt, R., Gaskill, H.V., Lancaster, J.L. and Stridbeck, H. (1984) Invest. Radiol. 19, 212–215.

Lote, K. (1981a) Acta Radiol. Oncol. 20, 91–96.

Lote, K. (1981b) Am. J. Roentgenol. 137, 909–914.

Lote, K. and Lekven, J. (1982) Acta Radiol. Oncol. 21, 461–462.

Lote, K. and Myking, A.O. (1982) Acta Radiol. Oncol. 21, 353–358.

Lote, K., Følling, M., Rosengren, B., Svanes, K. and Lekven, J. (1980) Acta Radiol. Oncol. 19, 343–351.

Lote, K., Følling, M., Lekven, J. and Rosengren, B. (1981) Am. J. Roentgenol. 136, 969–975.

Malmquist, M. (1982) Pharmacia Research Report, unpublished.

Malmquist, M. and Bodin, N.O. (1982a) Pharmacia Research Report, unpublished.

Malmquist, M. and Bodin, N.O. (1982b) Pharmacia Research Report, unpublished.

Malmquist, M. and Waller, T. (1983) Pharmacia Research Report, unpublished.

Malmquist, M., Bodin, N.O., Dougan, P., Rothman, U. and Teder, H (1982) Pharmacia Research report, unpublished.

Malmquist, M., Smedegård, G. and Waller, T. (1983) Pharmacia Research Report, unpublished.

Rothman, U., Arfors, K.-E., Aronsen, K.F., Lindell, B. and Nylander, G. (1976) Microvasc. Res. 11, 421.

Russell, G.F. (1983) Pharm. Int. 4, 260–262.

Teder, H., Aronsen, K.F., Lindell, B. and Rothman, U. (1978) Acta Chir. Scand., suppl., 487, 71.

Teder, H., Nilsson, B., Jonsson, K., Hellekant, C., Aspegren, K. and Aronsen, K.F. (1983) in Anthracyclines and Cancer Therapy (Hansen, H.H., Ed.), pp. 166–176, Excerpta Medica, Amsterdam.

Tuma, R.F., Forsberg, J.E. and Ågerup, B. (1982) Cancer 50, 1–5.

Wulff, K. (1975) Thesis, University of Lund, paper No. 3.

Young, A.E. (1981) Br. Med. J. 283, 1144–1145.

Microspheres and Drug Therapy. Pharmaceutical, Immunological and Medical Aspects
edited by S.S. Davis, L. Illum, J.G. McVie and E. Tomlinson
© 1984, Elsevier Science Publishers B.V.

The use of degradable starch microspheres for transient occlusion of blood flow and for drug targeting to selected tissues

Ronald F. Tuma

1. Introduction

The systemic administration of many types of drugs for the treatment of disease in localized areas has the disadvantage that the drug, in the concentration needed for treatment, may be toxic to healthy tissue. There have been many different approaches to this problem. One approach currently being investigated, both in the laboratory and in clinical trials, is the injection of degradable starch microspheres in conjunction with drugs into the arterial vessel supplying a targeted organ. The concept underlying this approach is that the microspheres, when suspended in a drug-containing solution and injected into the artery supplying a target organ, may trap the drug in the exchange vessels of the microcirculation. This would result in an increase in the time during which high concentrations of the drug would be available for exchange into the interstitial fluid and parenchymal tissue of the target organ.

The microspheres that were used in the investigations described in this chapter are made of cross-linked polysaccharide derivatives (Spherex®, Pharmacia AB, Sweden). They are degraded by plasma amylase. The rigidity, the size and the degradation rate of the microspheres can be varied by changing the degree of cross-linking of the molecule.

Arfors et al. (1976) were the first to demonstrate that intraarterial injection of degradable starch microspheres produced an occlusion of blood flow to the injected organ (pig intestines) and that this occlusion was reversible. Oxygen tension was reduced in the tissue area following the injection of microspheres, and returned to control values after degradation of the spheres. Lindell et al. (1977a) demonstrated in rats that blood flow to the liver could also be reduced temporarily following the injection of degradable starch microspheres into the hepatic artery. In a later study, Lindell et al. (1977b) provided evidence that, following injection of the microspheres into the hepatic artery, blood flow to liver tumors was reduced to a greater extent than blood flow to healthy liver tissue. Spherex has also been used in the clinical treatment of human hepatic tumors by Aronsen et al. (1979) and Dakhil et al. (1982). The results of the latter study indicated that the concentration of the cytostatic drug in the peripheral blood was decreased when the drug was administered with the microspheres.

The purpose of the studies described in this chapter was to evaluate the effects of intraarterial injection of degradable starch microspheres on blood flow, to study the behavior of the microspheres in the microcirculation and to determine their influence on local drug uptake in a target organ. For the studies of the effects on organ blood flow and drug uptake, the dog kidney was selected as the experimental model. Studies of the behavior of the microspheres in the microcirculation were conducted using the exteriorized hamster cheek pouch for direct in vivo microscopy. Part of these studies have been reported previously in Cancer (Tuma et al., 1982).

2. Dog kidney studies

The dog kidney was selected for the initial studies of the effect of intraarterial injection of the microspheres primarily because this organ, in most cases, has a single arterial vessel supplying blood to the organ. Dogs of mixed breed weighing between 20 and 30 kg were anesthetized with nembutal (30 mg/kg) administered intravenously. After tracheostomy a cannula was placed in a femoral vein for infusion of drugs and for supplemental infusion of anesthetics. Systemic blood pressure was measured via a cannula placed in an axillary artery. A renal artery was cannulated using a radio-opaque catheter which was introduced into a femoral artery and positioned in the renal artery under a fluoroscope to visualize the placement of the catheter. Blood flow to the kidney was measured by an electromagnetic flow probe placed around the renal artery. The flow was measured for at least 30 minutes prior to cannulation of the renal artery for injection of degradable microspheres. After injection of the spheres the cannula was immediately removed and continuous blood flow measurements were made for another 2 hours. Renal artery blood flow measurements were made on a total of 17 dogs. The amounts of microspheres injected into the kidney in four groups of experiments were 10.2×10^6 or 20.4×10^6 for the $36\text{-}\mu\text{m}$ microspheres and 2.6×10^6 or 3.5×10^6 for the $58\text{-}\mu\text{m}$ microspheres.

The alterations in renal blood flow that resulted from injection of the microspheres are illustrated in Figure 1. Following injection of the microspheres into the renal artery, blood flow decreased to less than 10% of the control flow. The duration of occlusion varied with the size and concentration of the microspheres used. The time required for full return to control flow was approximately 20 minutes with 10.2×10^6 of the $36\text{-}\mu\text{m}$ microspheres, 30 minutes with 20.4×10^6 of the $36\text{-}\mu\text{m}$ microspheres, and 60 minutes with 3.5×10^6 of the $58\text{-}\mu\text{m}$ microspheres. The duration of occlusion for different dogs was consistent for any given size and the amount of microspheres used. In a later analysis of these data, Lindberg (1983) found a very close correlation between the time required for blood flow to return to half the control value $(t_{1/2})$ and the product of the diameter of the microspheres and the dose in milligrams (Fig. 2). However, it should be kept in mind that quantitative changes in this relationship would result from changes in the properties of the microspheres, such as the degree of cross-linking between the starch molecules.

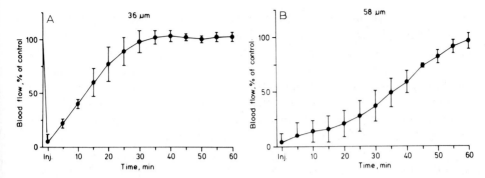

Figure 1. Change in kidney blood flow, expressed as a percentage of the control flow following the injection of (A) 20.4 × 10⁶ of the 36-μm microspheres and (B) 3.5 × 10⁶ of the 58-μm microspheres into the renal artery. The bars represent the standard deviation. From Tuma et al. (1982).

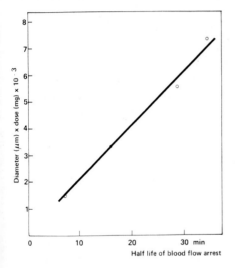

Figure 2. The correlation between the dose of microspheres injected, calculated as the product of the diameter and number of milligrams, and the time required for 50% return to control flow. From Lindberg (1983).

A preliminary investigation was also made on three dogs that received three consecutive injections of 3.5 × 10⁶ of the 58-μm microspheres into the renal artery to determine if any permanent damage was done to the kidney by injection of the microspheres alone. 1 month after the injections, the glomerular filtration rate, urine pH, osmolarity and output of the injected and non-injected kidney of each dog were compared. There were no significant changes in any of these parameters between the injected and non-injected kidneys.

An evaluation of the potential alterations in drug distribution that could result from the use of the degradable microspheres was made by comparing the tissue content of tritiated actinomycin D when the drug was injected alone and in combination with the microspheres. The modes of administration were as follows: intravenous injections of the drug were made in six dogs; injections of the drug alone into the renal artery were made in seven dogs; injections into the renal artery of the drug mixed with 20.4×10^6 of the 36-μm microspheres were made in eight dogs. This procedure was repeated with 3.5×10^6 of the 58-μm microspheres in eight dogs.

A total dose of 275 μg of actinomycin D was used for each injection. The total activity of the injected dose was 1.2 μCi. The drugs and the drug-microsphere combination were diluted in saline before injection. The dogs were killed 60 minutes after injection of the drug and tissue samples of cortex and medulla from both kidneys, skeletal muscle, liver and heart were taken for measurement of actinomycin D concentrations.

The results of these investigations showed that the use of the degradable starch microspheres could significantly alter the tissue distribution of the cytostatic drug. Intraarterial injection of actinomycin D alone resulted in a 6.4 times higher retention of the drug in the cortex and 3.4 times higher retention in the medulla as compared to the intravenous injection (Table 1). When the drug was mixed in a suspension with the 36-μm microspheres and injected into the renal artery the retention of the drug in the cortex was 15-fold higher and in the medulla 13-fold higher as compared to the intravenous administration of the same amount of drug in the absence of the microspheres (Table 1). When comparing the drug concentration in the kidney follow-

TABLE 1

Actinomycin D concentration in the injected kidney, contralateral kidney, heart, liver and skeletal muscle 60 minutes after administration of the drug intravenously (six animals), selectively into the renal artery (seven animals), and selectively into the renal artery in combination with the 36-μm and 58-μm degradable microspheres (eight animals)

	Actinomycin D concentration (μg/g)			
	Intravenous	Renal artery		
		Alone	36-μm microspheres	58-μm microspheres
Injected medulla[a]	—	0.166($\pm$0.043)	0.638($\pm$0.186)	0.698($\pm$0.300)
Injected cortex[a]	—	0.584($\pm$0.107)	1.378($\pm$0.662)	1.493($\pm$0.530)
Contralateral cortex	0.093($\pm$0.006)	0.074($\pm$0.010)	0.108($\pm$0.064)	0.075($\pm$0.011)
Contralateral medulla	0.048($\pm$0.015)	0.035($\pm$0.009)	0.051($\pm$0.030)	0.044($\pm$0.021)
Heart	0.030($\pm$0.066)	0.024($\pm$0.006)	0.021($\pm$0.006)	0.022($\pm$0.007)
Liver	0.084($\pm$0.011)	0.075($\pm$0.022)	0.066($\pm$0.022)	0.053($\pm$0.020)
Muscle	0.009($\pm$0.002)	0.008($\pm$0.003)	0.014($\pm$0.010)	0.006($\pm$0.002)

Values are mean and S.D. [a]Since this category does not apply to intravenous injection, the average concentrations in both kidneys are included under the category of contralateral kidney. From Tuma et al. (1982).

ing intraarterial injection of the drug alone with the concentration following injection of the drug mixed with the 36-μm microspheres, it was found that the cortex concentration was increased by a factor of 2.4 and the medullary concentration was increased by a factor of 3.8. Mixing the drug with the 58-μm microspheres caused a further increase in drug retention in the kidney. Calculations were made of the proportion of the total injected dose of actinomycin D that remained in the kidney 1 hour after injection (Table 2). These values were calculated from the product of the actinomycin D concentrations listed in Table 1 and the kidney weight, assuming 70% of the total kidney weight was comprised of cortex and 30% of medulla.

The amounts of actinomycin D found in heart, liver, skeletal muscle and the contralateral kidney were not significantly smaller after administration of the drug combination with the microspheres compared to the injection of the drug alone. This may be due in part to a reflux of a portion of the bolus of injected drug back into the aorta after blockage of the arterial tree of the kidney with the microspheres. This parameter was not controlled during the injection procedure. Furthermore, the amount of drug injected directly into the single organ was equivalent to the clinical dose used for systemic administration. This may have caused a saturation of the tissue. Although a significant reduction in the concentration of the drug in nontarget organs could not be demonstrated, it is important to realize that the ratio of concentration of the drug in the injected organ to the concentration in other organs was increased, implying that there is a possibility of increasing the therapeutic ratio by using degradable microspheres.

All of the above measurements of the tissue concentration of drug were made 60 minutes after injection of the microspheres, when normal blood flow was regained. Therefore, it was of interest to determine if the increased retention of drug in the target organ was sustained over a longer period of time. To answer this question,

TABLE 2

A calculation of the percentage of the total amount of injected actinomycin D that remains in the kidney 60 minutes after administration of the drug intravenously, selectively into the renal artery, and selectively into the renal artery in combination with the 36-μm and 58-μm degradable microspheres

	% of total injected actinomycin D remaining in the kidney			
	Intravenous	Renal artery		
		Alone	36-μm microspheres	58-μm microspheres
Cortex	1	8	18	20
Medulla	0.3	1	4	4
Total	1.3	9	22	24

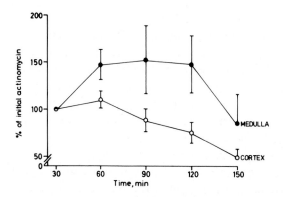

Figure 3. Changes in the kidney concentration of actinomycin D as a function of time following injection into the renal artery of the drug mixed with the 58-μm microspheres. The values are expressed as a percentage of the initial concentrations 30 minutes after the injection. Bars represent the standard deviation. Number of animals = 5. From Tuma et al. (1982).

275 μg of actinomycin D mixed in a suspension of the 58-μm microspheres were injected into the renal arteries of four dogs. Samples from the kidney cortex and medulla were taken with a biopsy drill 30, 60, 90, 120 and 150 minutes after injection. The actinomycin D concentration in each of the tissue samples was then measured. The results shown in Figure 3 demonstrate that the concentration of actinomycin D remained elevated over the period of measurement.

To test further the possibility that this technique could be used to alter the distribution of drugs a diuretic, ethacrynic acid, was injected either alone or in combination with microspheres into the renal arteries of dogs (Arfors et al., 1979).

The technique used for preparation of the animals was the same as that outlined in the experiments described above. In the initial portion of this experiment the effect of alterations in plasma amylase on the time of occlusion produced by the microspheres was examined. Following the injection of 60 mg of the 40-μm starch microspheres into the renal artery, renal blood flow approached zero. In dogs having a plasma amylase activity of approximately 2000 units/1, blood flow returned to the pre-injection values after approximately 15 minutes. In contrast, when the amylase activity was reduced to human values (200–300 units/l) the rate of degradation of the spheres was reduced so that it took 1 hour for blood flow to return to the pre-injection values. The results show, therefore, that the time of degradation of the spheres, and therefore the duration of the occlusion, is dependent upon plasma amylase concentration.

A comparison was made between the effect of ethacrynic acid injected into a renal artery when mixed with 60 mg of the starch microspheres and when injected in the same way without microspheres. The results of a typical experiment are illustrated in Figures 4 and 5. It can be seen from Figures 4 and 5 that the diuresis resulting from the drug-microsphere combination was four times greater in the injected kidney than when the diuretic was injected without microspheres. When injected without microspheres, the ethacrynic acid had a considerable effect on the non-injected kidney whereas there was very little effect on the non-injected kidney when the drug was mixed with microspheres.

Although the results obtained from these studies give support to the possibility that degradable starch microspheres can increase the local concentration of drugs in diseased areas, optimization of the technique is required before the full potential can be determined. A number of questions remain to be answered. Among these are the optimal size and degradation time for the microspheres in the tissue of interest, and the proper sequence of injection of the drug and microspheres. In order to answer these questions more information about the behavior of the microspheres in the exchange vessels of the microcirculation is necessary. This was the reason for initiating the direct in vivo microscopic studies in the hamster cheek pouch.

3. Microvascular studies

The purpose of this investigation was to observe directly the behavior of the degradable starch microspheres in the small blood vessels to provide additional insight into the precise way in which blood flow is occluded, to follow the spheres during degradation and determine their fate, and, finally, to determine the way in which blood flow is reinstated to the microcirculation following degradation of the spheres.

The exteriorized hamster cheek pouch is an experimental model that has been used for studies of the microcirculation by numerous investigators over the last three decades. A description of the structure and methods of preparation of the hamster cheek pouch for microvascular observation has been published previously by Duling (1973). Briefly, the hamster cheek pouch is an epithelial sac that has its origin at the corner of the mouth. Its function is the storage of food. The blood perfusing this tissue is supplied by branches of the external carotid artery. The neural innervation has its origin in the facial and spinal accessory nerves. Histologically, the proximal portion of the cheek pouch is composed of dense fibrous connective tissue, stratified squamous epithelium, skeletal muscle and a layer of loose areolar connective tissue. In the distal portions of the pouch the skeletal muscle layer is absent. The advantage of this structure for microvascular studies is that it has a rich supply of arterial vessels, venous vessels and capillaries and it can be prepared easily for direct, microscopic observation in the living animal.

Hamsters weighing approximately 100 grams were used in this investigation. The animals were anesthetized with sodium nembutal (0.6 mg/kg). A femoral vein was cannulated for supplemental injections of anesthetic and the trachea cannulated to facilitate breathing. The right carotid artery was cannulated for the injection of microspheres. The pouch was prepared for observation by introducing a cotton swab into the distal portion, twisting the swab and drawing the swab and the everted pouch out through the mouth. The pouch was then draped over a glass pedestal by pinning the borders of the pouch to a rubber ring surrounding the pedestal. During the pre-

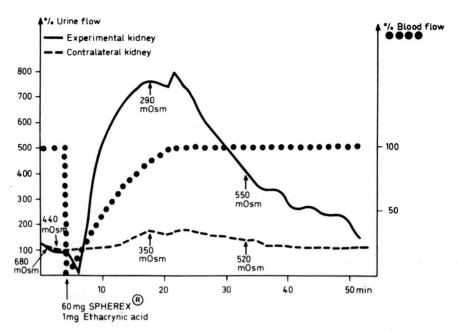

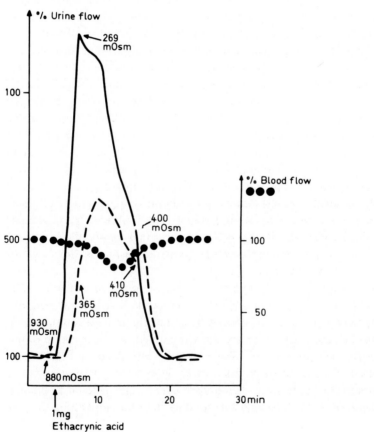

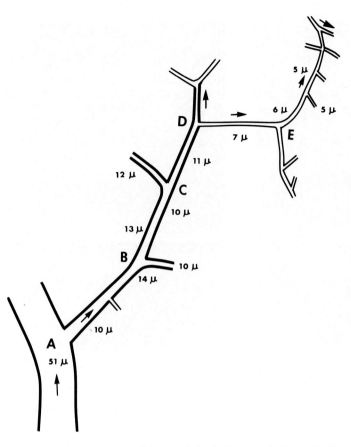

Figure 5. A sketch of an arterial network in the hamster cheek pouch. The diameters given are those of the vessels prior to the occlusion of the side branch, at point A, by a microsphere.

parative procedures the pouch was continuously bathed with a warm physiological saline solution. An incision was made through the top layer of the pouch. This layer was then pinned back to expose the bottom layer for observation. The loose areolar connective tissue was removed for optimal visualization. The tissue was covered with mineral oil to prevent drying. The animal was then placed on the stage of a microscope and the pouch transilluminated for observation. Blood vessels ranging in size from 100-μm arterial vessels to 5-μm capillaries could be observed in this preparation. The blood vessels were studied at magnifications of 250, 500 and 800 diameters. Recordings of the microcirculation were made using either 35-mm slides or video-

Figure 4. A. Changes in urine flow in the injected kidney (solid line) and contralateral kidney (dashed line) and blood flow in the injected kidney (dotted line) following injection of degradable starch microspheres mixed with ethacrynic acid into the renal artery. B. Changes in the same parameters when ethacrynic acid was injected into the renal artery without microspheres. From Arfors et al. (1979).

198

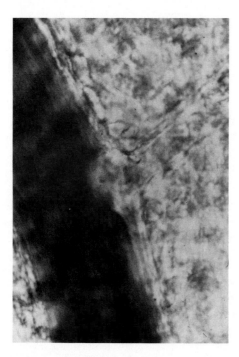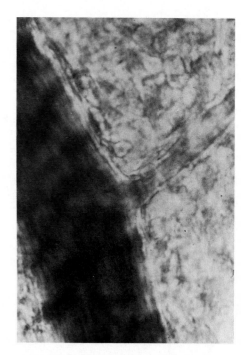

Figure 6. A photograph taken of area A in Figure 5. A microsphere can be seen occluding a side branch at this location.

Figure 7. Following partial degradation of the sphere, the sphere is moved to area B in Figure 5. Flow is now shown to be reinstated in area A.

tapes. Measurements of vascular diameter were made directly through the microscope using an eyepiece micrometer or from either the videotapes or 35-mm slides.

Prior to the injection of microspheres, one of the main arterial vessels supplying the pouch was selected for study. The diameter of this vessel and of the consecutive branches were measured. Degradable starch microspheres, 40 μm mean diameter (Spherex, Pharmacia AB), suspended in saline (30 mg/ml) were injected into the right carotid artery. Pilot investigations using fluoroscopy have shown that this injection procedure results in a retrograde flow of the injected solution into the root of the aorta. From this point the solution is carried by the flowing blood, in an antegrade direction, into the left carotid artery, where a portion of the solution enters the cheek pouch. The microsphere suspension was injected continuously (between 0.1 and 0.2 ml) until a microsphere was seen to lodge in the preselected area. The sphere was then followed as it degraded and was forced through a capillary into a venous vessel.

Approximately 3–5 seconds after injection, the microspheres were seen to enter the cheek pouch. The spheres moved rapidly with the flowing blood in the large arterial vessels in the pouch. The injection was continued until a microsphere was seen to

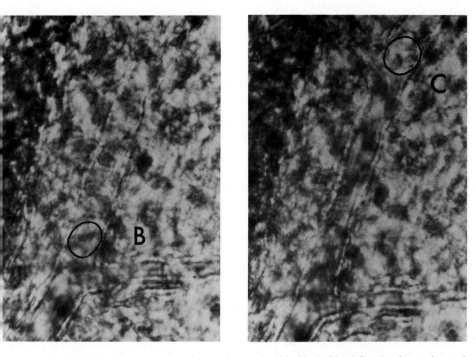

Figure 8. The location of the microsphere in area B is outlined in black. Blood flow has been reinstated to the remaining branches.

Figure 9. The microsphere, outlined in black, has been further degraded and pushed to location C shown in Figure 5. Flow to the upstream branches has been reinstated.

lodge in the preselected area. Figure 5 is a sketch of an arterial network selected for study in one of the experiments. Figures 6, 7 and 8, and 9 are photographs of areas A, B and C, respectively. In Figure 6 a sphere is shown occluding a side branch of the main arterial vessel in area A. As was the case in all the experiments the microsphere was seen initially to protrude into the lumen of the parent arterial vessel. The pressure gradient across the microsphere is presumably the force causing the sphere to remain lodged in the arterial side branch and is of sufficient magnitude to overcome the shear stress at this location. As can be seen in Figure 6, the flow of blood into the arterial side branch in area A is completely occluded, while flow continues through the parent vessel. As the sphere was degraded by plasma amylase it was forced into the side branch and moved along this vessel until, 8 minutes after injection, the sphere has moved to area B, as shown in Figure 8. As can be seen from Figures 7 and 8, the sphere was now occluding one of the daughter branches and flow was reinstated upstream and to the other branch. The photograph in Figure 9 was taken 10 minutes after injection, at which time the sphere had moved to area C and was now occluding one of the branches in this area. At this time blood flow was fully reinstated in areas A and B. Degradation of the sphere continued with the sphere being pushed through consecutive branches of this arterial tree until the sphere passed through a 5-μm capillary 20 minutes after injection. At this time flow was reinstated to all vessels.

The sequence of events described in this experiment is typical of what was seen in each of the animals. The movement and entrapment of the microspheres in progressively smaller arterial branches was seen as the pattern of microsphere behavior during degradation in all experiments. As the spheres moved in subsequently smaller arterial branches the unoccluded vessels upstream always became perfused with flowing blood. This pattern continued until the spheres passed through a capillary (5 μm in diameter) and flow was fully restored to all vessels. The average time required for the degradation and transit of a microsphere from the arterial side to the venous side of the circulation was 21 $\pm$ 4 minutes.

During degradation, the microspheres were seen to deform slightly and become somewhat egg-shaped when forced into an arterial branch. The spheres often caused a slight distention of the arterial vessels. Although the vessel immediately downstream from the microsphere was constricted, the vessel immediately upstream remained dilated. There was never any indication of vasospasm after passage of a microsphere through a vessel. The diameters of the arterial vessels were measured immediately after the microspheres were forced through a capillary. The diameters of these vessels were usually found to be greater than the preinjection diameter, as is indicated in Table 3.

Occasionally, when injected in large numbers, the microspheres were seen to form chains (a row of abutting spheres) in arterial vessels. These chains of spheres were not as effective in occluding blood flow as spheres lodged at the entrance of side branches. When the microspheres lodged in chains in an arterial vessel larger in diameter than that of the individual microspheres blood could usually be seen to flow around and between the microspheres, with the result that although flow was diminished it was not completely occluded. Eventually, as the microspheres degraded, the spheres forming chains in the arterial arcades were forced into smaller arterial vessels and, finally, through a capillary into the venous side of the circulation.

Platelets and leukocytes could be clearly seen at the higher magnifications used for observation. In none of the experiments were either of these cellular elements seen to be activated. Platelets were not seen to adhere to the spheres nor were platelet aggregates seen to form at any time during the experimental procedure. The adhesion or rolling of platelets and leukocytes to the endothelial cells of arterial vessels is a very sensitive indicator of damage to vascular endothelium and is seen in the initial stages of the inflammatory process. This phenomenon was never seen to result from microsphere injections. This would indicate that there was no gross damage to the vasculature of the target organ as a result of injection of the microspheres.

4. Discussion

The results of the studies described above show that the intraarterial injection of

TABLE 3

Post-injection diameters measured after the microsphere had passed through a capillary and flow was restored to all vessels

Hamster No.	Vessel No.	Effect of microspheres on vessel diameter		% change in diameter
		Pre-injection diameter (μm)	Post-injection diameter (μm)	
60681	1	43	47	+ 8
	2	18	25	+ 39
	3	9	25	+177
	4	12	22	+ 83
	5	13	22	+ 69
	6	11	15	+ 36
	7	6	12	+ 20
61081	1	88	74	+ 7
	2	22	28	+ 27
	3	10	24	+140
61181	1	74	74	0
	2	21	27	+ 29
	3	20	25	+ 25
61681	1	26	37	+ 42
	2	32	33	+ 3
	3	8	9	+ 13
62281	1	50	52	+ 4
	2	14	12	− 14
	3	13	14	+ 8
	4	10	10	0
72181	1	43	43	0
	2	41	45	+ 10
	3	29	37	+ 28

degradable starch microspheres causes a transient reduction of blood flow that is reproducible and dose-dependent. Although it might be technically easier to produce an occlusion of an arterial vessel supplying a target organ by using a balloon tip catheter, this type of occlusion would not prevent collateral flow to the target organ. The occlusion of the small arterial vessels produced by the degradable microspheres would eliminate this possibility so long as the diameter of the microspheres is smaller than that of the collateral vessels. The advantages of using starch microspheres over other substances that have been injected into the cardiovascular system for the purpose of occlusion are that the microspheres are degraded by an enzyme endogenous to the body and that this degradation process can take place relatively rapidly. The rate at which degradation takes place could be altered by varying the degree of cross-linking between the starch molecules, by predigesting the microspheres in amylase to produce a more rapid degradation, or by altering the amylase levels in the body. The direct extrapolation of the animal data for human evaluation is complicated by the fact that there is a large variation in plasma amylase levels between species. The amylase concentration in hamster and rat plasma is over 20 times greater than that in human plasma. The amylase concentration in the dog is approximately 10 times higher than that in humans. This would mean that the behavior of the microspheres should be qualitatively similar although the absolute times may be quite different.

The results of the microcirculatory studies indicate that flow is reinstated to upstream branches as the microspheres are forced further along the arterial tree. Since the occlusion of blood flow by the microspheres would result in an accumulation of vasoactive metabolites a reactive hyperemia can be expected in vessels when they are initially reperfused. This probably indicates that even when flow has returned fully to control values microspheres may still be occluding a portion of the arterial tree.

The results of the studies measuring tissue drug concentrations indicate that the concentration of a drug can be increased selectively in a target organ when that drug is injected in combination with the microspheres. These findings are supported by the ethacrynic acid studies showing that the pharmacological effect of the drug was increased in the injected kidney and decreased in the contralateral kidney when the drug was injected in combination with the microspheres.

As mentioned previously, although the results of these investigations give promising evidence that the use of degradable starch microspheres may provide a means to increase selectively the drug concentration in a target organ, the full potential of the technique remains to be evaluated. The results of the microcirculatory study indicate that the drug is probably trapped downstream from the microspheres and that the upstream trapping of the drug may be relatively ineffective. This would seem to be a desirable result since the majority of the exchange process should take place at the level of the capillaries and postcapillary venules. The optimal size of the microspheres that should be used to accomplish this goal has not been evaluated experimentally, although 40-μm spheres appear to be in the effective range. The finding that most of the drug seems to be trapped downstream from the microspheres raises some question about the sequence of the injection of the drugs and microspheres. If downstream trapping is indeed the only way that the drug is effectively retained in the tissue for prolonged periods of time, it is possible that the drug should be injected immediately before the microspheres rather than being mixed with the spheres. This suggestion remains to be tested.

It is also interesting to speculate how other measures may be used to increase further the effectiveness of the technique. It is possible that the inclusion of a substance that would increase vascular permeability in the drug-microsphere mixture would further increase the amount of drug that could reach the targeted tissue. The intravenous injection of a second drug that could inactivate a cytostatic drug previously injected into an artery in combination with microspheres may also make it possible to have the drug available in an active form only in the diseased area, and therefore decrease further untoward side effects in other tissues.

Although this chapter has dealt with potential uses of degradable starch microspheres in chemotherapy there are other potential uses for this technique in cancer therapy. Forsberg and his coworkers (1978a, b) have provided evidence that the hypoxia resulting from the transient ischemia caused by microsphere occlusion may be effective in protecting healthy tissue from radiation damage, and therefore increase the therapeutic ratio in some applications of this technique. It is also possible that the microspheres may be useful in hyperthermic treatment of tumors since the ability to heat selected tissues is greatly dependent upon the blood flow of the tissue.

Acknowledgments

This work was supported by Grant Number CA253156 awarded by the National Cancer Institute, DHEW. The author would like to acknowledge the valuable assistance of Lynn Heinel in the preparation of this manuscript.

References

Arfors, K.-E., Forsberg, J.O., Larsson, B., Lewis, D.H., Rosengren, B. and Odman, S. (1976) Nature 262, 500–501.

Arfors, K.-E., Tuma, R.F. and Agerup, B. (1979) Bibl. Anat. 18, 205–207.

Aronsen, K.F., Hellekant, C., Holmberg, J., Rothman, U. and Tedeer, H. (1979) Eur. Surg. Res. 11, 99–106.

Dakhil, S., Emsinger, W., Cho, K., Niederbuber, J., Doan, K. and Wheeler, R. (1982) Cancer 50, 631–635.

Duling, B. (1973) Microvasc. Res. 5, 423–429.

Forsberg, J.O. and Jung, B. (1978a) Acta Radiol. 17/5, 353–361.

Forsberg, J.O., Jung, B. and Larsson, B. (1978b) Acta Radiol. 17/6, 485–496.

Lindberg, B. (1983) in Proceedings of the International Conference on Commercial Applications and Implications of Biotechnology, pp. 863–876, Online Publications Ltd., Northwood.

Lindell, B., Aronsen, K.F. and Rothman U. (1977a) Eur. Surg. Res. 347–356.

Lindell, B., Aronsen, K.F., Rothman, U. and Sjogren, H.O. (1977b) Res. Exp. Med. 171/1, 63–70.

Tuma, R.F., Forsberg, J.O. and Agerup, B. (1982) Cancer 50, 1–5.

Microspheres and Drug Therapy. Pharmaceutical, Immunological and Medical Aspects
edited by S.S. Davis, L. Illum, J.G. McVie and E. Tomlinson
© 1984, Elsevier Science Publishers B.V.

Adriamycin-loaded albumin microspheres: Lung entrapment and fate in the rat

N. Willmott, H.M.H. Kamel, J. Cummings, J.F.B. Stuart and A.T. Florence

1. Introduction

A fundamental problem in cancer chemotherapy is the supply of drug in lethal concentrations to cells in a solid tumour. Tumours are seldom recognised until they are several centimetres in diameter, and, to be effective, the antineoplastic drugs must overcome several barriers. If the tumour is in the brain the drug must traverse the blood/brain barrier and capillary walls, and cross tissue into the tumour itself and diffuse to the target cells. At the same time, the drug is being metabolised, or bound, or otherwise inactivated, even though it is required at critical concentrations in the individual cells, and must remain for a certain duration at or above a certain minimum level to achieve the maximum destructive effect on the tumour cell. A simplified model of a tumour would be a sphere, considered as a central core of low permeability with a more permeable and probably well-perfused outer shell. An outer layer may also exist in brain tumours due to compression of surrounding tissues by the tumour expanding in a confined space (Levin et al., 1981).

The inadequacy of much conventional anticancer drug delivery dawns with the realisation that so few drugs are active because they perhaps never reach the target site. It is important in designing delivery systems to have an indication as to how long concentration gradients have to be maintained to achieve adequate drug penetration of tumours. The calculations of Levin et al. (1981) show that a concentration level of adriamycin (ADX) falls by 50% only 2 mm from the surface of a spherical tumour after 24 hours in contact with drug solution. Also, although methotrexate (MTX) achieves greater penetration, the level of drug falls to 50% over 5 mm in the same time. Even perfusion of a drug intraarterially — itself a hazardous operation — cannot maintain sufficiently high levels of drug bathing a tumour without producing toxic levels throughout the body.

The advantage of formulating drugs so that they are physically trapped in the capillary bed of certain tumour-bearing organs and there slowly release drug is that high concentrations of drugs are maintained locally (ideally in close proximity to the tumour).

In this paper we examine the entrapment, fate and drug release characteristics of albumin microspheres containing adriamycin after intravenous administration of the spheres to the rat. Microspheres offer the possibility of target selectivity through choice of appropriate size or surface characteristics (Illum and Davis, 1982), and also of slow release of drug, which may prevent metabolism or dilution in tissue fluids as well as minimising systemic toxicity.

2. Materials and methods

2.1. Preparation of microspheres

The method used by us is based on that of Lee et al. (1981), modified so as to permit administration of microspheres to animals on the day of preparation. 200 mg bovine serum albumin (BSA) were dissolved in the minimum volume of buffer and, from the commercially available vials, 10 mg ADX were added in a known volume of water. The disperse phase was completed by adding a known amount of glutaraldehyde immediately prior to emulsification in a 60:40 mixture of cottonseed oil and petroleum ether (120–160°C). The resulting microspheres were washed three times in petroleum ether, twice in isopropanol, and twice in phosphate-buffered saline containing 0.5% Tween 80 (PBS-Tween). Following filtration through 76-μm wire mesh, the microspheres were ready for use. Routinely, samples were taken to obtain: (a) particle size (50% weight average) (using a Coulter Counter); (b) weight of microspheres (by filtration through a 0.22-μm Millipore filter); (c) amount of native ADX in the microspheres (following digestion in 0.25% trypsin solution).

Selected preparations were used for intravenous administration to rats at a dose of 3–5 mg.

2.2. Quantitation of ADX and metabolites

Serum samples containing ADX were extracted with chloroform/isopropanol (2:1) and the organic layer separated. After evaporation to dryness samples were reconstituted in methanol and analysed using a reversed-phase high-performance liquid chromatography (HPLC) system having a fluorescence detector (excitation wavelength, 480 nm; emission, 560 nm). Retention times and extraction efficiencies (50–100%) were computed by reference to an internal standard (daunorubicin). Peaks in each sample were assigned a molecular identity by comparison with relative retention times of standards. Figure 1 illustrates the separation achieved by this technique.

To obtain the total amount of native ADX in each preparation of microspheres, a known weight of microspheres was digested with trypsin, the sample extracted in chloroform/isopropanol (2:1) and the extract analysed either by HPLC as described above or by fluorimetry.

2.3. In vitro release of drug

ADX-containing microspheres were washed twice further to remove Tween 80. Microspheres in aliquots of 6 mg were then suspended in 10 ml phosphate buffer, incubated at 37°C with shaking, and at intervals aliquots were taken, centrifuged, and

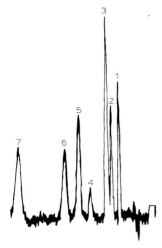

Figure 1. Separation by HPLC of ADX, five metabolites and daunorubicin used as internal standard. 1–7 are adriamycinol, adriamycin, adriamycinol aglycone, adriamycin aglycone, daunorubicin, adriamycinol 7-deoxyaglycone and adriamycin 7-deoxyaglycone, respectively.

the supernatants analysed for drug. Release of ADX is expressed as amount of drug in supernatant as a percentage of native drug in the aliquot of microspheres. This latter value was determined by HPLC or fluorimetry following trypsin digestion and solubilisation of microspheres.

2.4. Histology and microscopy

Transmission electron microscopy was performed as described elsewhere (Glauert, 1967). For scanning electron microscopy, microspheres were either critical point-dried or air-dried, their appearance being the same after both procedures.

For fluorescence and bright-field microscopy, formalin-fixed rat lungs were sliced into small tissue blocks, processed through alcohols and embedded in paraffin wax. 5-μm sections were cut and used unstained for fluorescence microscopy. Propyl gallate in glycerol was used to mount the section in order to prevent photobleaching (Giloh and Sedat, 1982). Under appropriate fluorescent illumination ADX in microspheres emitted light in the yellow-orange region (550–560 nm), which could readily be distinguished from background tissue fluorescence. The microspheres which appeared yellow-orange against a green background were enumerated by point counting.

3. Results

3.1. Characteristics of microspheres

By varying the stirring speed and the proportion of oil in continuous phase and using filters of known mesh size, glutaraldehyde cross-linked albumin microspheres were prepared in the size range 7–80 μm. The mean diameters of microspheres used in this work were in the range 11.8–15.3 μm, and appeared in light microscopy uniformly round, smooth and globular with very few aggregates. Using SEM, the surface of the spheres appeared textured, although there were some departures from sphericity (Fig. 2). The transmission electron microscope revealed microspheres to be solid structures, with few internal discontinuities (Fig. 3).

The stability of the microspheres was greatly influenced by the conditions used in their preparation. For example, if the concentration of glutaraldehyde was too low (under 0.3%) or the volume of disperse phase too high (over 3 ml) the microspheres were not stable enough to survive the washing procedure intact. Drug-loading of microspheres was also dependent to some extent on the reaction conditions. Thus, there was a tendency to achieve higher loadings of drug with lower disperse phase volumes. The maximum incorporation of ADX achieved was 10 μg ADX per mg microspheres, which represents an incorporation efficiency of 20%.

3.2. In vivo distribution of microspheres following systemic injection

To investigate loss of particles from the rat lung, microspheres were administered intravenously; at intervals, animals were killed, exsanguinated, and the organs processed for histology. These experiments used microspheres prepared with disperse-phase volumes of 2–3 ml and glutaraldehyde concentrations of 0.33–0.5%.

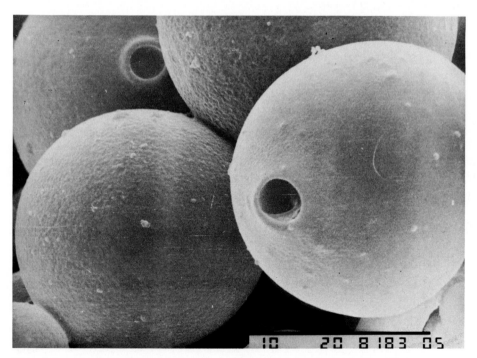

Figure 2. Scanning electron photomicrograph of ADX-containing microspheres. Bar, 10 μm.

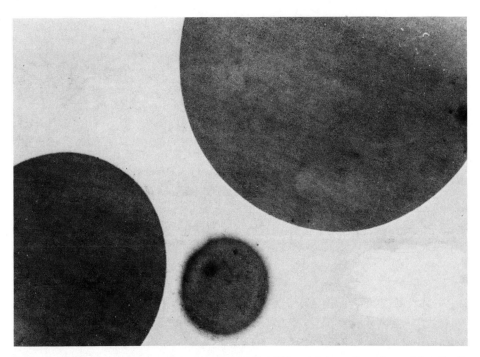

Figure 3. Transmission electron photomicrograph of ADX-containing microspheres. Magnification, × 10,175.

It can be seen from Figure 4 that microspheres were still present 24 hours after injection at approximately 50% of their initial value, but by 48 hours the density was considerably lower. By day 4 no particles were detected in lung sections. It is of considerable interest that degradation of microspheres was evident in the lung after 24

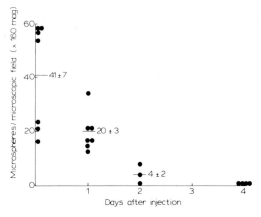

Figure 4. Loss of ADX-containing microspheres from the lung as a function of time. Values for each individual rat were the average of 20 fields from two lung sections. Each symbol represents one rat. Values shown are mean ± 1 S.E.

hours. Comparison of Figures 5a and b with Figures 6a and b illustrates the changes in morphology which occur during erosion.

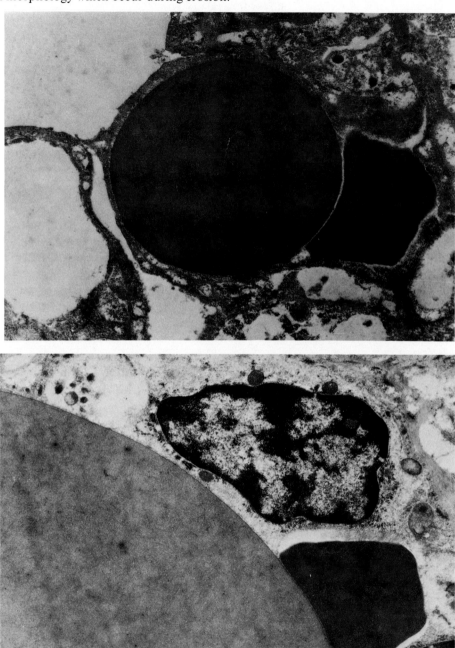

Figure 5a. Transmission electron photomicrograph of rat lung immediately after injection of microspheres. Formalin-fixed material. Magnification, × 12,935. b, As above; magnification, × 12,935.

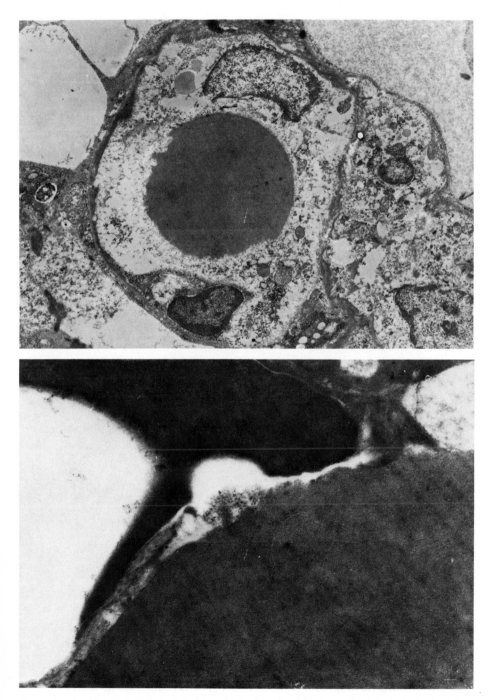

Figure 6a. Transmission electron photomicrograph of rat lung 24 hours after injection of microspheres. Formalin-fixed material. Magnification, × 7,415. b. As above. Magnification, × 31,050.

212

3.3. Serum levels of ADX after intravenous injection of microspheres

At intervals of 0 minutes, 6, 24 and 48 hours and 4 days following intravenous injection of microspheres, rats were killed, exsanguinated, and the serum of individual rats analysed for adriamycin using HPLC. In these experiments microspheres prepared using a low disperse-phase volume and glutaraldehyde concentrations of 0.5–1% were used. Results were similar with the different preparations studied.

From Figure 7 it can be seen that when incorporated into microspheres serum ADX levels were highest immediately after injection, whereupon they declined to a low but consistent level for at least 24 hours. This is in contrast to serum ADX levels following bolus injection of an equivalent amount (70 μg) of free ADX. Thus, despite initial levels some 6-fold higher than after microsphere injection, after 6 hours ADX was no longer detectable in serum. Metabolites of ADX were detected only at the zero time point. After bolus and microsphere administration only 7-deoxyadriamycinol aglycone and ADX, were detected.

It can be seen from Figure 8 that release of ADX is virtually complete after 3 hours, although the amount released was only 30–40% of the drug loading in the microspheres. Examination of trypsinates of microspheres by HPLC, coupled with a fluorescence detector, revealed only the ADX peak (Fig. 9).

4. Discussion

Limited penetration of solid tumour tissue by most cytotoxic anti-cancer drugs,

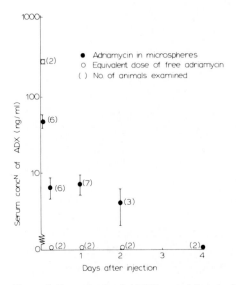

Figure 7. Serum levels of ADX in rats injected with drug-containing microspheres. Dose of native ADX was approx. 70 μg in each case. Error bars represent mean $\pm$ 1 S.E., or higher and lower value. Limit of detection, 2.5 ng/ml.

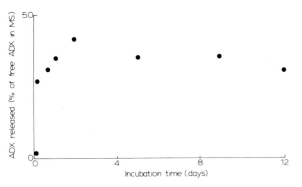

Figure 8. In vitro release of ADX from microspheres. Release expressed as % of native ADX in microspheres, as determined after trypsin digestion. Each point was mean of two determinations. Microspheres prepared using low disperse-phase volume and 1% glutaraldehyde.

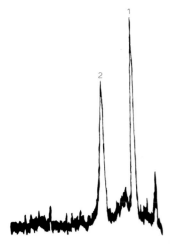

Figure 9. HPLC analysis of trypsin digest of microspheres. 1 and 2 are adriamycin and daunorubicin, respectively.

including ADX, has been repeatedly demonstrated (Durand, 1981; West et al., 1980; Nederman et al., 1981). Moreover, this phenomenon has been proposed as a reason for the meagre and usually transient effect of such drugs on solid tumours observed clinically (Levin et al. 1981). It can be shown on theoretical grounds that maintenance of drug levels in the vicinity of the tumour over a prolonged period of time can lead to increased penetration of solid tumour tissue (Levin et al., 1981). Therefore, it can be predicted that measures to deliver drug to the vicinity of the tumour and to release drug slowly at the site would produce an increased anti-tumour effect compared with both bolus injection and slow infusion (Cowsar, 1974).

In the present studies we have attempted to prepare a biodegradable, biocompatible drug carrier that by virtue of particle size will become entrapped in capillary beds. To investigate whether these aims were achieved (a) localisation of microspheres in the lung was examined following intravenous administration and (b) drug-release characteristics were examined both in vivo and in vitro.

Quantitation of microspheres in lung tissue was determined by point counting the number of microspheres in sections of lung tissue under fluorescent illumination. Point counting techniques are somewhat inaccurate, as reflected by the wide scatter of results; however, as currently practised the method is capable of detecting large differences in sphere deposition. It is apparent from Figure 4 that microspheres reside in the lung for at least 24 hours after injection, at which point they are clearly in the process of erosion (Figs. 6a and b). By 4 days they are no longer detectable. Preliminary observations of ours indicate that residence time in tissue can be increased by increasing the cross-linking of the microspheres, as expected from the results of others (Lee et al., 1981). Examination of sections from liver, spleen and kidney revealed very few microspheres.

The HPLC technique used is capable of resolving total fluorescence into that due to ADX and its metabolites, some of which, for example the aglycones, are inactive pharmacologically and biochemically (Bachur, 1975). In addition, its limit of detection was as low as 2.5 ng/ml. It is clear from Figure 7 that the pharmacokinetics of free and microsphere-entrapped ADX were very different. Thus, in the free form the drug was non-detectable after 6 hours. This is in accord with our own more detailed studies of the pharmacokinetics of ADX in rats and with other observations in experimental animals and humans (Reich, 1978; Wilkinson et al., 1979) that confirm a short serum half-life. ADX was detectable in serum for at least 24 hours following intravenous administration in microspheres. The system exhibited a 'burst effect' in vivo, a common characteristic of 'sustained' release systems (Baker and Lonsdale, 1974; Lee et al., 1981).

It is clear that the microspheres studied entrap in capillary beds and release drug at low concentrations, over a period of at least 24 hours. At first sight, the latter observation appeared to be at variance with in vitro release rates (Fig. 8) which showed that release was virtually complete after 3 hours. However, it is apparant from Figure 8 that by no means all of the drug was released in the in vitro assay. Moreover, protein assays revealed that microspheres remained over 90% intact over the period investigated (unpublished observations). These data, together with the observation that microspheres undergo degradation, are consistent with an in vivo release due to two mechanisms, namely, early release by diffusion and later sustained release by degradation of the protein matrix.

Further work is clearly necessary to increase the loading of microspheres with ADX before any testing in animal tumour systems. However, some speculation as to the future use of microspheres in cancer chemotherapy is possible. Thus, three modes of administration can be considered, i.e., local, intraarterial and intravenous. Local administration would involve direct injection of microspheres into tumour lesions, thus obviating the problems of tissue localisation, and rely solely on the sustained release characteristics. This technique appears to exclude internal tumour lesions, except, for example, those visible with the aid of a bronchoscope. Intraarterial injection should transport microspheres directly to the target organ (see Tomlinson et al., section 2, Ch.1). However, the presence of arterial collaterals, for example in the liver (Michels, 1953), may diminish the effect. On the positive side, tumour vessels generally lack the contractile elements of normal vessels. Therefore, it may be possible to use a vasoconstrictor to reduce blood flow to vessels supplying non-tumour tissue. Lung and liver are perfused by a dual blood supply; therefore, intravenous injection via the caval or portal circulation is possible here. A caveat regarding this mode of administration is that it will probably be effective only against micro metastases, because as secondary tumours of lung and liver enlarge they acquire a predominantly arterial blood supply (Ogilvie et al., 1964; Ackerman et al., 1969).

Acknowledgements

The authors acknowledge with gratitude the skilled technical assistance of Mrs. Agnes Hughes. They are grateful to Dr. Jeremy Thomas for providing tissue sections for analysis, Dr. Kate Carr for use of the scanning electron microscope (purchased with funds from the Scottish Home and Health Department), Professor Peter Toner for use of the transmission electron microscope, Professor K.C. Calman for use of the animal facility of the Department of Clinical Oncology, University of Glasgow, and the Medical Research Council of Great Britain who defrayed the costs of this research. Thanks are due to Mrs. E. Carruthers for typing the manuscript.

References

Ackerman, N.B., Lien, W.M., Kondi, E.S. and Silverman, N.A. (1969) Surgery 66, 1067.

Bachur, N.R. (1975) Cancer Chemother. Rep. 6, 153–160.

Baker, R.W. and Lonsdale, H.K. (1974) in Controlled Release of Biologically Active Agents (Tanquery, A.C. and Lacy, R.E., Eds.), pp. 15–71, Plenum Press, New York.

Cowsar, D.R. (1974) in Controlled Release of Biologically Active Agents (Tanquary, A.C. and Lacy, R.E., Eds.), pp. 1–13, Plenum Press, New York.

Durand, R.E. (1981) Cancer Res. 41, 3495–3499.

Giloh, H. and Sedat, J.W. (1982) Science 217, 1252–1254

Glauert, A.M. (1967) in Techniques for Electron Microscopy (Kay, D., Ed.), pp. 166–213, Blackwell, Oxford.

Illum, L. and Davis, S.S. (1982) J. Parenteral Sci. Tech. 36, 242–248.

Lee, T.K., Sokoloski, T.D. and Royer, G.P. (1981) Science 213, 233–235.

Levin, V.A., Patlak, C.S., and Lindahl, H.D. (1981) J. Pharmacokinet. Biopharm. 8, 257–296.

Michels, N.A. (1953) Cancer 6, 708–715.

Nederman, T., Carlsson, J. and Malmquist, M. (1981) In Vitro 17, 290–298.

Ogilvie, R.W., Blanding, J.D., Wood, M.L. and Knisley, W.H. (1964) Cancer Res. 24, 1418–1425.

Reich, D. (1978) Pharmacol. Ther. 2, 239–243.

West, G.W., Weichselbaum, R. and Little, J.B. (1980) Cancer Res. 40, 3665–3668.

Wilkinson, P.M., Israel, M., Pegg, W.J. and Frei, E. (1979) Cancer Chemother. Pharmacol. 2, 21–26.

Microspheres and Drug Therapy. Pharmaceutical, Immunological and Medical Aspects
edited by S.S. Davis, L. Illum, J.G. McVie and E. Tomlinson
© *1984, Elsevier Science Publishers B.V.*

217

CHAPTER 4

In vitro and in vivo evaluation of CCNU-loaded microspheres prepared from poly((±)-lactide) and poly(β-hydroxybutyrate)

Marie-Christine Bissery, Fred Valeriote and Curt Thies

1. Introduction

One approach to decreasing the host toxicity of anticancer agents such as 1-(2 chloro-ethyl)-3-cyclohexyl-nitrosourea (CCNU), while maintaining or even increasing the cytotoxic effect on the tumor cells, is to target the drug to the specific location of the tumor. A way to reach this goal is to use drug-loaded, biodegradable, injectable microspheres which are targeted to specific organs on the basis of their size. Much work has centered on the preparation and characterization of such microspheres and this work has recently been reviewed (Heller, 1980; Thies and Bissery, 1984). A few investigators have tested these particles in vivo (Sugibayashi et al., 1979; Couvreur et al., 1979; Sjöholm and Edman, 1979).

In the present study, two types of microspheres have been evaluated, i.e., poly-((±)-lactide) (PLA)-CCNU microspheres and poly(β-hydroxybutyrate) (PHB)-CCNU microspheres. The microspheres were designed to fall within the 1–15 μm size range. Their in vitro drug release characteristics, host toxicity and distribution in the mouse have been examined.

2. Materials and methods

2.1 Preparation of microspheres

Poly(β-hydroxybutyrate) (PHB) and ^{14}C-labelled PHB were generously supplied by I.C.I., Agricultural Products Division, Billingham, U.K. Poly((±)-lactide) (PLA) was supplied by Dr. Norbert Mason, Washington University, St. Louis, MO. 1-(2 Chloroethyl)-3-cyclohexylnitrosourea (CCNU) was obtained from the National Cancer Institute, Bethesda, MD. Poly(vinyl alcohol) (PVA) (Vinol 205®), 88% hydrolysed, was supplied by Air Products Corporation, Allentown, PA. Methocel, grade A-15LV, was obtained from Dow Chemical, Midland, MI. Reagent grade methylene chloride and chloroform were purchased from Fisher Scientific, Pittsburgh, PA.

The microspheres were prepared by a solvent evaporation process carried out at atmospheric pressure. Polymer (1.2 mg) was dissolved in 50 ml of $CHCl_3$ (PHB) or CH_2Cl_2 (PLA). CCNU (0.3 g) was added to the organic phase, which was subsequently emulsified with 375 ml of 0.25% PVA solution in a Waring blender. The resulting suspension was stirred in a 1000-ml beaker with 125 ml of a 1% Methocel solution until the solvent was completely evaporated. The microspheres obtained were centrifuged, washed, filtered through a 20-μm filter and lyophilized. The lyophilized samples were kept at $-20°C$ until used in order to minimize CCNU degradation during storage.

2.2. Microsphere characterization

2.2.1. Surface topography
Microsphere size range was estimated by optical microscopy (Leitz Laborlux 12 microscope). The surface of the microspheres was examined with a scanning electron microscope (Hitachi Model HHS-2R, SEM, Tokyo, Japan).

2.2.2. CCNU content
The amount of CCNU in the microspheres used was assayed by HPLC. The microspheres were dissolved in 4 ml of $CHCl_3$ (PHB-CCNU microspheres) or 2 ml of Dioxane (PLA-CCNU microspheres). Ethanol was added, thereby precipitating the polymer and leaving a polymer-free CCNU solution. The CCNU content of the clear solution was determined by injecting 10-μl samples into a Varian Model 5000 HPLC unit (Varian Corp., Walnut Creek, CA) equipped with a variable wavelength UV Detector set at 254 nm. HPLC operating conditions were: column, MCH-10 reserve phase; solvent, 50:50 water/acetonitrile; solvent flow rate, 1.0 ml/min; temperature, 31°C. Under these conditions, CCNU eluted at 10.4 minutes. Freshly made standards containing known amounts of CCNU were run each day. All samples were kept in the dark and on ice before analysis.

2.2.3. Release characteristics
In vitro release of CCNU from microspheres was determined at 37°C in Tris buffer (pH 7.2). Drug-loaded microspheres (20 mg) were placed in the appropriate medium (17 ml) and rotated in a rotating bottle apparatus (Ernest Menhold, Lester, PA) at 40 rpm. Agitation was then stopped and the microspheres were isolated by centrifugation at $1000 \times g$ for 10 minutes. The amount of CCNU left in the microspheres was determined by the HPLC procedure described in section 2.2.2.

2.3. In vivo evaluation
All in vivo experiments were conducted in 8–12-week-old AKR mice or 8–12-week-old BD_2F_1 mice. The mice were kept 20 per cage and allowed free access to food and water.

2.3.1. Dose preparation
Known amounts of microspheres were weighed and suspended in 5% dextrose in water (D5W). The suspension was vortexed for 2 minutes and filtered through a

15-μm filter. In some cases, Tween 80 (to a final concentration of 5%) was added and the sample sonicated. The suspension was then immediately injected using a 1-ml plastic syringe. All volumes injected, unless otherwise mentioned, were 0.5 ml.

Standard CCNU solutions for injection were prepared by dissolving the drug in a mixture of ethanol, polyethoxylated oil (POE$_{40}$) and D5W in a 1:1:8 ratio.

Except for the toxicity studies, the weight of polymer-CCNU microspheres injected was calculated so as to deliver 0.3 mg of CCNU per mouse.

2.3.2. Toxicity studies

In order to determine the toxic response of the mice to various microsphere preparations, increasing weights of particles were injected through the tail vein in groups of 5–15 mice. PHB and PLA microspheres (5, 10, 15, 20 and 30 mg), PHB-CCNU microspheres (5, 7.5, 10, 15 and 20 mg) and PLA-CCNU microspheres (5, 10, 15 and 20 mg) were tested. The toxicity of CCNU injected intravenously was also checked at various doses, ranging from 0.2 to 1.2 mg. Mortality observations were made daily and continued for 60 days after treatment.

2.3.3. Distribution of microspheres

An aqueous suspension (0.5 ml) of ^{14}C-labelled PHB microspheres (5 mg per ml, 0.1 mCi per gram of polymer) was injected into mice intravenously. At 0.5, 1 and 24 hours and 7 days thereafter, one mouse was killed and the organs assayed for radioactivity. Organs or tumors were weighed, and minced in a glass counting vial fitted with a polyethylene-lined cap. The tissues were solubilized in a water bath at 55°C by Protosol® at 1 ml per 100 mg of tissue, except for the liver, which was at 1 ml per 150 mg of tissue. After 16 hours, 10 ml of Econofluor® were added to a known amount of the previously solubilized sample. The samples were counted in a scintillation counter for 10 minutes (Searle Analytic — Liquid Scintillation System, Model 81). Protosol and Econofluor were purchased from New England Nuclear, Boston, MA.

2.3.4. Verification of the biological activity of encapsulated CCNU

The biological activity of encapsulated CCNU was checked by extracting CCNU from PLA-CCNU microspheres and testing it against a murine leukemia. Standard unencapsulated CCNU solutions of 0.2 and 0.3 mg were also evaluated. CCNU was dissolved as described in section 2.3.1.

For extraction of CCNU from CCNU-PLA microspheres, a known amount of spheres (100.15 mg) was added to 1.25 ml of ethanol and kept for 10 minutes in an ice water bath. The sample was sonicated for 2 minutes, centrifuged, and the supernatant removed. It was assayed by the HPLC procedure described above (section 2.2.3). POE$_{40}$ and D5W were added (in the same ratio as described above) in order to achieve the necessary volume.

2.3.5. AKR leukemia passage and assay

The AKR leukemia used is a transplantable lymphocytic leukemia kept viable in our laboratory by weekly passage. The spleen colony assay procedure has been described previously by Valeriote et al. (1973). Mice received 5×10^5 leukemia cells by tail vein injection on day 0, and 4 days later the CCNU sample (0.5 ml) was administered via the tail vein. 24 hours later, the mice were killed and a monodisperse cell suspension was prepared from their femoral marrow. A fraction of this suspension was injected into recipient AKR mice. 8 days later, these recipient mice were killed and their spleens removed and placed in Bouin's fixative. The macroscopic colonies on the spleen were counted and the fractional survival calculated by comparison to an untreated control. The untreated control at 4 days had approximately 10^5 leukemic colony forming units (LCFU) per femoral marrow.

2.3.6. Increase in lifespan (ILS) assay

Mice received 5×10^5 AKR leukemia cells by tail vein injection. 4 days later, groups of 10 mice received either PHB, PLA, PHB-CCNU, PLA-CCNU microspheres or an unencapsulated CCNU solution (0.15 and 0.3 mg). Survival was checked daily for 60 days after treatment.

2.3.7. Histological evaluation

Lungs and liver were removed 2 or 24 hours, and 14 days after intravenous injection of PLA or PHB microspheres. Tissues were processed through formaldehyde fixative and paraffin embedding. Sections of 5 μm thickness were prepared and stained with hematoxylin and eosin.

3. Results

3.1. Microsphere characterization

All the PLA and PHB microsphere samples used in this study contained a range of different particles. Figure 1 illustrates the variation in particle size and shape found for one PHB sample. Most particles have considerable sphericity. Deviations from sphericity are most noticeable with PHB microspheres. Neither PLA nor PHB microspheres have macroscopic surface pores that scanning electron microscopy (10,000 magnification) can detect. PHB microspheres often have a shrivelled appearance.

If the PLA or PHB particles in the various microsphere samples were fully dispersed, all such particles would be less than 15 μm in diameter. However, all microsphere samples contain a mixture of single polymer particles and small aggregates of polymer particles. The aggregates consist of a number of small particles irreversibly fused together. Thus, the microsphere samples used for this study were complex mixtures of various individual particles and assorted aggregates.

Table 1 lists the various microspheres used, their drug loading and their size range. The size range given was determined by optically sizing about 50 particles. Microspheres that contained CCNU carried drug loadings of less than 10 wt.%. Attempts to prepare small microspheres with higher CCNU payloads consistently led to formation of free CCNU crystals in the aqueous phase.

3.2. Release characteristics

Figure 2 shows the change in CCNU content of two microsphere samples as a function of incubation time in 37°C Tris buffer. CCNU disappears rapidly from PHB-

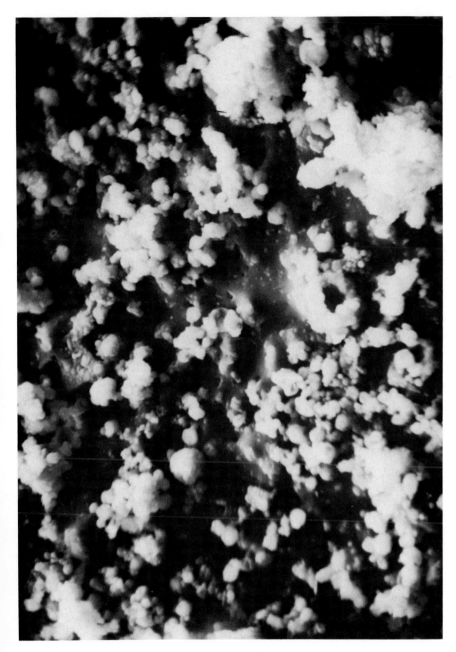

Figure 1. Scanning electron micrograph of CCNU-loaded PHB microspheres. × 500.

CCNU microspheres under these conditions. CCNU disappears much more slowly from PLA-CCNU microspheres. In the latter case, there is a rapid initial loss of CCNU, after which the CCNU content decreases slowly in a nearly linear manner.

The data in Figure 2 were determined by measuring the amount of CCNU left in

TABLE 1

Characteristics of microspheres

Type of microsphere	Size range (μm)	CCNU content (wt.%)	Type of experiment[a]
PLA	1– 4	0	2, 5, 6
PHB	1– 5	0	2
	1– 5	0	5, 6
	1–12	0	6
[14]C-labelled PHB	1–12	0	3
PLA-CCNU	1– 5	7.4	2
	1–10	7.2	1, 5
	3–18	5.9	6
PHB-CCNU	1– 7	5.6	1, 2, 5
	1–11	2.5	6

[a] Experiments were: 1, release; 2, toxicity; 3, time distribution; 4, bioassay; 5, survival; 6, histology.

the microspheres after various incubation times, because CCNU is unstable in aqueous media (Colvin, 1982). HPLC analyses established that non-degraded CCNU is released by the microspheres into the aqueous phase, but analyses of the aqueous phase for CCNU are complicated by its instability.

3.3. Toxicity of the microspheres

Mice tolerated intravenous injections of up to 20 mg of drug-free PLA or PHB microspheres. No deaths were recorded at this dose level over a period of 60 days. Injection of 30 mg of microspheres caused 100% mortality. At this dose, most mice died within minutes after injection, due to severe respiratory problems. PLA-CCNU microspheres containing 7.5 wt.% CCNU gave an LD_{50} of 14.5 mg. This corresponds to a CCNU dose of 1.1 mg. PHB-CCNU microspheres containing 5.4 wt.% CCNU gave an LD_{50} of 8.5 mg. This corresponds to a CCNU dose of 0.48 mg. The LD_{50} of unencapsulated CCNU injected intravenously in the same strain of mice was found to be 0.66 mg.

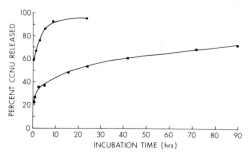

Figure 2. Release profile of CCNU-loaded microspheres in Tris buffer, pH 7.2, at 37°C. ●, PHB-CCNU (7.4%) microspheres; ■, PLA-CCNU (5.6%) microspheres.

3.4. Tissue distribution of microspheres

The distribution of ^{14}C-labelled PHB microspheres was followed in AKR mice for 7 days following injection. Table 2 shows the distribution of ^{14}C radioactivity in various organs, including heart, brain, lung, liver, spleen and kidney. The values are expressed as percentage of administered dose as well as in counts per minute (cpm) per gram of tissue. 30 minutes after injection, 47% of the radioactivity was found in the lungs, 14% in the liver and 2.1% in the spleen. All other organs and tissues contained less than 1% of the injected dose.

1 hour later, the radioactivity in the lungs and liver increased to 62 and 16%, respectively, while it remained almost stable in the spleen. By 24 hours, 60% of the radioactivity was found in the lungs, 24% in the liver, 1.6% in the spleen, and 0.1% in the kidneys. Finally, at 7 days the radioactivity was similar in amount and distribution to that noted at 24 hours, except for the lungs, where the amount decreased from 60 to 44%.

3.5. Biological activity of the encapsulated CCNU

Unencapsulated CCNU and CCNU extracted from PLA-CCNU microspheres were tested against AKR leukemia. The response was measured by the clonogenic assay for LCFU. Doses of 0.2 and 0.3 mg unencapsulated CCNU and 0.21 mg extracted CCNU were administered. The results are shown in Figure 3, in which the effect of

TABLE 2

Distribution of ^{14}C-labelled PHB microspheres after intravenous injection

Sample	30 minutes		1 hour		24 hours		7 days	
	% dose	cpm per g of tissue ($\times 10^4$)	% dose	cpm per g of tissue ($\times 10^4$)	% dose	cpm per g of tissue ($\times 10^4$)	% dose	cpm per g of tissue ($\times 10^4$)
Blood	—	0.04	—	—	—	0.01	—	0.03
Heart	—	0.91	—	0.85	—	0.83	—	0.30
Lungs	46.5	136	61.9	125	59.6	133	43.6	86.0
Liver	14.2	4.62	16.1	4.79	24.3	8.25	24.9	6.03
Spleen	2.19	13.5	2.37	12.8	1.57	8.58	2.55	9.46
Kidneys	0.83	1.06	1.02	1.05	0.12	0.18	0.12	0.17
Femoral marrow from left femur	—	1.22	—	1.95	—	3.48	—	4.11
Brain	0.06	0.07	0.09	0.09	0.06	0.06	0.04	0.04
Muscle around left femur	—	—	—	0.16	—	0.15	—	0.07
Gut wall, 2 cm	—	1.19	—	—	—	0.10	—	0.06

One mouse per time period was injected with a sample of ^{14}C-labelled PHB microspheres containing 47×10^4 cpm.

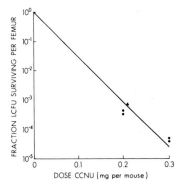

Figure 3. Survival fraction of leukemic colony-forming unit following treatment with CCNU: ●, CCNU that had never been incorporated in microspheres; ▲, CCNU extracted from microspheres.

CCNU is represented by a circle and the effect of extracted CCNU is represented by a triangle. The results for CCNU extracted from the microspheres coincided well with those found for unencapsulated CCNU. This indicates that both CCNU samples have similar activity against leukemia cells.

3.6. Survival experiment

In order to assess the systemic activity of encapsulated CCNU, CCNU-loaded microspheres were injected into tumor-bearing mice and survival times were determined. The results were compared to free CCNU. Table 3 lists the different treatments examined, as well as mean survival times and ILS. These data indicate that PHB-CCNU and PLA-CCNU microspheres containing a total of 0.3 mg of CCNU cause, respectively, an increase in lifespan of 43 and 30%. This is significantly less than the

TABLE 3

Effect of various types of microspheres administered on day 4 on the survival of AKR leukemia-bearing mice

Sample	Dose (mg)		Survival time (days, ± S.D.)	ILS (%)
	Microspheres	CCNU[a]		
Control	—	—	6.0±0	0
PHB	5.3	0	6.1±0.3	2
PLA	3.9	0	6.0±0	0
CCNU	—	0.15	11 ±3.8	85
	—	0.30	18 ±4.5	198
PHB-CCNU	5.6	0.30	8.6±1.8	43
PLA-CCNU	4.3	0.30	7.8±0.9	30

[a] Amount of CCNU delivered to the mouse (mg).

85 and 198% increases caused, respectively, by 0.15 and 0.3 mg of free CCNU. Drug-free PHB and PLA microspheres had no effect on life span.

3.7. Histological data

As the tissue distribution studies revealed that most of the spheres were concentrated in the lungs and the liver, only these two organs were studied. In normal mice, none of the polymers studied gave any sign of inflammatory reaction. The lungs presented some congested areas and occasional vascular engorgement. The microspheres, within the 1–5 μm range, were observed more easily in the lungs and appeared as well-defined spherical transparent particles phagocytized by the lung cells. No cell damage was observed.

It was more difficult to locate microspheres in the liver. However, they were found in the tissues surrounding the capillaries.

4. Discussion

The size of drug-loaded microspheres is an important factor affecting their fate when administered. Microspheres smaller than about 7–8 μm diameter injected intravenously pass through the lung and concentrate in the reticulo-endothelial system (RES) (Kanke et al., 1980). Microspheres above 7–8 μm injected intravenously become entrapped in the lung. Accordingly, by exerting precise control over the size of drug-loaded microspheres, one can target such particles to either the lungs or the RES. Monodisperse spheres with perfect spherical geometry are preferred.

The PLA and PHB microspheres used in this study do not meet the above requirements. For example, all PLA and PHB samples examined by scanning electron microscopy contained a variety of particle sizes and shapes. One source of the size variation is the normal variation in oil-phase drop size that occurs when an oil phase is mechanically emulsified into an aqueous phase. A second, more troublesome, source of particle size variation is the slight particle-particle aggregation that occurred during the solvent evaporation and particle isolation steps. Such aggregation caused permanent particle-particle fusion and formation of relatively large, irregularly shaped clusters of particles. It is believed that these aggregates were a primary factor causing mouse mortality to increase from 0% at a 20 mg dose of drug-free microspheres to 100% at a dose of 30 mg. At present, steps are being taken to reduce the extent of aggregation that occurs during the particle formation process and to eliminate more effectively from the final formulation any aggregates that do form.

Figure 1 shows that PHB microspheres are often somewhat irregular in shape, even if they are discrete, unaggregated particles. This characteristic feature of PHB is attributed to its high crystallinity. PLA, an amorphous polymer, consistently forms spherical microspheres. The small PLA and PHB microspheres used in this study did not contain macroscopic pores visible by scanning electron microscopy at 10,000 magnification. Nevertheless, there was a significant difference in the rate at which the two types of microspheres release their drug. Figure 2 indicates that CCNU is extracted in vitro much more quickly from PHB microspheres than from PLA microspheres. The difference in CCNU-release rate from microspheres of similar size caused by changing the material of fabrication is an asset, since it offers a means of examining how altering the CCNU-release profile affects microsphere performance in vivo. Another means of altering release rate is to vary drug payload carried by the microspheres. All small CCNU-containing microspheres evaluated thus far have contained less than 10% drug. Attempts to prepare microspheres with higher CCNU loading have consistently resulted in formation of free CCNU crystals.

The rapid release of CCNU from PHB microspheres undoubtedly contributed to the finding that the LD_{50} of such microspheres is approximately half that of PLA-CCNU microspheres. Interestingly, the LD_{50} of CCNU caused by PHB microspheres is somewhat less than that of unencapsulated CCNU. Whether the difference is significant remains to be determined. The toxicity of CCNU-loaded PLA and PHB microspheres is well below the toxic dose of such microspheres free of drug. This indicates that the toxicity is due to the CCNU carried by the microspheres and not to the microspheres alone.

The fate of PHB microspheres has been examined by injecting radioactively labelled PHB microspheres into mice. 7 days post-injection, most of the radioactivity from such microspheres was located in the lungs, liver and spleen. The amount of radioactivity in these organs was quite constant over the 7-day period. The slight decrease observed in the lungs may reflect biodegradation of the PHB and recirculation of the smallest microspheres. The increase in radioactivity in the lungs and liver observed in the first 24 hours is attributed to clearance of microspheres from the blood, as reported by Kanke et al. (1980).

The survival studies showed that PHB-CCNU and PLA-CCNU microspheres had little effect on ILS of leukemia-bearing animals relative to that observed for equivalent amounts of free CCNU alone. This is not unexpected, since the leukemia cells in the lungs and liver are not what determines animal survival for this systemic leukemia. Our present studies are directed towards quantitating the survival of the leukemia cells in individual organs, to determine whether targeting leads to differential cell killing.

Acknowledgements

The authors would like to thank J. Benett for making the microspheres and B. Sunier for the scanning electron microscopy. This work was supported in part by grants from the Fondation pour la Recherche Medicale, Paris, France, PHS grant CA-34144 from the National Cancer Institute, DHHS, and the Wayne State University Ben Kasle Trust for Cancer Research.

References

Colvin, M. (1982) in Pharmacologic Principles of Cancer Treatment (Chabner, G., Ed.), pp. 276–308, W.B. Saunders Co., Philadelphia.

Couvreur, P., Kante, B., Lenaerts, V., Scailteur, V., Roland, M. and Speiser, P. (1979) J. Pharm. Sci. 69, 199–202.

Heller, J. (1980) Biomaterials, 1, 51–57.

Kanke, M., Simmons, G., Weiss, D., Bivins, B. and De Luca, P.P. (1980) J. Pharm. Sci. 69, 755–762.

Sjöholm, J. and Edman, P. (1979) Rat. J. Pharmacol. Exp. Therm., 211, 656–662.

Sugibayashi, K., Akimoto, M., Morimoto, Y., Nadai, T. and Kato, Y. (1979) Chem. Pharm. Bull. 27, 204–209.

Thies, C. and Bissery, M.C. (1984) in Biomedical Applications of Microencapsulation (Lim, F., Ed.), CRC Press, Boca Raton, pp. 53–74.

Valeriote, F., Vietti, T. and Tolen, S. (1973) Cancer Res. 33, 2658–2661.

Microspheres and Drug Therapy. Pharmaceutical, Immunological and Medical Aspects
edited by S.S. Davis, L. Illum, J.G. McVie and E. Tomlinson
© *1984, Elsevier Science Publishers B.V.*

229

CHAPTER 5

Microencapsulation of anticancer drug for intraarterial infusion, and its clinical application

Ryosuke Nemoto and Tetsuro Kato

1. Introduction

An effective chemotherapeutic regimen for treatment of cancer could be facilitated by exposing the cancerous lesions to high concentrations of anticancer drugs for periods long enough to kill all of the cancer cells. Although anticancer drugs come from many different classes of chemicals and act by different mechanisms, the majority are specifically toxic to actively proliferating cells, regardless of whether they are malignant or normal, and are rapidly cleared from the circulation.

If an anticancer drug were associated with an appropriate carrier material, the drug-carrier complex would accumulate or be retained at its desired site of action and release the drug in active form at a suitable rate. This pharmaceutical route seems simple, practical and attractive, and it is expected to play a crucial role in cancer chemotherapy.

Although the carrier systems of anticancer drugs have been widely discussed, the majority of them remain of limited pharmaceutical and experimental interest. The systems which have been applied to a considerable number of cancer patients are limited to emulsions (Takahashi et al., 1976) and ethylcellulose microcapsules (Kato and Nemoto, 1978). Both were originally developed by surgeons, with encouraging results. In this chapter, we present the experimental and clinical use of microencapsulated drugs for intraarterial infusion chemotherapy.

2. Ethylcellulose microencapsulation

Ethylcellulose microcapsules were prepared, based on the principles of coacervation (Speiser, 1976) with certain modifications. Mitomycin C (MMC) was chosen as a prototype drug for several reasons. MMC has been widely used as an antibiotic agent in cancer chemotherapy in Japan for more than 20 years. MMC exhibits good stability against heat and chemicals, and is inexpensive.

2 grams of MMC crystalline powder with a mean particle diameter of approximately 1 μm (Kyowa Hakko Kogyo Co. Ltd., Tokyo) were dispersed in a solution

containing 0.5 g ethylcellulose, 0.5 g polyethylene and 50 ml cyclohexane at 80°C, and the mixture was gradually cooled to room temperature with gentle stirring. In this process, aggregated MMC particles were encapsulated with a thin layer of ethyl-cellulose. MMC microcapsules prepared in this way were rinsed several times with n-hexane containing 1% hydrogenated castor oil and air-dried at 45°C for 6 hours so that the phase-separated polyethylene, cyclohexane and n-hexane were completely removed. The microcapsules were collected through a 45-mesh screen and sterilized at 140°C for 2 hours. MMC microcapsules thus prepared were expected to consist, on average, of 80% (w/w) MMC as the core and 20% (w/w) ethylcellulose as the shell (Kato and Nemoto, 1978).

3. In vitro properties of MMC microcapsules

Scanning electron microscopic observation showed that MMC microcapsules are irregular particles with rough, invaginated surfaces (Fig. 1). This indicates that ethyl-cellulose forms a thin coating over the aggregated MMC particles, which are needle-like crystals, during the process of microencapsulation. The mean particle size was 224.6 ± 54.9 μm (mean $\pm$ S.D., $n = 100$). The microcapsules suspended in saline or 5% glucose solution can be readily infused through an 18-gauge needle as well as

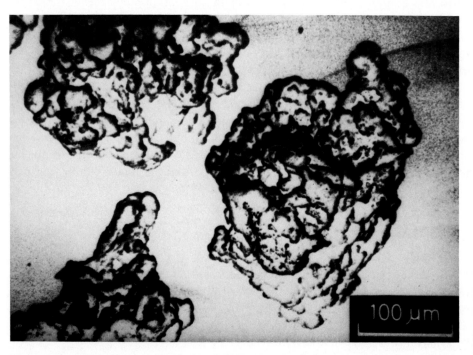

Figure 1. Scanning electron microscopic view of MMC microcapsules forming an irregular particle, with rough surface. Fron Kato et al. (1980), with permission.

through a fine catheter commonly used for selective arterial catheterization (Kato and Nemoto, 1978; Kato et al., 1980).

Duplicated bioassay for MMC microcapsules revealed that 50 mg of MMC microcapsules contained 40.5 mg (81%, w/w) and 42.0 mg (84%, w/w) of biologically active MMC, respectively. This result was in good agreement with the prescribed MMC content (80%, w/w) of the microcapsules.

Sustained release of MMC from MMC microcapsules was clearly demonstrated by the in vitro assay (Fig. 2). The amount of MMC released from the microcapsules after 6 hours of stationary incubation in 37°C saline was 31 ± 1.5% (mean ± S.D., $n = 3$) while non-encapsulated MMC was completely dissolved by this time. After 1 hour of rotating incubation, 48 ± 2.3% MMC was released from the microcapsules, while the non-encapsulated MMC was entirely dissolved. It took 3 hours for the MMC within MMC microcapsules to be released completely into the rotating saline.

4. Animal experiments for intraarterial use of microcapsules

Sustained drug release is one of the most prominent advantages of encapsulated drugs. This can be achieved, whatever dosage forms are employed. However, the most important problem of drug-delivery systems is their selectivity to tumor lesions. MMC microcapsules were designed to be transported to a desired site via selective arterial catheterization and trapped by small vessels in tumor tissues. The feasibility and effectiveness of this approach were demonstrated as follows.

4.1. Distribution of intravascular microcapsules and drug release
The kidneys were isolated from six mongrel dogs and the renal arteries were intu-

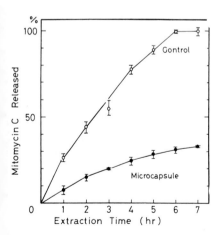

Figure 2. Release rates of MMC from MMC microcapsules (●) and non-encapsulated MMC crystalline particles (○) after stationary incubation in saline at 37°C. Data are expressed as percentage of MMC dissolved in the filtrate of saline. Bars, mean ± S.D. ($n = 3$). From Kato et al. (1980), with permission.

bated with a polyethylene catheter. Following preliminary irrigation with 100 ml saline containing heparin, 12.5 mg of MMC microcapsules containing 10 mg (80%, w/w) of MMC were suspended in 40 ml saline and infused into the left renal artery through the catheter, and further irrigation with 100 ml saline at an infusion pressure of 100 mmHg followed. For the control, 10 mg of non-encapsulated MMC in usual dosage form for injection use was infused into the right renal artery in the same manner (Kato and Nemoto, 1978).

The kidneys of three dogs were photographed immediately after the infusion with soft X-ray following intraarterial infusion of barium sulfate-gelatin solution. The angiograms revealed a moderate decrease of fine vascularity in the kidneys infused with MMC microcapsules, indicating embolization of small branches of the intrarenal arteries. Serial slices of the kidneys showed that MMC microcapsules remained mainly at the junction of the interlobular artery and the arterial arch.

The kidneys obtained from three other dogs were immersed in 10% formaldehyde for 48 hours after the drug infusion, and serially sliced to examine the drug diffusion into the renal parenchyma. Multiple purple spots were observed in the tissue at the cortico-medullary junction of the kidneys infused with MMC microcapsules, while no colored areas were detected in the kidneys infused with non-encapsulated MMC. The coloration in the kidney tissue indicates a diffusion of highly concentrated MMC from the intravascular microcapsules.

These findings proved that the intravascular MMC microcapsules occlude small vessels with a diameter corresponding to the particle size of the microcapsules in the early stage of infusion and then release highly concentrated MMC into the surrounding tissue.

4.2. Drug activity in target organs and systemic circulation

Mongrel dogs weighing approximately 10 kg were anesthetized with intravenous pentobarbital and a catheter was inserted into the left renal artery through the right femoral artery. In each of five dogs, 12.5 mg of MMC microcapsules containing 10 mg of MMC suspended in saline was infused into the left renal artery through the catheter. For the control, each of three dogs received 10 mg of non-encapsulated MMC in the same manner. Blood samples were obtained from the right common iliac vein at the determined intervals and bilateral nephrectomy was done 6 hours after the drug infusion. Three tissue specimens were sampled from the upper, middle and lower sections of each kidney. Bioassay for MMC in the serum and the kidney tissue homogenate was performed by the agar diffusion method using *Escherichia coli* (Kato et al., 1980).

Bioassay of the tissue homogenate revealed that the kidneys infused with MMC microcapsules retained biologically active MMC (mean value, 0.046 ± 0.014 $\mu g/g$) 6 hours after the infusion, while MMC could not be detected in the control kidneys infused with non-encapsulated MMC (Fig. 3).

MMC levels in the circulating blood of the animals infused with MMC microcapsules were significantly lower than those of the control animals ($P < 0.01$) through

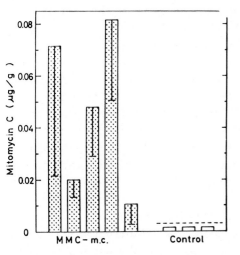

Figure 3. MMC activity in the kidney tissue 6 hours after intraarterial infusion of MMC microcapsules (five dogs) and non-encapsulated MMC (control, three dogs). Bars, mean ± S.D.; -----, limitation of bioassay (0.003 μg/g). From Kato et al. (1980), with permission.

30 minutes after the drug infusion (Fig. 4). The peak MMC level, observed 5 minutes after the infusion, was 0.580 ± 0.159 μg/ml in the MMC microcapsule group, while that in the control group was 2.166 ± 0.340 μg/ml ($P < 0.005$). In terms of bioavail-

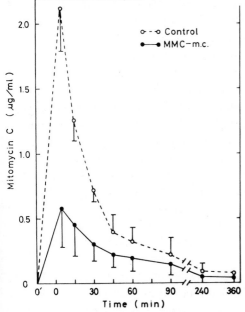

Figure 4. Blood levels of MMC after intraarterial infusion of MMC microcapsules (●) ($n = 5$) and non-encapsulated MMC (○) ($n = 3$) into the kidney, 0'–0, infusion time (15 minutes); bars, mean ± S.D. From Kato et al. (1980), with permission.

ability, calculated by the area under the blood level curve, the amount of MMC released from the kidneys into the circulating blood by the MMC microcapsule group was estimated to be approximately 40% that of the control group.

Intraarterial infusion of anticancer drugs in the usual dosage form has been employed as a mode of selective cancer chemotherapy, but the bulk of the infused drugs tends to be rapidly eliminated from the target lesion, as shown in the present experiment. In contrast, MMC in the form of ethylcellulose microcapsules proved able to sustain its biologic activity for more than 6 hours, even in the kidney, which has a potent enzyme system inactivating MMC. This implies that the ethylcellulose microcapsules protect the encased MMC from enzymatic inactivation and slowly release MMC, and so prevent its rapid clearance from the kidney.

4.3. Morphological evaluation of intravascular MMC microcapsules

Various modes of transcatheter arterial treatments were performed using the dog kidney as the target organ (Nemoto et al., 1980). The left renal artery in each animal was catheterized through the right femoral artery and 18 animals were divided into five experimental groups according to the materials infused through the catheter: three dogs received 10 mg non-encapsulated MMC (group 1), four dogs received 12.5 mg placebo microcapsules which contained lactose instead of active drugs (group 2), four dogs received 10 mg non-encapsulated MMC immediately after the infusion of 12.5 mg MMC microcapsules (group 3), four dogs received 12.5 mg MMC microcapsules containing 10 mg MMC (group 4) and three dogs received 60 ml saline (control). The animals were killed 5 days after the treatments and their kidneys were submitted to gross, microscopic and angiographic evaluation (Fig. 5).

In group 1 kidneys infused with non-encapsulated MMC, gross appearance showed partial mild subcapsular hemorrhage, rather diffuse in the outer medulla, but no apparent focal necrosis. Microscopic observation revealed occasional necrosis and desquamation of the tubular epithelium in the subcapsular outer cortex. The inner cortex and the medulla appeared to be intact except for patchy focal hemorrhage. The glomeruli remained unaltered. Angiography indicated no remarkable change. As a whole, morphological changes were minimal in this group.

Group 2 kidneys infused with placebo microcapsules showed multiple spotty, mottled hemorrhagic foci, mainly in the outer cortex, in gross view. Microscopic findings confirmed that small foci of necrosis were scattered mainly in the cortex and also in the subcortical outer medulla. The absence of cortical vessels and several partially obstructed branches in arcuate arteries were shown in angiography. These histological changes in the individual foci were evident, but still confined to the small, scattered portions.

Group 3 kidneys infused with placebo microcapsules and non-encapsulated MMC had irregular pale lesions of infarction involving the entire width of the cortex and partially extending into the medulla with marginal congestion. Angiography revealed complete obstruction of arcuate arteries and small avascular areas mainly at the corticomedullary junctions. However, microscopic observation showed considerably large areas of intact tissue.

Group 4 kidneys infused with MMC microcapsules showed the most extensive changes of ischemia as well as infarction or necrosis, irregular congestion and focal hemorrhages involving both the cortex and the medulla. Only a focal remnant of intact parenchyma was scattered throughout the kidneys. The interlobar and arcuate arteries and their more peripheral branches were often thromboembolized, with fibrin thrombi occasionally containing brownish-gold crystalloid particles, indicating the fragments of the microcapsules. Thromboangitis of some interlobular arteries and afferent arterioles extending in the glomeruli was particularly evident. Angiography revealed marked obstruction of the peripheral cortical arteries and extended avascular areas, but major branches of arteries were shown to be not embolized. The control kidneys infused with saline were proved to have no detectable changes.

The results clearly demonstrated that selective intraarterial infusion of MMC microcapsules produces the most intensive histological damage in the target organ as compared with other kinds of treatment examined. Non-encapsulated MMC causes only minimal cytotoxic changes and placebo microcapsules induce small foci of infarction, but the large part of the renal parenchyma remained unaffected. Though the combination of non-encapsulated MMC and placebo microcapsules enhances the cytotoxic effects, the degree and extent of morphological changes are far less than those obtained from MMC microcapsules.

The markedly enhanced cytotoxic effects of intraarterial MMC microcapsules must result from a function of infarction and prolonged drug action. Edematous changes in the surrounding tissues must occur at the same time in the early stage of infarction and may increase the extent of intraparenchymal migration of the released drug from the microcapsules.

4.4. Toxicity of MMC microcapsules

MMC microcapsules containing 80% (w/w) MMC were injected into the bilateral internal iliac arteries of mongrel dogs under intravenous pentobarbital anesthesia. The dose of MMC microcapsules, which is expressed as the MMC content of the microcapsules, ranged from 0.25 to 2 mg/kg in each experimental group. For the controls, non-encapsulated MMC was injected in the same manner. All four dogs which had received 0.5 mg/kg MMC microcapsules survived for more than 60 days, but those injected with 1 and 2 mg/kg MMC microcapsules died within 7 days. On the other hand, all dogs which had received 0.5 and 1 mg/kg of non-encapsulated MMC died within 9 days, and only the dogs injected with 0.25 mg/kg non-encapsulated MMC survived for more than 60 days. Consequently, the maximum tolerated dose of MMC microcapsules was estimated to be 0.5 mg/kg, while that of non-encapsulated MMC was 0.25 mg/kg (Nemoto et al., 1979). This finding, indicating that intravascular MMC microcapsule reduces by half the toxicity of non-encapsulated MMC, is consistent with the results from pharmacokinetic studies presented earlier.

236

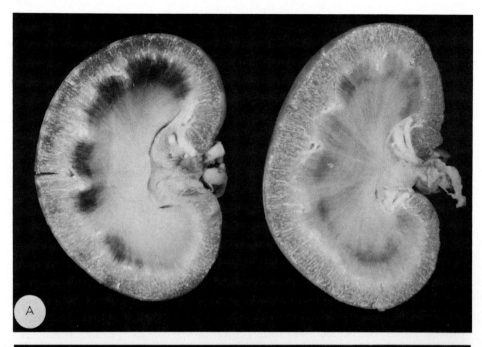

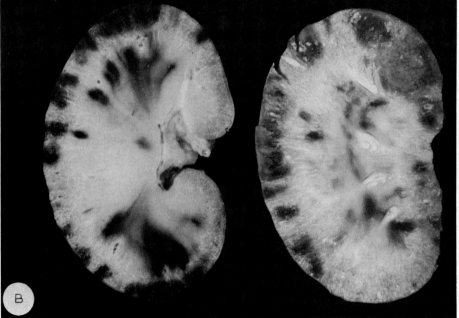

4.5. Summary

In view of our findings from animal experiments, it can be concluded that microencapsulated MMC infused into a cancerous lesion through arterial catheterization exerts two antitumor actions against the surrounding tumor tissues: one is selective

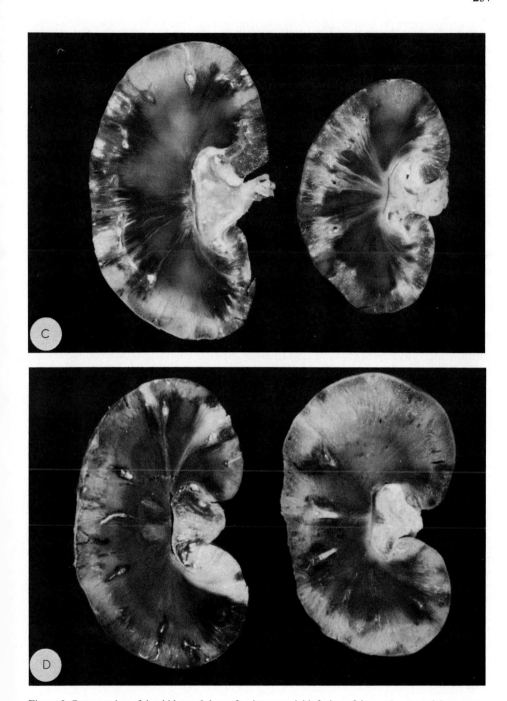

Figure 5. Cross-section of dog kidneys 5 days after intraarterial infusion of drugs. A, group 1 (non-encapsulated MMC). B, group 2 (blank capsules). C, group 3 (blank capsules and non-encapsulated MMC). D, group 4 (microencapsulated MMC). From Nemoto et al. (1980), with permission (© 1980, Williams and Wilkins Co., Baltimore).

necrosis of the tumor caused by occlusion of the supplying artery and the other is intensive chemotherapy with minimum systemic toxicity. In other words, transcatheter arterial infusion of microencapsulated MMC into the malignant region causes a therapeutic infarction of malignant tissue together with a topical regional anticancer chemotherapy, called chemoembolic therapy.

5. Clinical application of microencapsulated MMC

Arterial chemoembolization with the microencapsulated anticancer drugs may be applied to a variety of tumor lesions where selective arterial catheterization is possible. Encouraged by the experimental results described above, this mode of treatment has been used since March 1978 in patients with malignant tumors in various organs.

These included primary or secondary tumors in the liver, kidney, urinary bladder, prostate, uterus and bone (Kato et al., 1979a, 1981a; Nemoto et al., 1981). Recently, tumors in the lungs and neck were submitted to this treatment. Early experiences with MMC microcapsules were summarized as follows.

5.1. Subjects

From March 1978 to March 1982, 285 patients with invasive or nonresectable malignant tumors were subjected to arterial chemoembolization using MMC microcapsules (Table 1). These included 71 renal cell carcinomas, 117 primary or metastatic hepatic carcinomas, 49 urinary bladder carcinomas, 20 prostatic carcinomas and 28 other malignant tumors. 134 patients had several metastases or were in a far-advanced stage.

TABLE 1

Patients subjected to microcapsule therapy (March 1978–March 1982)

Diseases	No. of cases
Renal cell carcinoma	71 (35)
Hepatoma	67 (8)
Metastatic hepatic carcinoma	50 (50)
Bladder carcinoma	49 (18)
Prostatic carcinoma	20 (11)
Miscellaneous[a]	28 (12)
Total	285 (134)

Figures in brackets represent the number of patients with recurrent or metastatic tumors.

[a] Gastrointestinal tract, bone, female genital organs, lung.

TABLE 2

Frequency of microcapsule therapy in individual patients (March 1982)

No. of treatments	No. of cases
1	190 (67%)
2	60 (21%)
3	23 (8%)
4	12 (4%)
Totals	285 (100%)

The mean interval of repeated infusion was 35.8 ± 19.2 (S.E.) days. The mean dose was 21 mg.

5.2. Methods

MMC microcapsules suspended in saline were infused into the arteries supplying the tumors through a catheter, which was inserted into the femoral artery under local anesthesia and guided under fluoroscopy into the target arteries. The catheter was removed immediately after the infusion so that the patients could enjoy a catheter-free condition until the next infusion was due. Of 285 patients, 190 received a single infusion, 60 received two infusions and 35 received three or four infusions (Table 2). The mean value of total MMC doses expressed by MMC content of the microcapsules was 21 mg and the mean interval of repeated infusion was 35.8 days.

5.3. Results

Responses to the treatment were tumor reduction, pain relief, hemostasis of massive bleeding, and adjuvant effects on radical surgery. Objective tumor reduction greater than 50%, which was expressed by the product of two diameters, was found in 74 of 211 measurable tumors. Of the remaining 137 tumors, 77 showed a moderate tu-

TABLE 3

Tumor response to microcapsule therapy (March 1982)

Reduction rates (%)	No. of cases	
100	6 (3%)	
>75	31 (15%)	74 (36%)
>50	37 (18%)	
>25	27 (12%)	77 (37%)
≤25	50 (24%)	
0	60 (28%) —	60 (28%)
Totals	211 (100%)	

The reduction rates are expressed by the products of the two diameters.

240

mor reduction of less than 50% and only 60 (28%) had no definite tumor reduction (Table 3). In general, tumor size began to decrease a few days after the infusion and reached a minimum approximately 1 month later (Figs. 6 and 7).

Improvement of symptoms and signs, such as pain, anorexia, dysuria, constipation, edema, massive hemorrhage or hydronephrosis, was often observed. Pain was relieved in 24 (80%) of 30 painful lesions, including four bone mestastases resistant to radiotherapy. Gross hematuria and massive genital bleeding were improved in all of 15 patients with primary or secondary lesions in the kidney, urinary bladder, cervix or vagina.

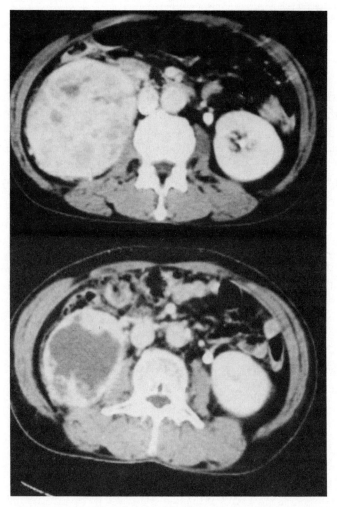

Figure 6. Computerized tomograms of right renal cell carcinoma before (top) and after (bottom) mitomycin microcapsule infusion with gelatin sponge embolization. Estimated reduction rate with central necrosis is 30% in diameter. From Kato et al. (1981a) J. Am. Med. Assoc. 20, 1123–1127. © 1981, American Medical Association.

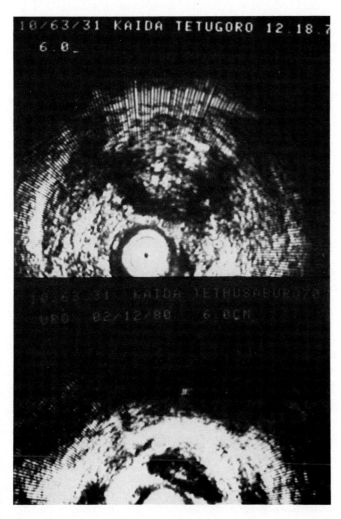

Figure 7. Echograms of highly invasive prostatic carcinoma before (top) and after (bottom) the mitomycin microcapsule infusion. Indistinct enlarged echo indicating extracapsular invasion is reduced to normal-sized prostatic echo. From Kato et al. (1981) J. Am. Med. Assoc. 20, 1123–1127. © 1981, American Medical Association.

Tumor reduction induced by the treatment satisfactorily facilitated surgical manipulations followed by radical operation. These included four renal cell carcinomas involving the vena cava, four urinary bladder carcinomas extending to the pelvic wall or the sigmoid colon and two cervical carcinomas invading the urinary bladder and the pelvic wall. MMC microcapsule therapy did not affect the postoperative course.

Considering the fact that all of the patients had invasive tumors, half of which had failed to respond to previous treatment, and the majority of the tumors received semiselective treatment with MMC microcapsule infusion, these results are encouraging.

TABLE 4

Side effects and complications of microcapsule therapy (March 1982)

Symptom or sign	Cases
Bone marrow depression	35% (8%)
Local pain	28% (6%)
Fever	25% (9%)
Anorexia	19% (3%)
Skin ulcer	9% (9%)
Infection	2% (2%)
Others	4% (3%)

Figures in brackets represent the percentage of cases required for treatment.

Systemic toxicity of MMC microcapsules was found to be mild. For example, hematological toxicity occurred in 100 (35%) of 285 patients, but blood transfusion or steroid administration was needed in only 8%. No other notable toxic effects were experienced (Table 4), except skin necrosis in the gluteal area, which occurred in 18 patients who had received semiselective MMC microcapsule infusion into the internal iliac arteries. The same complication was reported to occur in 90% of the patients continuously infused with 5-fluorouracil (Nevin and Hoffman, 1975). This complication might be caused by MMC microcapsules infused into nontarget arteries, such as superior and inferior gluteal arteries. Since percutaneous superselective catheterization into the branches of the internal iliac artery is frequently unsuccessful in elderly patients, transient artificial occlusion of the nontarget arteries with absorbable gelatin sponge is recommended to avoid skin necrosis.

5.4. Summary

Arterial chemoembolization with microencapsulated drugs has been submitted to clinical use since March 1978, about half of the patients being treated during the last 1.5 years. It has been proved that this mode of treatment can be applied to a variety of tumor lesions, providing remarkable therapeutic effects with minimal systemic toxicity. The majority of patients have been treated with only one or two infusions, repeated, if indicated, at intervals of 1 month or more.

The clinical experiences have shown that approximately one fourth of the treated tumors fail to respond to arterial chemoembolization. This may be attributable to either inadequate catheterization, inadequate dose relative to tumor size, insufficient tumor vascularity or low drug sensitivity. The practice of catheterization technique, detailed optimization of dose schedule and use of microcapsules with multiple drug actions may further improve the response rate to this treatment.

6. Conclusion

It had been emphasized that the major problem of drug-delivery systems in cancer chemotherapy is the area-specificity of the drugs. To solve this problem, the idea of arterial chemoembolization with the microencapsulated drugs was introduced, illustrating the experimental background and promising clinical results. This method is simple and practical in respect to clinical use, but it still has the technical problem of selective arterial catheterization. Subsequently, a magnetic control system was presented as an adjunct to transcatheter arterial chemoembolization (Kato et al., 1979b). This approach represents the possibility of extending the indication of arterial chemoembolization and also the feasibility of effective intracavitary chemotherapy.

Acknowledgments

The research summarized in this article was performed in cooperation with Drs. Yoshiharu Tamagawa (Department of Radiology), Masaoki Harada (Department of Pathology), Katsuo Unno (Department of Pharmacy) and Akio Goto (Department of Pharmacy) in Akita University School of Medicine.

The authors thank Drs. Masaaki Shindo, Hisashi Mori and Ryoetsu Abe for their critical reading of this work. We appreciate the technical assistance of Mrs. E. Nemoto, Miss A. Ino and M. Kondo in the preparation of the manuscript.

References

Kato, T. and Nemoto, R. (1978) Proc. Jpn. Acad. 54, 413–417.

Kato, T., Nemoto, R., Mori, H. and Kumagai, I. (1979a) Lancet 2, 479–480.

Kato, T., Nemoto R., Mori, H. and Unno, K. (1979b) Proc. Jpn. Acad. 55, 470–475.

Kato, T., Nemoto, R., Mori, H. and Kumagai, I. (1980) Cancer 46, 14–21.

Kato, T., Nemoto, R., Mori, H., Takahashi, M., Tamakawa, Y. and Harada, M. (1981a) J. Am. Med. Assoc. 20, 1123–1127.

Kato, T., Nemoto, R., Mori, H., Takahashi, M. and Harada, M. (1981b) Cancer 48, 674–680.

Kato, T., Nemoto, R., Mori, H., Takahashi, M. and Tamakawa, Y. (1981c) J. Urol. 125, 19–24.

Nemoto, R., Mori, H., Kumagai, I. and Kato, T. (1979) J. Jpn. Soc. Cancer Ther. 14, 1150–1157.

Nemoto, R., Kato, T., Mori, H. and Harada, M. (1980) Invest. Urol. 18, 69–73.

Nemoto, R., Kato, T., Iwata, K., Mori, H. and Takahashi, M. (1981) Urology 17, 315–319.

Nevin, J.F. and Hoffman, A.A. (1975) Am. J. Surg. 130, 544–549.

Speiser, P. (1976) in Microencapsulation (Nixon, J.R., Ed.), pp. 1–11, Marcel Dekker, New York.

Takahashi, T., Ueda, S., Kono, K. and Majima, S. (1976) Cancer 25, 1507–1514.

Microspheres and Drug Therapy. Pharmaceutical, Immunological and Medical Aspects
edited by S.S. Davis, L. Illum, J.G. McVie and E. Tomlinson
© *1984, Elsevier Science Publishers B.V.*

CHAPTER 6

The use of biocompatible microparticles as carriers of enzymes and drugs in vivo

Ingvar Sjöholm and Peter Edman

1. Introduction

Carrier systems for drugs have been the subject for increasing explorative research in the last years, and several excellent reviews have already discussed the developments in the field (e.g., Juliano, 1980). In fact, the drug carrier concept represents a completely new approach to drug formulation with the purpose of transporting drugs — both low-molecular-weight substances and macromolecules such as enzymes — to specific cells or organs in order to attain a more distinct or higher local concentration. As far as macromolecular systems (e.g., liposomes, albumin microspheres, synthetic small-sized particles) are concerned, one can foresee at least two targets for such carriers injected intravenously, namely specific cells in the circulation to which the carrier can be actively directed and cells belonging to the reticuloendothelial system (RES). In addition, different carrier systems, to which drugs can be immobilized, might be used, e.g., to protect easily metabolized biologically active compounds, with the aim of installing them parenterally as controlled release preparations or as locally acting depots. However, the present paper will discuss only microparticles, which are to be used as drug carriers for intravenous (or intraperitoneal) injection.

Thus far, no solid drug carrier system has been approved by any drug control agency, and it is obvious that much more work has to be performed on several important aspects. One of the most important problems to be solved before a carrier can prove useful is to design a system with controlled biodegradability. The carrier has to be degradable in order not to create a storage disease, but has to be stable in the circulation for long enough to be able to carry its load of drugs to the correct target. It also has to be non-immunogenic. Moreover, a procedure for the immobilization of the drugs has to be chosen, which does not render the immobilized drugs immunogenic by exposing new antigenic determinants on autologous proteins or giving low-molecular-weight drugs hapten properties. The carrier has to be biocompatible and not induce any lasting inflammatory processes or any other toxic reactions. The retention of biological properties of the immobilized drugs within the carrier or after release is a necessity, as well as a small size for any particulate system in order to avoid the blocking of capillaries. Practical advantages would be reproducible properties, simple production and high carrier capacity.

2. Preparation and properties of microparticles of cross-linked poly-saccharides

Polyacrylamide is easy to prepare in the laboratory and has found wide applications for different purposes. It can be prepared easily in bead form as microparticles by emulsion polymerization and can then also be used for the immobilization of proteins (Fig. 1). The microparticles of polyacrylamide with different immobilized proteins are excellent tools for different purposes in vitro, but cannot normally be used in man, since polyacrylamide is metabolized very slowly in vivo. However, soluble poly-saccharides can also be used for the preparation of microparticles after derivatization

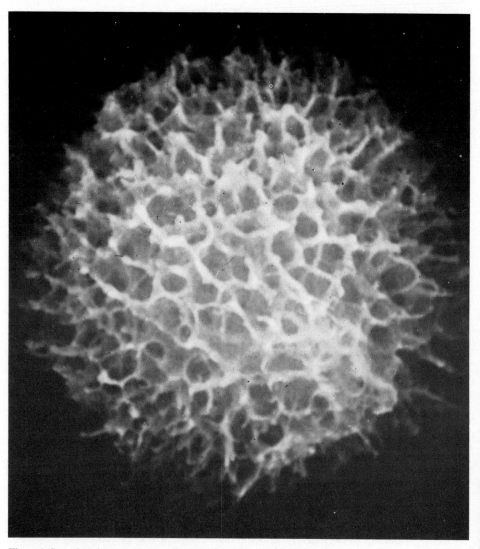

Figure 1. Scanning electron micrograph of a polyacrylamide microparticle.

with, e.g., acrylic acid glycidyl ester, which will introduce acrylic groups in the mono-saccharide moieties. Upon polymerization, these will form cross-linking hydrocarbon chains between the polysaccharides forming the microparticles (Fig. 2).

2.1. Preparation of acrylic polysaccharides

The reaction between the acrylic acid glycidyl ester and polysaccharides is a slow process, when carried out at room temperature and in an aqueous medium at pH 11 (Edman et al., 1980), partly due to the poor solubility of the ester. The derivatization degree (D.D.), e.g., with maltodextrin, can vary between three and twelve acrylic groups per 100 glucose units by increasing the reaction time from 3 to 15 days. In addition to maltodextrin, dextran, glycogen and hydroxyethyl starch (Lepistö et al., 1983) have been modified successfully with acrylic acid glycidyl ester. The ester is partly hydrolyzed during the derivatization, and consequently the products have been purified in our later work by toluene extraction and gel filtration on Sephadex G-25.

Bromination has been used for the determination of the D.D., but the method is imprecise and is perturbed by side reactions with the polysaccharides. Therefore, a sensitive and convenient NMR method was developed by which the signals from the double bonds could be directly related to those from the anomeric protons of the polysaccharide. Thereby a figure of the D.D. can be obtained directly without a separate determination of the polysaccharide concentration (Lepistö et al., 1983).

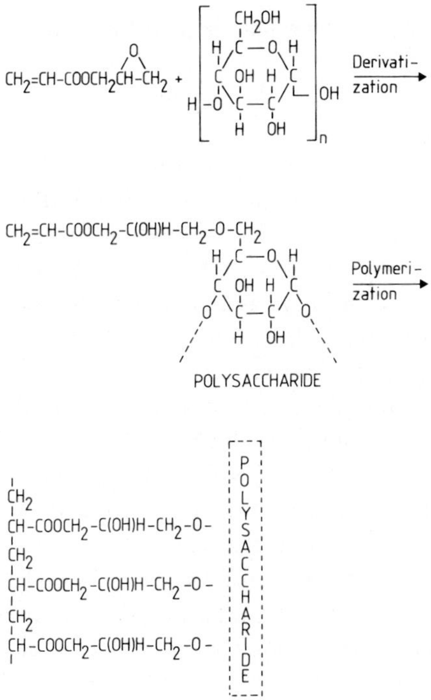

Figure 2. Principal reaction scheme for preparation of polyacryl starch.

2.2. Preparation of starch and dextran microparticles

Microparticles are prepared by emulsion polymerization in a water-in-oil-emulsion. The acrylic polysaccharides are dissolved in the water phase at neutral pH up to a concentration of about 30% (Edman et al., 1980; Artursson et al., 1984). The protein to be immobilized is also dissolved in the water phase together with the catalyst, ammonium peroxidisulphate. The pH is controlled after the addition of the catalyst. The water phase is then homogenized (under nitrogen) with a powerful homogenizer (e.g., an Ultraturrax) with Pluronic F68 as detergent in a chloroform/toluene mixture (4:1). The composition of the organic phase is chosen to give a density of 0.98 g/ml in order to facilitate a stable emulsion. The polymerization is initiated by the addition of N,N,N',N'-tetramethylethylenediamine after formation of an emulsion with a suitable degree of dispersion. For some applications, an extra cross-linker in the form of N,N'-methylenebisacrylamide may be added to the water phase, when a more metabolically stable and more porous microparticle is required.

The microparticles are isolated by centrifugation and extensively washed with buffer. Careful exclusion of oxygen and good quality reagents are needed for a successful polymerization. Generally, the lowest concentration of acrylic groups to allow the formation of particles is about 0.6% (w/v).

The composition of the microparticles is defined by the concentration of the different components in the water phase (Edman et al., 1980). The D-T-C code is then used, in which D means the total concentration of the polysaccharide (in g/100 ml), T denotes the total concentration of acrylic groups (expressed as acrylamide equivalents in g/100 ml) and C the fraction of added extra bisacrylamide (percent, w/w, of total amount acrylic monomers).

2.3. Immobilization of proteins in microparticles

The mechanisms determining the immobilization of proteins in polyacrylamide particles have been discussed in some detail by Ekman et al. (1976). The immobilization is due partly to entrapment by the polymeric network and partly to physical fixation within the polymeric bundles. In polysaccharide microparticles the yield of immobilized proteins is much improved by comparison with polyacrylamide particles, despite the fraction of acrylic polymer being substantially decreased, generally to less than 4% of the dry weight. The addition of polysaccharides means that the pore size is decreased and the amount of protein which is immobilized by entrapment is significantly increased. The influence of the particle composition on the immobilization of serum albumin is illustrated in Table 1. It is obvious that the yield of microparticles during the polymerization and, consequently, also the yield of immobilized proteins are increased with increasing concentration of acryloylated starch (D) and with increasing concentration of acryloyl groups (T), i.e., the degree of derivatization. The amount of immobilized protein can reach about 35–40% of the particle dry weight. If extra bisacrylamide is added, the pore size of the polymeric particle will increase, resulting in an impaired yield of immobilized protein and a smaller protein content.

The biological properties of proteins immobilized in polyacrylamide microparticles

TABLE 1

Immobilization of ^{125}I-labelled human serum albumin in maltodextrin microparticles

Microparticle composition (D-T-C)	Total yield of microparticles (%)	Total protein yield (%)	Total protein content (mg/mg dry weight)	Leakage in 6 weeks (%)
5-0.2-0	7.9	2.2	0.218	34
7-0.2-0	5.4	3.4	0.386	34
10-0.2-0	28.1	7.3	0.206	62
10-0.3-0	58.1	13.8	0.192	52
10-0.4-0	46.2	27.5	0.373	38
10-0.4-5	44.6	9.8	0.180	43
10-0.4-25	19.4	3.8	0.164	56
10-1.2-60	55.6	22.4	0.287	40

are essentially fully retained and the proteins are also stably bound in the particles (Ekman and Sjöholm, 1978). However, the functional capacity of albumin when bound in the starch microparticles is only about 50%, when the binding of salicylic acid is measured. A larger leakage from the particles, when stored in buffer, can also be detected, resulting in a total loss of about 40–60% of the protein from the particles in 6 weeks, depending on the composition (Table 1).

2.4. Immobilization of low-molecular-weight drugs

Low-molecular-weight drugs cannot be entrapped effectively in starch or dextran microparticles, but have to be bound covalently to the particles, e.g., via the glucose residues. In principle, immobilization may be carried out by copolymerization of acrylic acid derivatives obtained by coupling the drugs via the carboxylic group, e.g., as amides. In vivo, the complexes may then be hydrolyzed in the lysosomes, releasing an active drug. However, such experiments have not yet been performed, but ready-made starch microparticles have been used as starting material for the immobilization of drugs.

Several methods can be applied, but it is essential to choose a linkage between the drug and the polysaccharide which is readily cleaved in vivo. Moreover, the reaction used for the immobilization should not change the structure of the polysaccharide to such an extent that the saccharide moiety is no longer metabolized via normal carbohydrate pathways. Periodate can be used to produce an aldehyde function, to which drugs with free amino groups can bind, whereupon the Schiff's base formed can be stabilized with, for example, sodium cyanoborohydride (Jentoft and Dearborn, 1979). Such experiments have been performed, but it is uncertain to what extent the starch residues of such preparations can be metabolized intracellularly. In our hands, carbonyldiimidazole has given promising results (Laakso, T., Stjärnkvist, P. and Sjöholm, I., preliminary results, 1983). The method was suggested by Bethell et al. (1979) and has been used to prepare activated matrices for biospecific affinity chromatography (Bethell et al., 1981). After activation of the starch microparticles, the imidazole bond to the carbamate function is attacked by drugs with nucleophilic groups, e.g., amino groups. The bonds formed should be hydrolyzed in vivo, leaving the carbohydrate unmodified, but extensive studies in vitro with lysosomal enzymes and in vivo tests should be performed to confirm these theories.

3. Distribution and elimination of microparticles

3.1. Elimination kinetics

It is well known that when injected intravenously, particles in the submicron range (< 1 μm) are rapidly cleared from the circulation by the normal reticuloendothelial defence mechanism irrespective of particle composition (Juhlin, 1960; Sjöholm and Edman, 1979). However, when the particles are not dispersed sufficiently prior to injection, aggregation can occur. Such aggregates or large particles (those greater than 7 μm in diameter) will be trapped in the lung capillaries and cause pulmonary embolism. Such embolisms have been seen accidently in our studies and also by Schroeder et al. (1978a,b), where polystyrene microspheres of a mean diameter of 3 μm given intravenously to dogs resulted in the death of three out of four animals.

Upon intravenous injection in mice and rats, the microparticles are rapidly cleared from the circulation with a $t_{1/2}$ of 20–90 minutes, dependent on the surface characteristics and composition of the particle. The blood concentration-time profiles show that the clearance of the microparticles from the blood follows an exponential relationship. Protein-containing microparticles are rapidly extracted from the circulation, with a $t_{1/2}$ of about 20 minutes compared to 40 minutes for empty microparticles. However, when the protein-containing particles are coated with poly(ethylene glycol), the survival time in blood is restored, and also significantly increased up to 90 minutes (Artursson et al., 1983). These results clearly demonstrate the importance of surface charge and surface modification in controlling the survival time of particles in the blood stream. However, the results from our studies with protein-containing, empty and poly(ethylene glycol)-coated particles showed that the surface characteristics of the polyacrylamide microparticles did not significantly affect their final deposition in the mouse or rat. The particles were deposited largely in the liver and spleen irrespective of surface characteristics; 60–80% of injected dose was recovered in these organs 1 day post-injection. The elimination of particles from the blood stream was not delayed by repeated intravenous injections of particles, indicating that the phagocytic activity of the reticuloendothelial cells is difficult to block.

3.2. Distribution

As mentioned above, after intravenous injection the particles are rapidly cleared from the blood stream by the fixed macrophages belonging to the reticuloendothelial system (RES). The particles were thus found in the liver, spleen and bone marrow. The

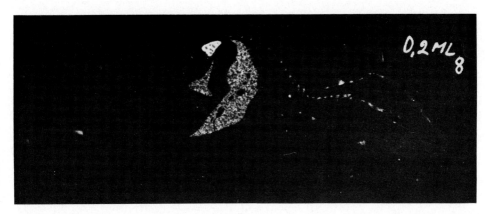

Figure 3. Whole body autoradiograph of a mouse after intravenous injection of ^{14}C-labelled microparticles of polyacryldextran (DTC = 11-1-75).

autoradiograph in Figure 3 shows the qualitative distribution of the particles. Quantitatively, approximately 60–80% of the dose was concentrated in the liver and spleen (Sjöholm and Edman, 1979). The apparent half-life of the microparticles in these organs depends, as expected, on the type of particle. Polyacrylamide microparticles are very slowly degraded, showing terminal half-lives of about 20–25 weeks. Particles made from dextran containing a small number of acrylic groups are eliminated more rapidly, showing half-lives of 4–12 weeks (Edman and Sjöholm, 1982a, 1983b), while starch particles have even shorter half-lives (Laakso, T., Artursson, P. and Sjöholm, I., preliminary results, 1983).

The findings indicate that the rate of metabolism of microparticles in vivo can be controlled by the composition of the particles (type of polymer and cross-linking degree). The stability and rate of metabolism of the microparticles can be studied conveniently in vitro with serum and isolated lysosomal fractions. The results from such studies show especially that metabolism of polyacryl starch microparticles is related to the protein content and the degree of cross-linking (Table 2).

After intravenous injection of large amounts of ^{14}C-labelled polyacrylamide microparticles into mice, significant quantities of radioactivity were detected in the bile and gallbladder after 3, 9 and 27 weeks (Edman and Sjöholm, 1983b). The particles used had a T-C value of 8–25 and a diameter of 0.1–0.4 μm (92.8% of the particles had a diameter within this range, 2.2% were smaller and 5.2% had a diameter of 0.4–0.5 μm). This finding indicates that particles or fragments thereof are partly eliminated from the liver into the intestines by biliary excretion.

3.3. Intracellular localization of microparticles

Intravenous injection of particles of different materials (polyacrylamide, polyacryldextran and polyacryl starch) will, as mentioned above, result in their uptake by the fixed macrophages of the reticuloendothelial system in liver, spleen and bone marrow. In our studies, it is shown clearly that after phagocytosis the particles are intro-

TABLE 2

Degradation of starch microparticles in serum and in a lysosome-enriched fraction

Microparticle composition (D-T-C)	Solubilized radioactivity (cumulative values)	
	Incubation in serum (1 hour)	Incubation in lysosomal fraction (6 hours)
Empty microparticles		
10-0.2-0	21.8±1.8	51.1±3.2
10-0.4-0	12.6±0.8	36.4±3.2
10-0.4-20	10.8±2.3	53.5±7.8
Protein-containing microparticles[a]		
10-0.2-0	38.0±0.9	83.5±2.4
10-0.4-0	28.5±2.3	54.3±3.4
10-0.4-20	40.6±1.5	73.8±2.4

The ^{14}C-labelled starch particles were preincubated for 1 h in serum before further incubation in the lysosomal fraction. This was done to simulate the biological conditions in which the microparticles will exist after intravenous injection. Values are mean ± S.D. from 3–6 experiments.
[a] Human serum albumin, 100 mg per ml water phase.

duced into the lysosomal vacuome, as seen indirectly in the transmission electron microscope (TEM), by the markedly increased number of secondary lysosomes and their swelling (Fig. 4).

Since the particles themselves have a very low electron density, they had to be labelled with ferritin to allow visualization in the electron microscope. By using ferritin-loaded microparticles it is possible to show directly by TEM the lysosomal accumulation of microparticles after intravenous injection (Edman et al., 1983b).

In vitro investigations of unstimulated peritoneal macrophages which had been exposed to ferritin-labelled microparticles showed an increased number of secondary lysosomes, containing material with tiny electron-dense particles corresponding to the ferritin of the microparticles (Fig. 5). This finding provides further evidence that the microparticles are lysosomotropic (Edman et al., 1983b).

4. Morphological consequences of the localization of microparticles to the RES

4.1. Studies in mice

Intravenous injections of large doses of microparticles (> 160 mg/kg body weight) into mice produced a hepatosplenomegaly (Sjöholm and Edman, 1979). The enlarge-

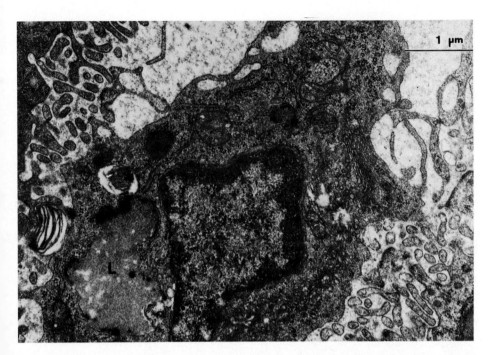

Figure 4. Kupffer cell 2 months after intravenous injection of polyacrylamide microparticles. L denotes a large secondary lysosome filled with material (presumably microparticles).

ment of these organs was very rapid. The liver weight reached its maximum after 5–8 days but returned essentially to normal after 1–2 months. The effects on the spleen were relatively greater than on the liver. The spleen weight was about 220% of that of the control after 3–5 days. The engorgement was partially reduced, but the organ weight did not return to normal within the 8-week study period. Injections of smaller doses of particles (40–80 mg/kg) produced a smaller enlargement of the liver and spleen, while doses under 40 mg/kg of starch particles did not produce any detectable morphological changes (Edman et al., 1983b; Laakso, T., Artursson, P., Edman, P. and Sjöholm, I., preliminary results, 1983).

Histological studies (light and transmission electron microscopy) of the liver showed a vacuolization of the parenchymal cells 1–2 days after injection of 4 mg microparticles. The vacuoles were due to mitochondrial swelling, followed by rupture of the cristae (Fig. 6). After a few more days, necrotic areas developed, corresponding to the initial vacuolization, followed by an invasion of inflammatory cells. After 1–2 weeks granulomas were formed which replaced the necrotic areas. The same phenomena were observed in the spleen and bone marrow. In the spleen, 1–3 days after injection, the limits between the white and red pulps were blurred and the sinusoids were dilated. Later, there was a heavy infiltration of inflammatory cells under formation of abscesses and granulomas. The bone marrow showed an infiltration of polymorphonuclear cells and macrophages with formation of granulomas. After 1 week, the

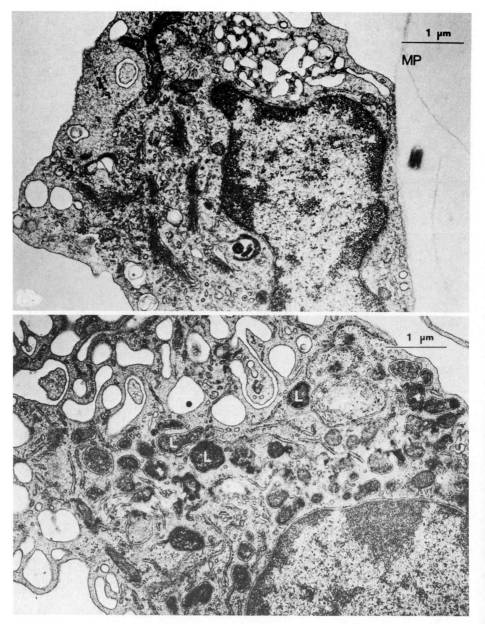

Figure 5. Mouse peritoneal macrophage 72 hours after exposure to ferritin-loaded polyacrylamide micro-particles. Note large number of secondary lyosomes (L) containing microparticles labelled with ferritin. The top is a normal mouse peritoneal macrophage cultured in vitro. MP denotes the microprecipitate to which the cells have attached.

bone marrow showed a normal appearance (Edman et al., 1983b).

The weight changes of the liver and spleen followed the morphological changes

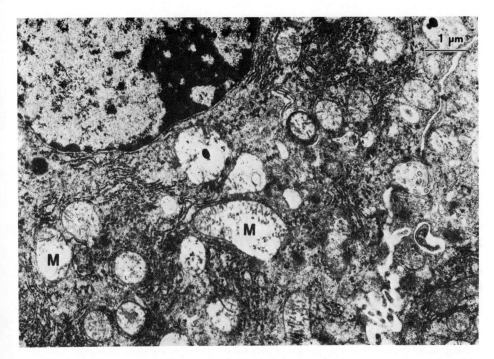

Figure 6. Liver parenchymal cell 2 days after intravenous injection of 4 mg polyacrylamide microparticles into mouse. Swollen mitochondria (M) with ruptured cristae can be seen.

seen in the light and electron microscopes and reached maxima at the same time as the maximum in tissue damage. Organs not containing cells of the reticuloendothelial system are not affected and showed no histological alterations. The effects detected are dose-dependent and are not seen in mice after injection of moderate doses (< 40 mg/kg). Even readily degraded liposomes given intravenously in massive doses to mice produce a hepatosplenomegaly (Gregoriadis et al., 1983; Poste, 1983).

4.2. Studies with isolated macrophages

The adverse effects on the reticuloendothelial system caused by massive doses of microparticles enountered in mice, as described above, can be studied in much greater detail in vitro using cultures of mouse peritoneal macrophages (unstimulated). The toxic reactions detected in these cultures are strictly dose-dependent. From our studies with small polyacrylamide microparticles (mean diameter, 0.25 μm) it is concluded that the ratio between the number of particles and macrophages is about 4000 when ultrastructural alterations are first encountered. Results from mice indicate that about 5000–6000 particles have to be taken up per phagocytic cell before any reaction can be seen in the tissue. This means that cultured peritoneal macrophages are more sensitive to particle exposure than the fixed macrophages of the reticuloendothelial system (Edman et al., 1984). Of interest among the ultrastructural changes seen in the exposed macrophages was a great number of cytoplasmic por-

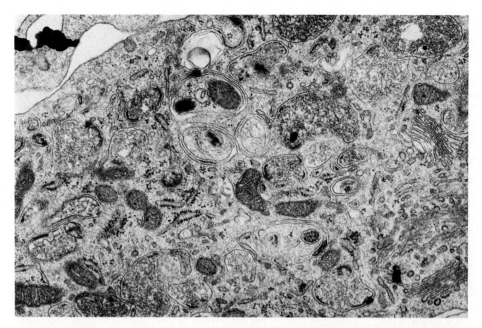

Figure 7. Macrophage 72 hours after exposure to polyacrylamide microparticles showing an excessive formation of multilayer membranes wrapping around cytoplasmic areas (autophagic vacuoles).

tions surrounded by membrane-bound flattened saccules or vacuoles (Fig. 7). These structures were interpreted as being autophagic vacuoles involved in autophagocytosis (Hamberg and Edman, 1983). It appears that a massive dose of particles induces a wave of autophagosome formation in the macrophages and that the vacuoles are converted to autolysosomes through the mixture of the vacuolar contents with lytic enzymes. It is well known that autophagocytosis is a normal process and is enhanced by cell damage. Another interesting finding, encountered after exposure to high doses of particles, is that some cells did not reveal any content of acid phosphatase (Edman et al., 1984). About the same number of cells failed to accumulate acridine orange, which normally accumulates in the lysosomes. This means that the cells have lost completely the normal content of their lysosomal vacuome as a result of particle phagocytosis. From the literature it is known that macrophages exposed to external stimuli are subjected to secretion of lysosomal enzymes during phagocytosis, termed regurgitation (Schlorlemner et al., 1977).

5. The immunological consequences of entrapment of proteins in microparticles

The use of particulate carriers for the in vivo delivery of enzymes is intimately associated with immunological consequences such as enhancement of antibody production and amplified cellular immunity. Experiments have shown that parenteral injection of liposome-entrapped enzyme produces higher antibody titres than soluble enzymes (Allison and Gregoriadis, 1974; Heath et al., 1976). Particles made up from different acrylates, e.g., polymethylacrylate, polyacrylamide, have also been shown to increase the immunogenic properties of simultaneously administered antigens (Kreuter et al., 1976).

The microparticle itself is a macroporous bead, in which entrapped and immobilized proteins are partly localized on the particle surface (Ljungstedt et al., 1978; Artursson et al., 1984), and consequently the antigenic determinants of the protein will be exposed to immunocompetent cells. In our studies, we have shown that intravenous and intraperitoneal injections of L-asparaginase-containing microparticles in mice elicit an enhancement of the humoral antibody response compared to a soluble enzyme given by the same route (Edman and Sjöholm, 1982b). Intramuscular or subcutaneous injection of microparticles gave a much weaker immune response. From these experiments it can be concluded that the microparticles act as an immunological adjuvant. Preliminary results (Artursson, P., Edman, P. and Sjöholm, I., 1983) with polyacryl starch microparticles containing human serum albumin administered to mice have confirmed our earlier observation that the particles work as a pure adjuvant, amplifying the cellular and humoral response.

The antigenicity (here meant, the ability to react with an antibody) of entrapped enzyme in microparticles has also been investigated using a modified Arthus reaction in the foot pad of preimmunized mice. The animals pretreated with L-asparaginase parenterally were challenged by injection into the left hind foot pads of either soluble L-asparaginase or entrapped L-asparaginase in microparticles. Physiological saline or 'empty' microparticles were injected as controls into the right foot pad. The degree of oedema produced was compared with the control and the calculated ratio was compared for soluble and entrapped enzyme. The conclusion is that the antigenicity of microparticle-entrapped enzyme is decreased compared to the soluble enzyme (Edman and Sjöholm, 1982b).

6. Microparticles as enzyme carriers

The passive targeting to the RES and the lysosomotropic character of the microparticles are factors which suggest that they might be used as enzyme carriers in replacement therapy for hereditary storage diseases afflicting the RES. Several groups of such diseases are now well known (see, for example, Desnick et al. (1976) for a review), but no specific treatment has been successful hitherto. Soluble enzymes injected intravenously are not active since the enzyme cannot pass the different membranes and reach the specific cell compartment, the lysosomal vacuome, where the undigested substrate is stored. Some clinical trials are in progress with β-glucocerebrosidase immobilized in liposomes and erythrocyte ghosts for the treatment of the symptoms accompanying Gaucher's disease (Belchetz et al., 1977; Beutler et al.,

1977), but the final reports are not yet available. Inherited storage diseases in laboratory animals are not well known, but such conditions can be induced artificially in mice or rats with, for example, dextran, which is taken up and stored in the macrophages of the RES (Colley and Ryman, 1976).

6.1. Dextranase in polyacryldextran microparticles

Positive effects of dextranase carried in microparticles were demonstrated in mice, to which large amounts of ^{14}C-labelled, cross-linked dextran T40 (molecular weight 40,000) had been administered (Edman and Sjöholm, 1982a). The dextran was injected in the form of polyacryldextran microparticles ($DTC = 11$-1-75), which were taken up essentially in the liver (about 60%) and spleen (about 15%). The half-life of these particles in the liver is about 8–10 weeks without treatment, as shown in Figure 8. Injection of 0.1 unit of dextranase had no influence on the elimination of the stored dextran. However, when the enzyme was injected in immobilized form in a polyacryldextran particle ($DTC = 11$-2-75), the half-life was significantly decreased to 3–4 weeks. Dextranase was effectively immobilized in the microparticles, if the preparation was carried out at high pH and low temperature since the maximum for enzyme activity is on the weakly acid side of neutrality. The enzyme-carrying microparticles were rapidly eliminated from the circulation, with a $t_{1/2}$ of about 40 minutes, and taken up by the same cells storing the labelled polyacryldextran. In the acid environment of the lysosomes, the dextranase broke down the carrier and subsequently was able to metabolize the stored dextran. In this application, the carrier and enzyme functioned as a 'metabolic bomb' (Edman and Sjöholm, 1982a).

6.2. The relation between the metabolism of the carrier and the denaturation of the carried enzyme

It is generally considered necessary that the carriers for enzymes or other drugs have

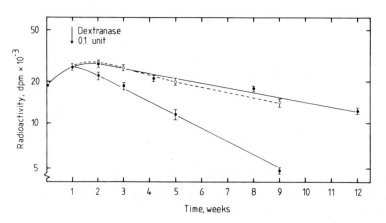

Figure 8. Degradation and elimination of ^{14}C-labelled polyacryldextran from livers of mice after an intravenous injection of 0.1 IU dextran in polyacryldextran microparticles (■) or in free solution (□). The control was given physiological saline intravenously (●).

to be metabolized completely in vivo. In the example discussed above, the enzyme digested its own carrier before it fulfilled its task in the lysosomes. This principle can be applied only exceptionally. In vitro experiments have shown (Artursson et al., 1984) that polyacryl starch microparticles can be prepared, which are degraded rapidly in serum and by lysosomal enzymes (Table 2). The rate of metabolism can be decreased by increasing the content of hydrocarbon chains (T), but is increased with increasing amounts of immobilized protein.

The starch microspheres have also been shown to be metabolized rapidly in vivo (Laakso, T., Artursson, P. and Sjöholm, I., unpublished, 1983) and to be active in the dextran storage disease in mice presented above (Artursson, P., Edman, P. and Sjöholm, I., preliminary results, 1983). Immobilized dextranase was then released rapidly from the starch microparticles in vivo and was able to metabolize the stored dextran particles. The enzyme also had a significant effect on the degradation of injected dextran, if administered 1 day prior to the injection of the substrate, but not if the dextran particles were given 3 days after the injection of the immobilized dextranase. It is thus clear that the degradation of the starch carrier is a rapid process and that the enzyme is released easily from the starch particles. However, the stability of the dextranase in the lysosomal milieu must be relatively limited, since no enzymatic activity could be detected after 3 days. If the observation also holds true for other enzymes, it means that lysosomal enzymes have a rapid metabolic turnover and that a metabolically more stable enzyme carrier might be needed, when a more prolonged duration is wanted.

6.3. Immobilized asparaginase in microparticles given intramuscularly

L-Asparaginase has been used for more than 10 years for the treatment of lymphatic leukemia (Oettgen et al., 1969; Ohnuma et al., 1970). Good effects are achieved through the deprivation of L-asparagine from the growing cells, but the immunogenicity of the enzyme and other side effects, chiefly the induction of asparagine-producing enzymes (Edman and Sjöholm, 1983a), prevent repeated and prolonged treatment. However, the efficacy of the enzyme can be improved significantly by immobilization in polyacrylamide microparticles as shown in rats (Edman and Sjöholm, 1979) and in mice (Edman and Sjöholm, 1983a). An L-asparagine-dependent Gardner lymphoma cell line, 6C3HED, was then inoculated as an ascites tumor, in C3H mice. The effect on the serum level of L-asparagine and on the survival time was studied after treatment by different routes with soluble or immobilized L-asparaginase. It was shown that the best effect was obtained with two injections of enzyme-containing microparticles given intramuscularly, which could keep the L-asparagine level close to zero values for up to 10 days. Moreover, 10 out of 12 mice survived the observation period (50 days), in contrast to the control group in which the members survived 10 days.

Polyacrylamide particles injected intramuscularly are not metabolized to any appreciable extent, but are eventually encapsulated in the tissues. However, any immobilized enzyme is well protected from proteolytic enzymes, which cannot penetrate the microparticles through the pores. On the other hand, these are large enough to allow the substrate to reach the enzyme and to be reacted upon so long as the collagenous, non-vascularized capsule around the microparticles is not formed. Barvic et al. (1967) and Sprincl et al. (1971) have noted the same phenomena after implantation of other acrylic polymers in rats.

7. Conclusions

The targeting of drugs to specific cells or tissues has long been an attractive thought, with the purpose of improving the therapeutic index of a drug, especially in cancer therapy. Today, the goal seems to be achievable following the developments in biotechnology (e.g., the production of specific immunoglobulins) which might be used to target actively drug carriers such as liposomes to a specific cell. However, theory has not yet been realised in practice and it is more realistic to restrict the discussion on the use of carriers to those applications where the normal cleaning system of the circulation, the reticuloendothelial system, is operating.

The present review has discussed starch microparticles as carriers for enzymes and drugs and it has been shown that such a carrier system is capable of directing an enzyme to lysosomes of the RES and is able to accelerate significantly the degradation and elimination of material stored in the lysosomes. The starch microspheres do not cause any respiratory problems when injected intravenously, and so far they have not produced any toxic reactions in mice and rats, when used in moderate doses. The carrier itself is not immunogenic.

Soluble starch (or any other biocompatible polysaccharide) can be used for the preparation of the microparticles in which the starch molecules are cross-linked via hydrocarbon chains. These are formed from acryloyl ester side chains, which are polymerized at room temperature and at neutral pH in an emulsion polymerization process. The fraction of the hydrocarbon chains is small, 2–4% of the particle dry weight, but is probably metabolized only slowly. The metabolism has not yet been studied in detail, due to methodological problems, but Couvreur and Aubry (1984) stat that the size of the polymer in polyisobutylcyanoacrylate nanoparticles is less than 1,000 daltons. It is probable that such a small polymer will be metabolized reasonably fast in the lysosomes and that the more simple polymer present in the starch particles in a much lower concentration will also be eliminated without giving rise to a new storage disease. This point has to be studied in more detail before any definite conclusions can be drawn.

Recent studies have shown that the starch component is rapidly metabolized in serum and in the lysosomal milieu. The rate of metabolism can be controlled by adjusting the hydrocarbon chain content, which in addition will influence the porosity of the particles. Entrapped enzymes are rapidly released from the particles. Also, the release rate can be controlled by the polymeric component and it has become obvious that a correct balance between the starch component and the hydrocarbon chain is essential to ensure an optimal effect in the in vivo compartment. When dextranase was used in our artificial storage disease model, the enzyme was released relatively quickly and inactivated, and no activity was detected after 3 days. In this case, the substrate was a macromolecule, and in such a situation the enzyme has to be released from the carrier to exert its activity in free solution. Thus, the degradation of the carrier is an important factor that controls the release of the enzyme and has to be correlated to the denaturation of the enzyme in the lysosomes in order to obtain an optimal duration. If the substrate is a low-molecular-weight substance a more metabolically stable particle might be the better alternative (i.e., the proportion of cross-linking hydrocarbon chains should be larger) which will also facilitate the penetration of the substrate into the carrier. Nevertheless, the porosity is small enough to prevent the lysosomal enzymes entering the microparticle to denature the carried enzyme.

The starch microparticle has thus proven its potential value as an enzyme carrier in vivo, but even more attractive are future applications, in which the microparticles might be used as carriers for low-molecular-weight drugs. Then, the drugs will have to be covalently bound to the starch (or to a polymer, which can be carried entrapped in the particles). Several widely spread diseases afflicting a large proportion of the world's population are connected with the RES. The cause of leishmaniasis, schistozomiasis and many other subtropical and tropical diseases is parasites, which reside in the lysosomes of RES for at least some time in their life cycle. No drug formulation has yet shown efficacy for the treatment of these, in many cases fatal, diseases. The starch in the microparticles can be chemically activated, with, for example, carbonyldiimidazole used for coupling amino group-containing drugs (and, with some modifications, other functional groups). The potential of the starch microparticles is therefore high, but extensive studies in animal systems have to be performed to prove their usefulness.

References

Allison, A.C. and Gregoriadis, G. (1974) Nature 252, 252.
Artursson, P., Laakso, T. and Edman, P. (1983) J. Pharm. Sci. 72, 1415–1420.
Artursson, P., Edman, P., Laakso, T. and Sjöholm, I. (1984) J. Pharm. Sci., in press.
Barvic, M., Kliment, K. and Zavadil, M. (1967) J. Biomed. Mater. Res. 1, 313–323.
Belchetz, P.E., Braidman, I.P., Crawley, J.C.W. and Gregoriadis, G. (1977) Lancet ii, 116–117.
Bethell, G.S., Ayers, J.S., Hancock, W.S. and Hearn, M.T.W. (1979) J. Biol. Chem. 254, 2572–2574.
Bethell, G.S., Ayers, J.S., Hearn, M.T.W. and Hancock, W.S. (1981) J. Chromatog. 219, 361–372.
Beutler, E., Dale, G.L., Guinto, E. and Kuhl, W. (1977) Proc. Natl. Acad. Sci. U.S.A. 74, 4620–4623.
Colley, C.M. and Ryman, B.E. (1976) Biochim. Biophys. Acta 451, 417–425.
Couvreur, P. and Aubry, J. (1984) in Topics in Pharmaceutical Sciences, Vol. 11 (Breimer, D.D., Ed.), Elsevier Science Publishers, Amsterdam, in press.
Desnick, R.J., Thorpe, S.R. and Fiddler, M.B. (1976) Physiol. Rev. 56, 57–99.
Edman, P. and Sjöholm, I. (1979) J. Pharmacol. Exp. Ther. 211, 663–667.
Edman, P. and Sjöholm, I. (1982a) Life Sci. 30, 327–330.

262

Edman, P. and Sjöholm, I. (1982b) J. Pharm. Sci. 71, 576–580.

Edman, P. and Sjöholm, I. (1983a) J. Pharm. Sci. 72, 654–658.

Edman, P. and Sjöholm, I. (1983b) J. Pharm. Sci. 72, 796–799.

Edman, P., Ekman, B. and Sjöholm, I. (1980) J. Pharm. Sci. 69, 838–842.

Edman, P., Nylén, U. and Sjöholm, I. (1983a) J. Pharmacol. Exp. Ther. 225, 164–167.

Edman, P., Sjöholm, I. and Brunk, U. (1983b) J. Pharm. Sci. 72, 658–665.

Edman, P., Sjöholm, I. and Brunk, U. (1984) J. Pharm. Sci. 73, 153–156.

Ekman, B. and Sjöholm, I. (1978) J. Pharm. Sci. 67, 693–696.

Ekman, B., Lofter, C. and Sjöholm, I. (1976) Biochemistry 15, 5115–5120.

Gregoriadis, G., Kirby, C. and Senior, J. (1983) Biol. Cell. 47, 11–18.

Hamberg, H. and Edman, P. (1983) Acta Path. Microbiol. Immunol. Scand. Sect. A, 91, 1–8.

Heath, T.D., Edwards, D.C. and Ryman, B.E. (1976) Biochem. Soc. Trans. 4, 129–131.

Jentoft, N. and Dearborn, D.G. (1979) J. Biol. Chem. 254, 4359–4365.

Juhlin, L. (1960) Acta Physiol. Scand. 48, 78–87.

Juliano, R.L. (1980) Drug Delivery System. Characteristics and Biomedical Applications. Oxford University Press, New York.

Kreuter, J., Mauler, R., Gruschkau, H. and Speiser, P. (1976) Exptl. Cell. Biol. 44, 12–19.

Lepistö, M., Artursson, P., Edman, P., Laakso, T. and Sjöholm, I. (1983) Anal. Biochem. 133, 132–135.

Ljungstedt, I., Ekman, B. and Sjöholm, I. (1978) Biochem. J. 170, 161–165.

Oettgen, H.F., Old, L.J., Boyse, E.A., Campbell, H.A., Philips, F.S., Clarkson, B.D., Tallal, L., Leeper, R.D., Schwartz, M.K. and Kim, J.H. (1969) Cancer Res. 27, 2619–2631.

Ohuma, T., Holland, J.F., Freeman, A. and Sinks, L.F. (1970) Cancer Res. 30, 2297–2305.

Poste, G. (1983) Biol. Cell. 47, 19–38.

Schlorlemner, H.U., Burger, B., Hylton, W. and Allison, A.C. (1977) Br. J. Exp. Pathol. 58, 313–326.

Schroeder, H.G., Bivins, B.H., Sherman, G.P. and De Luca, P.P. (1978a) J. Pharm. Sci. 67, 508–513.

Schroeder, H.G., Simmons, G.H. and De Luca, P.P. (1978b) J. Pharm. Sci. 67, 504–507.

Sjöholm, I. and Edman, P. (1979) J. Pharmacol. Exp. Ther. 211, 656–662.

Sprincl, L., Kopecek, J. and Lim, D. (1971) J. Biomed. Mater. Res. 4, 447–458.

Microspheres and Drug Therapy. Pharmaceutical, Immunological and Medical Aspects
edited by S.S. Davis, L. Illum, J.G. McVie and E. Tomlinson
© *1984, Elsevier Science Publishers B.V.*

The characterization of radiocolloids used for administration to the lymphatic system

Lennart Bergqvist, Sven-Erik Strand and Per-Ebbe Jönsson

1. Introduction

There is considerable need for a method of examining the lymphatic drainage and lymph nodes in the diagnosis and treatment of malignant diseases. Although radiographic lymphography with contrast media is a clinically accepted method for investigating the lymphatic system, it is not always applicable because the medium must be injected into a suitable lymph vessel.

Lymphoscintigraphy is currently performed after interstitial injection of inert colloids. Foreign particles that are transported with the lymph are mostly phagocytized in the lymph nodes. It is believed that the particles can pass through the junctions between the endothelial cells of the lymphatic capillaries and/or be transported in vesicles through the cells by pinocytosis (Gangon, 1979; Yoffey and Courtice, 1970).

The size dependence for interstitial particle absorption has been verified in both animal and human studies (Ege and Warbick, 1979; Kaplan et al., 1979; Strand and Persson, 1979). Particles with small diameters (i.e., less than a few nanometers) will mostly be exchanged through the blood capillaries. Larger particles, with diameters up to a few tens of nanometers, will be absorbed into the lymph capillaries. Large particles (hundreds of nanometers) will be trapped in the interstitial space for a long time.

The colloid particles in the lymph nodes must be recognized by the macrophages in order to be phagocytized. Receptors on the macrophages recognize the particles either through coated opsonins or by the nature of the surface itself (Frier, 1981). The cell membrane is capable of phagocytic response which is proportional to the size and number of particles presented to it. If all available sites of uptake become saturated, the rate of clearance from the lymph will be determined by the rate of regeneration of absorbing sites, comprising the ingestion of the occupied site, followed by resynthesis of the plasma membrane. The surface charge of the particle as well as the agent with which the colloid is stabilized has also been reported to influence phagocytosis (Frier, 1981; Wilkins and Myers, 1966).

2. Particle characterization in vitro

Particle sizes of colloids proposed for interstitial lymphoscintigraphy are in the range of a few nanometers up to hundreds of nanometers. However, most colloids in clinical use are less than 100 nm. The most common techniques for sizing colloid particles are listed in Table 1, together with the measurable parameters.

2.1. Experimental studies

2.1.1. Radiopharmaceuticals
Previously we have investigated different radiocolloids (Bergqvist et al., 1983; Strand and Persson, 1979). In this chapter data are reported for four technetium-labeled radiocolloids, of which the two with the smaller particle sizes are recommended for lymphoscintigraphy. Data for the radiopharmaceuticals are summarized in Table 2.

2.1.2. Electron microscopy
Scanning electron microscopy was conducted in order to evaluate the particle size and shape. The sample was spread on a polycarbonate filter (Nuclepore®, 0.4 μm), dried and coated with a thin layer of AuPd. Pictures of ^{99m}Tc-antimony sulfide colloid and ^{99m}Tc-sulfur colloid are shown in Figure 1.

2.1.3. Microfiltration
The proportion of radioactivity in different size ranges of colloid particles was studied with microfiltration. Small samples (approximately 30 μl) of the colloid were passed through polycarbonate filters (Nuclepore®) held in Swinnex 25 (Millipore®)

TABLE 1

Sizing techniques

Technique	Resolution	Measurable parameters				
		Shape	Size distribution	Activity/ size distribution	Chemical composition	Charge
Electrophoresis	molecular weight			X		X
Gel chromatography	molecular weight			X		
Electron microscopy						
Transmission	0.2 nm	X	X		X	
Scanning	10 nm	X	X		X	
Ultrafiltration	15 nm			X		
Photon correlation						
spectroscopy	2 nm		X			
Microcentrifugation	100 nm			X		
Light microscopy	200 nm	X	X			
Coulter Counter®	400 nm		X			

TABLE 2

Radiopharmaceuticals investigated

Radiopharmaceutical	Manufacturer	Content			Pertechnetate	Boiling time
		Precolloid	Stabilizer	Buffer		
^{99m}Tc-Sb$_2$S$_3$(Labelaid)	Byk-Mallinckrodt	Sb$_2$D$_3$(1.3 mg)	PVP (8.0 mg)	Potassium bitartrate (1.5 mg)	2–4 ml	15–30 min
^{99m}Tc HSA-colloid (AlbuColl-Scintimed)	Banna	HSA colloid (5 mg)	–	–	1–8 ml	–
^{99m}Tc-sulfur colloid	In house preparation	Sodium thiosulfate (12 mg)	Gelatin (13 mg)	Sodium phosphate (0.2 M, 4 ml)	5 ml	3 min
^{99m}Tc-HSA-colloid (ALBU-RES)	Solco	HSA colloid (2.5 mg)	–	–	1–5 ml	–

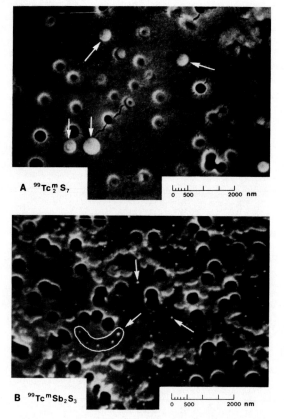

Figure 1. Scanning electron microscopy of colloids (A) $^{99m}Tc_2S_7$ and (B) $^{99m}TcSb_2S_3$. Some of the colloid particles are indicated with arrows.

filter holders. The pore size of the filters was between 0.015 and 2 μm. The filter was rinsed after the application with 2 ml distilled water and set under air pressure. The filter and the filtrate were then measured for radioactivity.

The percentage activity retained on each filter was thus obtained and the relative frequency (percent activity per size interval) was estimated. Relative frequency distributions of the four colloids are given in Figure 2 and the median values of the activity distributions are given in Table 3.

2.1.4. Photon correlation spectroscopy

By using a laser light-scattering spectroscopy technique (Coulter Nano-Sizer), the mean particle size of the colloids (>20 nm) was determined. This technique is based on measurements of the Brownian motion of particles in a solution causing a changing frequency of a scattered laser beam. The results for the colloids measured with this technique are given in Table 3.

2.1.5. Number of particles

The number of coloid particles injected interstitially will influence the rate of outflow

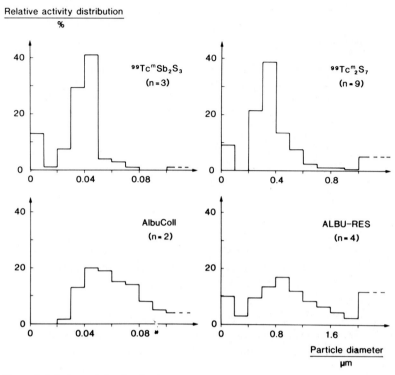

Figure 2. Relative activity distribution as obtained by ultrafiltration given as mean values for the different experiments (*n*) for each colloid.

from the injection site (Zum Winkel, 1972) and the phagocytosis in the lymph nodes (Griffin et al., 1975). In Table 4, the particle concentrations for the four colloids have been calculated with the assumptions of spherical, uniform particles and particle density.

TABLE 3

Results of particle sizing of radiocolloids with different techniques

Radiopharmaceutical	Particle size (nm)			
	Manufacturer's quoted value	Light scattering	Scanning electron microscopy	Micro-filtration (median value)
$^{99m}TcSb_2S_3$	3–30	43 (3)	< 50	40
^{99m}Tc-μAA (AlbuColl)	Mean, 50	–	–	60
$^{99m}Tc_2S_7$	–	375 (3)	300–600	350
^{99m}Tc-μAA (ALBU-RES)	200–1000	250 (3)	–	1200

Figures in parentheses are the polydispersity index.

TABLE 4

Calculated particle concentration

Colloid	Amount of colloid-forming substance	Assumed mean particle size (nm)	Assumed particle density (g·cm^{-3})	Volume of suspension (ml)	Number of particles per ml
$^{99m}TcSb_2S_3$	1.3 mg Sb_2S_3, 8 mg PVP	40	1	6.0	$\sim 5 \times 10^{13}$
^{99m}Tc-μAA (AlbuColl)	5 mg HSA	60	1	5.0	$\sim 10^{13}$
$^{99m}Tc_2S_7$	12 mg $Na_2S_2O_3 \cdot 5\,H_2O$	350	2	11.5	$\sim 10^{10}$
^{99m}Tc-μAA (ALBU-RES)	2.5 mg HSA	500	1	5.0	$\sim 10^{10}$

2.2. Results

Table 3 and Figures 1 and 2 show that the mean size of the labeled particles is between 40 and 1200 nm in diameter for the four preparations investigated. Our results in Table 3 show good agreement between the different sizing techniques for all of the colloids, except ALBU-RES.

The number of particles in the colloid suspensions will range from 10^{10} to 10^{14} per ml of solution. The labeling efficiency, measured by the GCS technique (Strand and Persson, 1979), was found to be better than 90% for all the preparations.

2.3. Discussion

The range in particle sizes can vary considerably between the different preparations. For, e.g., ALBU-RES, one preparation had a mean particle size of 500 nm and a narrow size distribution whereas three other preparations had mean particle sizes of about 1200 nm and wide size distributions. These latter values are considerably different from the values given by the manufacturer (range, 200–1000 nm). An explanation for this was recently given by Chia and Schrijver (1983), who showed with microfiltration that the amount of Al^{3+} in the generator eluate will drastically influence the particle size of ALBU-RES.

3. Particle characterization in serum

When a colloid is injected interstitially it will be in contact with the interstitial fluid, which resembles the composition of serum. In the literature, very few data have been published concerning changes in particle size after contact with serum. In a study by Dornfest et al. (1977), where a sulfur colloid was incubated with serum, the particle size decreased in anemic serum and increased in normal serum.

To investigate further the nature of the change of particle size in serum an extensive study with the four colloids has been undertaken and some preliminary results are given below.

3.1. Experimental studies

To study the change of particle size, microfiltration was performed on the colloid suspensions. Nuclepore filters with pore diameter between 0.015 and 2 μm were used; the number of holes per filter being between 5×10^9 and 5×10^7, respectively.

The colloid (0.2 ml) was incubated with 2 ml serum for 1 hour at $37°C$ in a water bath equipped with a sample whipper. A 0.1 ml sample of the solution was applied on the filter, rinsed and set under air pressure as described in section 2.1.3. In each experiment the non-incubated colloid preparation was also filtrated as a control.

3.2. Results

The mean particle size of $^{99m}TcSb_2S_7$ increased after incubation with normal rat serum from 320 to 450 nm (Fig. 3). Three experiments were made and the ranges of filtrate activity shown in the figure is ascribed to a combination of the uncertainty with the microfiltration technique and slight differences in the colloid preparations.

3.3. Discussion

To increase knowledge of the lymphatic transport of colloids, particle sizing in serum is of great importance.

A decrease of particle size for sulfur colloids may be due to decomposition of the particle, with release of sulfur (Frier, 1981) while increase of size may be due to plasma protein coating and particle aggregation.

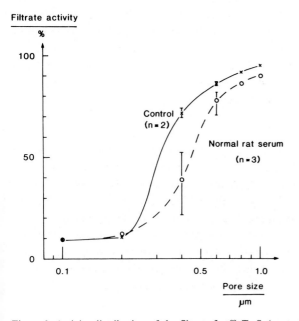

Figure 3. Activity distribution of the filtrate for $^{99m}Tc_2S_7$ (control) and for $^{99m}Tc_2S_7$ incubated in normal rat serum. Ranges of filtrate activity are given for the filter pore sizes 0.4 and 0.6 μm.

4. Biokinetics in rabbits

Different animal models have been reported in the literature in order to study the biokinetics of radiocolloids proposed for lymphoscintigraphy (Dunson et al., 1973; Ege and Warbick, 1979; Gallagher et al., 1980; Strand and Persson, 1979; Warbick et al., 1978). The species most commonly used is the rabbit. In most cases subcutaneous injection of the colloid has been performed, either on the dorsum of the hind feet or at the xiphoid process.

When the colloid is injected in the lower extremities, the popliteal, inguinal and lumbar nodes are studied; when injected below the xiphoid process the parasternal lymph nodes become visible.

4.1. Experimental studies

Experiments have been carried out on eight rabbits (weight, 1.3–2.4 kg). The animals were anesthetized with pentobarbitone sodium (ACO, Sweden) and fixed in supine position. This particular model was chosen because dynamic studies could be carried out and reproducible lymph flow could be established. The colloid (0.2–0.4 ml) was mixed with 100 IU hyaluronidase (Leo, Sweden) and was injected subcutaneously bilaterally just below the xiphoid process. Images were taken with a gamma camera equipped with a low-energy parallel hole collimator, every 90 seconds for the first 30 minutes and then every 180 seconds during the following 90 minutes. The data were stored in a computer. Static images of 5 minutes duration were also taken 4–5 hours after injection. Regions of interest were selected over the injection sites and the lymph nodes, and time-activity curves were generated. To illustrate this, the activity distribution and dynamic curves of the $^{99m}TcSb_2S_3$ colloid in a rabbit is shown in Figure 4.

After completion of the gamma camera studies, the animals were killed and dissected. Samples from different organs were taken and measured for activity in an automatic sample-changing NaI(Tl) well-counter.

4.2. Results

The percentage uptake in the parasternal lymph nodes and the remaining activity in the injection sites were calculated from the gamma camera measurements 2 and 4–5 hours after injection and results shown in Figure 5. The results show that the small-particle $^{99m}TcSb_2S_3$ colloid has the highest uptake in lymph nodes.

The range of specific activity in different tissues and the mean specific activity in parasternal lymph nodes about 5 hours after injection are given in Figure 6. The specific activity in most of the dissected tissues, except the kidneys, ranges from about 0.001 to 0.03%/g. In kidneys, the specific activity was up to 0.3%/g. The mean specific uptake in the lymph nodes was found to range between 5 and 50%/g.

4.3. Discussion

Depending on anatomical variations and difficulties in exactly reproducing the injec-

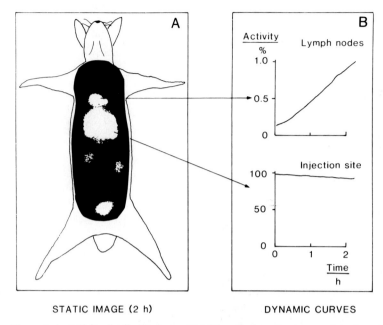

STATIC IMAGE (2 h)   DYNAMIC CURVES

Figure 4. A, Activity distribution in a rabbit 2 hours after subcutaneous injection of ^{99m}TcSb$_2$S$_3$. B, Time-activity curves for parasternal lymph nodes, and injection sites.

tion technique, the rate of colloid uptake in lymph nodes may vary. This is clear from Figure 5 and is supported by previously published data (Strand and Persson, 1979; Bergqvist et al., 1983). The main conclusion is that small particle colloids of less than 100 nm in size are the most suitable for interstitial lymphoscintigraphy.

The specific activity in different tissues is very low for most organs, with much higher uptake in the lymphatic tissue, of the order of 10^3. This ensures that a high contrast is obtained for lymph node imaging. The apparently similar mean specific uptake in the lymph nodes for the four preparations may partly be due to the difficulties in removing all the lymph nodes at the time of dissection.

5. Biokinetics in humans

In melanoma patients dissections of the regional lymph node are often performed for prophylactic or curative purposes. A simple and accurate method of predicting the lymphatic uptake from any given site of the primary lesion is lymphoscintigraphy, where a radioactively labelled colloid with suitable physical and chemical properties is injected subcutaneously or intradermally (Dworkin, 1982). An image of the lymph flow from the injection site to regional lymph nodes can then be obtained.

The aims of the investigation summarized below were to evaluate the possibilities of lymphoscintigraphy for exploring the lymph flow and regional lymph nodes as

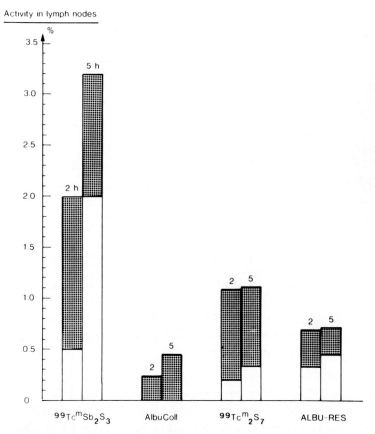

Figure 5. Range of uptake of activity in the parasternal lymph nodes measured in vivo with the scintillation camera 2 and 5 hours after injection.

well as for correlating the uptake of activity in isolated lymph nodes with the histopathology (Bergqvist et al., 1984).

5.1. Experimental studies

32 patients with malignant melanoma were examined after subcutaneous injections of about 40 M Bq $^{99m}TcSb_2S_3$ (Labelaid DRN 4333, Byk-Mallinchrodt) in a volume of 0.3–0.5 ml. No hyaluronidase or equivalent material was used. The preparations were tested for free pertechnetate with the GCS technique (Strand et al., 1981). The labeling yield was always better than 95%.

The injections were made around the scar of the biopsy site (12 patients), outside the skin graft (two patients), or above and below the site of the wide excision (six patients) of the primary lesion (peritumoral injections, PTI) in 20 of the 22 patients with truncal lesions. In the leg melanoma patients, in a patient with an unknown primary tumour site, and in two patients with vulva and anorectal melanoma, respectively, injections were made on the dorsum of the feet over the metatarsal bones (dorsopedal injections, DPI).

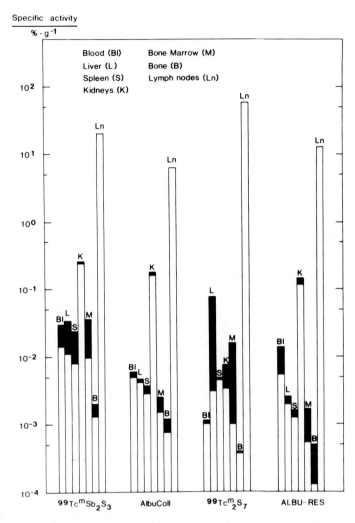

Specific activity

% · g⁻¹

Blood (Bl)   Bone Marrow (M)
Liver (L)   Bone (B)
Spleen (S)   Lymph nodes (Ln)
Kidneys (K)

Figure 6. Range of specific activity in different tissues and the mean specific activity in the parasternal lymph nodes at 5 hours after injection.

Dynamic and static images were recorded with a gamma camera (Searle, LFOV, Siemens) equipped with a parallel hole collimator. The images were stored in a computer (Gamma-11, Digital Eqp.) in a 64 × 64 matrix for later evaluation. Regions of interest were selected over each lymph-node region as well as over adjacent regions for background subtraction.

In 16 patients regional lymph-node dissections were performed the day after the lymphoscintigraphy. In ten DPI patients ilio-inguinal nodes were removed and in six PTI patients the regional lymph nodes draining the primary tumor site were removed. The specimens were carefully examined and the lymph nodes isolated. Each lymph node was weighed, inserted into a plastic test tube containing formalin, and

274

measured for ^{99m}Tc activity in an automatic sample-changing (NaI(T1)) well-counter.

5.2. Results

In the DPI patients the range of total percentage lymph node uptake after 4–6 hours was 0.5–5.9%, with a mean of 2.3%, whereas in the PTI patients the range was 0.0–5.6%, with a mean of 1.1%. The maximum activity uptake in a single lymph node the day after injection was found to be 0.75% (weight, 0.5 g). Lymph flow to ilio-inguinal nodes was shown in all the DPI patients. In the PTI patients, lymph flow to axilla and/or groin was shown in all but two.

Of 239 isolated lymph nodes, 29 were found to be tumor-involved. An activity uptake (>0.001%) was recorded in 17 of these nodes. Furthermore, the highest lymph node uptake was found in a node with metastatic disease in five of the 11 patients with lymph node metastases.

A correlation between the histological reports of the cancerous nodes and the activity uptake, as given in Figure 7, shows that several lymph nodes with microscopical metastases had high activity uptake. This was also found in some of the nodes that were massively tumor-involved.

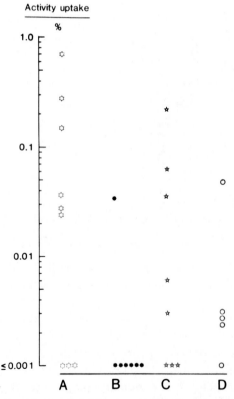

Figure 7. Correlation between uptake of activity and pathology of lymph nodes. A, Microscopical metastases; B, microscopical metastases with periglandular growth; C, massive metastases; D, unclassified.

The specific activity uptake was calculated and the results are given in Figure 8. The distribution of activity uptake in iliacal lymph nodes in the DPI patients was found to be log-normally distributed (Fig. 8A).

5.3. Discussion

The log-normal distribution of specific activity in the iliacal lymph nodes from the DPI patients indicates a complete saturation of the colloid particles. In the PTI patients no such distribution was found and the explanation for this may be that lymph flow to distant lymph nodes is smaller, thus giving an incomplete saturation

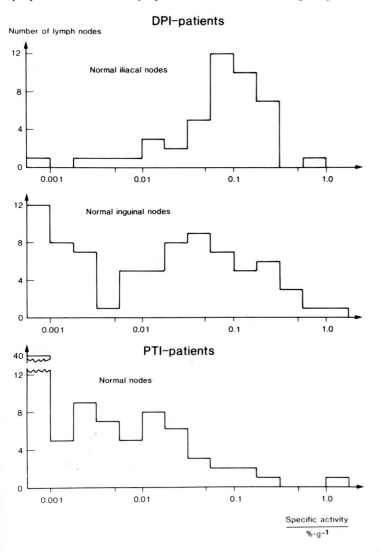

Figure 8. Distribution of specific activity of normal lymph nodes from patients injected dorsopedally (DPI) and peritumorally (PTI).

TABLE 5

Time for a 10% reduction of activity in the injection site after subcutaneous injection

Radiopharmaceutical	$T_{90\%}$(h)
$^{99m}TcSb_2S_3$	2.8
AlbuColl	2.8
$^{99m}Tc_2S_7$	a
ALBU-RES	7.5

[a] Only 1–2% outflow 5 h after administration.

of colloid particles. The occurrence of no or decreased activity uptake in some of the resected inguinal lymph nodes verifies that other areas, such as the lower trunk and perineum, are also drained by this nodal group. Almost all of the iliacal nodes show a complete saturation by colloid particles. This would be expected because these are secondary draining nodes.

No lymph node metastases have been found in areas not identified by lymphoscintigraphy during a follow-up period of 1–5 years.

In conclusion, lymphoscintigraphy with $^{99m}TcSb_2S_3$ in truncal melanoma patients reveals the lymphatic drainage from the primary tumour site when injections are made peritumorally. This information is of great importance if regional lymph node dissections are planned.

6. Dosimetry

6.1. Absorbed dose

Calculations of absorbed doses in injection sites, individual lymph nodes, gonads, liver and whole body have been made from data for 22 patients with primary malignant melanoma. The colloid, $^{99m}TcSb_2S_3$, was injected subcutaneously and investigated with lymphoscintigraphy (Bergqvist et al., 1982), as described in section 5.1.

Measurements at the injection site reveal that the tracer leaves the site with an approximately monoexponential outflow. The mean absorbed doses at the injection site for various final volumes are plotted in Figure 9, showing the rapid decrease of the absorbed dose with increasing final volume. The final activity volume was estimated to be about 10 cm³, giving a probable mean absorbed dose to the injection site of about 10 mGy/MBq ^{99m}Tc.

The maximum absorbed doses calculated for other tissues were: lymph nodes, 1 mGy/MBq; liver, 4 μGy/MBq; gonads, 20 μGy/MBq; and whole body, 5 μGy/MBq.

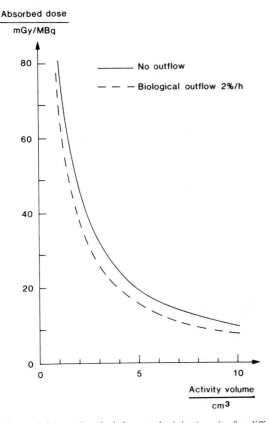

Figure 9. Mean absorbed dose at the injection site for different final activity volumes. Values are given for no outflow and for 2%/hour outflow of ^{99m}Tc.

6.2. Skin effect

Of particular interest is the estimation of the possible biological effects of different radionuclides in the skin after a subcutaneous injection. A method of assessing and comparing biological effects of ionizing radiation is provided by calculating the cumulative radiation effect (CRE); a concept often used in radiotherapy.

The CRE at the injection site was estimated when 40 MBq of different proposed radionuclides were injected subcutaneously under the assumption of similar biokinetics to the ^{99m}TcSb$_2$S$_3$ colloid. The final activity volume was assumed to be 10 cm^3 and calculations were made for the rate of outflow of 2%/h and for no outflow. The results are given in Figure 10.

7. General conclusions

Good quality control and the use of a well-defined colloid preparation constitute the basic criteria for any quantitative interpretation of lymphoscintigraphic investiga-

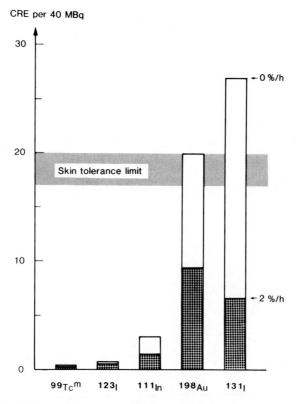

Figure 10. CRE at injection site for 40 MBq for different subcutaneously injected radionuclides, assuming a final activity volume of 10 cm³ and an outflow of activity of 0 and 2%/hour, respectively.

tions. The results presented in this chapter confirm earlier studies which showed that the optimal particle size for interstitial lymphoscintigraphy with inert colloids is of the order of tens of nanometers. Routine quality control of colloids can easily be performed with an microfiltration technique. However, electron microscopy, although more cumbersome, provides information about particle size as well as particle number.

The relation between activity and particle size can only be obtained with microfiltration. It should be remembered that the activity distribution obtained with this technique does not give the size distribution since the activity content in the particles may be related to either the particle volume or the particle surface area.

The eventual change in particle size in vivo must be known, if quantification of the in vivo kinetics is required.

In order to keep the absorbed dose at the injection site as low as possible, the outflow from the injection site should be fast. However, the cumulation of the released activity in other tissues should be small, thus preventing the background activity from affecting detection of activity in nearby lymph nodes.

The present chapter has been concerned only with radiocolloids that are incorporated in the lymph nodes. These radiopharmaceuticals give an anatomic outline of the lymphatics draining the injection site.

During the last years proposals have been made for the use of radioactively labeled antibodies for imaging metastases in the lymph nodes. This is being investigated by our group and is reported elsewhere (Strand et al., 1983). This new approach adds further possibilities for the evaluation of the lymphatic system.

Acknowledgements

This study was supported by grants from the John and Augusta Persson Foundation for Scientific Medical Research, Lund; Åke Wiberg Foundation, Stockholm; and the Swedish Medical Research Council, Project No. B83-17X-06573-01.

References

Bergqvist, L., Strand, S.-E., Persson, B., Hafström, L. and Jönsson, P.-E. (1982) J. Nucl. Med. 23, 698–705.

Bergqvist, L., Strand, S.-E. and Persson, B.R.R. (1983) Sem. Nucl. Med. 13, 9–19.

Bergqvist, L., Strand, S.-E., Hafström, L. and Jönsson, P.-E. (1984) Eur. J. Nucl. Med. 9, 129–135.

Chia, H.L. and De Schrijver, M. (1983) Eur. J. Nucl. Med. 8, 450–453.

Dornfest, B.S., Lenehan, P.F., Reilly, T.M., Mestler, G.E., Steigman, J. and Solomon, N.A. (1977) J. Reticuloendothel. Soc. 21, 317–329.

Dunson, G.L., Thrall, J.H., Stevenson, J.S. and Pinsky, S.M. (1973) Radiology 109, 387–392.

Dworkin, H.J. (1982) J. Nucl. Med. 23, 936–938.

Ege, G.N. and Warbick, A. (1979) Br. J. Radiol. 52, 124–129.

Frier, M. (1981) in Progress in Radiopharmacology (Cox, P.H., Ed.), Vol. 2, pp. 249–260, Elsevier/North-Holland, Amsterdam.

Gallagher, B.M., Delano, M.L., Watt, R. and Camin, L.L. (1980) J. Nucl. Med. 21, P36.

Gangon, W.F. (1979) Review of Medical Physiology, pp. 443–456, Lange, Los Altos.

Griffin, F.M.Jr., Griffin, J.A., Leider, J.E. and Silverstein, S.C. (1975) J. Exp. Med. 142, 1263–1282.

Kaplan, W.D., Davis, M.A. and Rose, C.M. (1979) J. Nucl. Med. 20, 933–937.

Strand, S.-E. and Persson, B.R.R. (1979) J. Nucl. Med. 20, 1038–1046.

Strand, S.-E., Persson, B., Christoffersson, J.O. and Knöös, T. (1981) in Progress in Radiopharmacology (Cox, P.H., Ed.), Vol. 2, pp. 231–248, Elsevier/North-Holland, Amsterdam.

Strand, S.-E., Bergqvist, L., Ingvar, C., Jönsson, P.-E., Brodin, T. and Sjögren, H.-O. (1983) in Radioimmunoimaging and Radioimmunotherapy (Rhodes, B.A. and Bruchiel, S.W., Eds.), pp. 307–322, Elsevier, New York.

Warbick, A., Chan, A.S.K. and Ege, G.N. (1978) in Proceedings of First International Symposium on Radiopharmacology, p. 55, Innsbruck.

Wilkins, D.J. and Myers, P.A. (1966) Br. J. Exp. Path. 47, 568–576.

Yoffey, J.M. and Courtice, F.C. (1970) Lymphatics, Lymph and the Lymphomyeloid Complex, pp. 519–522, Academic Press, London.

Zum Winkel (1972) Lymphologie mit Radionukliden, Verlag Hildegard Hoffman, Berlin.

Microspheres and Drug Therapy. Pharmaceutical, Immunological and Medical Aspects
edited by S.S. Davis, L. Illum, J.G. McVie and E. Tomlinson
© *1984, Elsevier Science Publishers B.V.*

Specific delivery of mitomycin C: Combined use of prodrugs and spherical delivery systems

Mitsuru Hashida and Hitoshi Sezaki

1. Introduction

The optimization of drug delivery and the resulting improvement in drug efficacy imply an efficient and selective delivery of a drug substance to its site of action and a reduction of the drug exposure of nontarget sites. This is the basic rationale for the concept of controlled drug delivery, that is, the use of systems and techniques for altering and controlling the absorption, blood levels, metabolism, organ distribution, and cellular uptake of pharmacologically active agents. In cancer chemotherapy, it seems particularly important to find ways to control the pharmacokinetic behaviour of the drug, since most anticancer agents show unselective cytotoxicity and severe side effects. Therefore, considerable research effort has been made to develop delivery systems for anticancer agents.

Among different approaches, the use of a physical device or the chemical transformation of a drug molecule into an inactive or latent form (prodrug design) appears to be promising for improving the delivery of anticancer agents. For the past decade, therefore, we have been engaged in studies on drug delivery systems for cancer from the viewpoints of utilization of physical devices such as emulsions (Hashida et al., 1977a, 1979; Yoshioka et al., 1982; Sezaki et al., 1982) and gelatin microspheres (Yoshioka et al., 1981), as well as the chemical modification of drug molecules (Hashida et al., 1978, 1981, 1983; Kojima et al., 1978, 1980; Kato et al., 1982; Sasaki et al., 1983a, b). Some of them have been investigated clinically and positive results have been achieved (Tanigawa et al., 1980; Sezaki et al., 1982).

Most attention has been focused on the spherical delivery systems, such as polymeric microparticles, liposomes and emulsions, due to their potential for delivering drugs to the desired site by parenteral administration, as discussed in other chapters of this book. The basic concept underlying the use of these delivery devices is that a sustained drug level can be obtained in a certain body compartment by balancing the drug-release characteristics of the delivery systems against the biological processes of drug elimination and metabolism. To achieve the goal of optimized drug delivery by using spherical carriers, a delivery system made up of carrier particles and the payload of drug should satisfy the following criteria: 1, it must include a sufficient amount of active drug in a latent manner until it reaches the site of action; 2, it must accumulate or remain at its desired site of action in the body; 3, it must release the drug at a suitable rate at the desired site; 4, it must have pharmaceutically acceptable characteristics with regard to stability, ease of sterilization and administration, and biodegradability. However, it is not easy to satisfy all these criteria for certain drugs incorporated into spherical carriers, since some drugs do not have suitable physicochemical properties for their incorporation into the carrier particles, nor for the control of their rate of release.

In order to accomplish ideal drug delivery, we tried to combine a sequence of pharmaceutical modifications in an integrated manner. On the basis of this consideration, we have designed several delivery systems for anticancer agents by combining physical and chemical approaches. In the present report, two representative delivery systems for the antitumour antibiotic, mitomycin C (MMC), will be described to demonstrate the potential utility of this approach.

2. Gelatin microspheres entrapping MMC in the form of a dextran conjugate

2.1. Preparation of gelatin microspheres and their biopharmaceutical characteristics

Microspheres containing the drug were prepared by a modified emulsifying method (Yoshioka et al., 1981). An aqueous solution of gelatin (30% w/v) and drug was added to sesame oil, with or without surfactants, and emulsified by vortex mixing or sonification at 70–80°C. The emulsions obtained were cooled to induce the complete gelation of spheres, diluted with cold acetone, and then filtered through a polycarbonate membrane. The spheres were hardened by chemical cross-linking with formaldehyde. The final products obtained were in the form of free-flowing powders of discrete spherical units. The size of spheres can be controlled by selecting the surfactant contents and the dispersion procedure in a primary emulsification process. Three kinds of spheres were prepared with mean diameters of 280 nm, 15 and 50 μm.

The in vivo behaviour of the microspheres after parenteral administration was examined in rats by incorporating ^{131}I-labeled human serum albumin into the microspheres as a tracer. Intramuscular injection of microspheres with a diameter of 280 nm resulted in their accumulation in the regional lymph nodes, suggesting their potential use as a lymphotropic carrier. Intravenous administration of these microspheres showed a predominant uptake by the reticuloendothelial system in the liver and spleen. On the other hand, microspheres with a diameter of 15 μm accumulated rapidly in the lung after intravenous injection (Yoshioka et al., 1981; Sezaki et al., 1982). Microspheres with a diameter of 50 μm were used in preliminary clinical trials. Transcatheter arterial infusion into the liver of microspheres incorporating MMC resulted in a prompt and persistent devascularization of the tumour region, indicating embolization of the small branches of the hepatic arteries. Significant therapeutic effects were observed in patients with a primary hepatic carcinoma.

In these spherical dosage forms, MMC was incorporated to extents between 15 and

60%, depending on the preparation conditions. On the other hand, MMC was released rapidly from smaller microspheres and more than 50% of the initial amount of MMC was recovered in the incubation medium at 30 minutes after the start of the incubation at pH 7.4 and 37°C. MMC was also released rapidly from microsphere systems with average diameters of both 15 and 50 μm, and it took about 2 hours for the release of 50% of the initially entrapped MMC. The relatively high water solubility and low molecular weight of MMC may be responsible for this phenomenon. The rapid release of MMC appears to be disadvantageous in supplying the tumour site with a sufficient amount of MMC as well as giving difficulties in the handling of the injections containing microspheres loaded with MMC.

2.2. Improvement of the entrapping efficiency and the release rate of MMC using macromolecular derivatives of MMC

In previous studies (Kojima et al., 1980; Kato et al., 1982), we developed a polymeric derivative of MMC, MMC-dextran conjugate (MMC-D), by coupling MMC to dextran employing ω-amino carboxylic acids as spacers (Fig. 1). MMC-D linked via ε-amino caproic acid (MMC-C6-D) by itself showed increased activities against various murine tumours following intraperitoneal administration (Hashida et al., 1981). Stability tests revealed that MMC-C6-D is more stable than free MMC against acid-catalysed degradation, and that MMC is released from the conjugate by a base-catalysed hydrolysis with a half-life of about 24 hours in a pH 7.4 phosphate buffer solution at 37°C. Pharmacokinetic analysis showed that MMC is also released from the conjugate in the body with a release rate similar to that of the in vitro release experiment. Thus, MMC-D is proved to act as a reservoir of MMC which behaves charac-

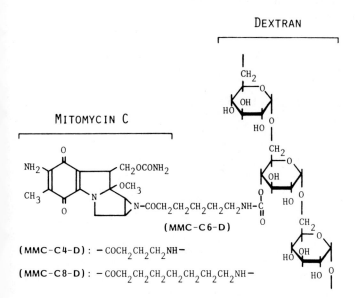

Figure 1. Chemical structures of mitomycin C-dextran conjugates with spacer arms of different lengths.

teristically as a macromolecule while supplying active drug in the body. Furthermore, MMC-D synthesized using spacers of different length, γ-aminobutylic acid (MMC-C4-D) and ω-aminocaprylic acid (MMC-C8-D), showed an alteration in the release rates depending on the length of the spacer, and the release half-lives were 10.8 and 42.8 hours, respectively.

Therefore, in order to improve the entrapping efficiency and to lower the release rate of MMC we attempted to incorporate MMC into microspheres in the form of the dextran conjugate. Since MMC-D is insoluble in acetone, unlike free MMC, most MMC was efficiently entrapped in the spheres as the conjugated form when MMC-D was incorporated into the microspheres. In contrast to the rapid release of free MMC from the microspheres, three kinds of MMC-D entrapped in microspheres showed a markedly slow release of MMC, which followed mono-exponential kinetics, with half-lives relatively similar to those of hydrolytic cleavage of the linkages between MMC and the spacers obtained under the same conditions (Fig. 2). Furthermore, no significant difference was observed in the release of MMC from microspheres of different sizes for which MMC was incorporated in the form of MMC-C6-D. These results indicate that the process of hydrolytic cleavage is a rate-limiting step in the release of MMC from microspheres incorporating MMC in the form of a macromolecular derivative. In this approach, dextran, the backbone of the conjugate, plays the role of an anchor which could hold MMC to the polymeric matrix of the microspheres. The in vivo experiments also proved the gradual release of MMC from dextran fixed in the spheres, because an enhanced accumulation and a subsequent slow disappearance of MMC from the lung were observed after the injection of microspheres (15 μm) containing MMC-C6-D. The possibility of enhancing the entrapment efficiency and controlling the release rate by combining chemical modifications of MMC with microspheres is demonstrated.

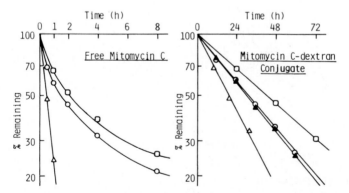

Figure 2. In vitro release of mitomycin C from microspheres of different sizes and entrapping free (left) or dextran-conjugated (right) mitomycin C. Left: microspheres with mean diameters of 280 nm (△), 15 μm (○), and 50 μm (□). Right: microspheres with a mean diameter of 15 μm entrapping MMC-C4-D(△), MMC-C6-D(○) and MMC-C8-D(□) and microspheres with a mean diameter of 280 nm entrapping MMC-C6-D(▲). Release was determined in pH 7.4 phosphate buffer solution maintained at 37°C.

3. Development of lipophilic prodrugs of MMC and their application to lipidic delivery systems

Recently, the use of lipid dispersion systems such as liposomes and oil/water (O/W) emulsions as carriers of antitumour drugs has been developed extensively and has attracted special interest in cancer chemotherapy (Gregoriadis, 1980; Patel and Ryman, 1981). A number of chemotherapeutic agents have been encapsulated in the lipidic carriers, and the abilities of these preparations in overcoming drug resistance (Kosloski et al., 1978), altering in vivo tissue distribution (Juliano and Stamp, 1978), reducing drug toxicities (Rahman et al., 1982; Forssen and Tökès, 1981), and prolonging retention in the injection site (Segal et al., 1975) have been demonstrated following systemic and local administration. However, there is a drawback to the use of certain drugs with these lipid dispersion systems, i.e., amphiphilic compounds such as MMC are poorly entrapped in these carrier systems while more lipophilic compounds can be incorporated efficiently in them. Although numerous attempts to improve the low entrapment efficiency have been made (Szoka and Papahadjopoulos, 1978; Fendler, 1980), by manipulating lipid compositions, buffer contents, or preparation procedures, no conclusive results have been reported for these standard pharmaceutical approaches. In the present study, an attempt has been made to overcome these difficulties by introducing chemical approaches to the design of lipidic delivery systems of MMC.

3.1. Development of lipophilic prodrugs of MMC

In order to increase the incorporation efficiency of MMC into liposomes or oil droplets of an O/W emulsion, MMC was derivatized to a more lipophilic form by linking it to lipidic disposable moieties. In Figure 3, the basic strategy for designing lipophilic prodrugs of MMC is represented. The process of prodrug design was divided into two parts: the selection of linkage structure ('X') and carrier moiety ('R') (Sasaki et al., 1983a,b). In the first step, studies were focused on the chemical stability and the enzymatic lability of the linkage (Sasaki et al., 1983c). The physicochemical properties, such as lipophilicity and lipid solubility, were examined for prodrugs having different disposable moieties. Parallel to these experiments, the pharmacological activities and biopharmaceutical properties of the prodrugs were examined. The structures and physicochemical properties of MMC prodrugs synthesized in the present study are summarized in Table 1.

In order to design the linkage structure between MMC and the disposable moiety, MMC was derivatized to more lipophilic forms by the introduction of a model lipophilic functional group, a benzene ring, via various linkages (II–VI). As shown in Table 1, they showed a relatively uniform increase in the lipophilicity due to the promoiety. Biological tests revealed that they exhibited characteristic antitumour activities after being regenerated to the parent drug. A close relationship was observed between their activities and chemical or enzymatic labilities. Among the five linkage structures, the alkoxycarbonyl-type linkage (carbamate linkage, compound VI) was

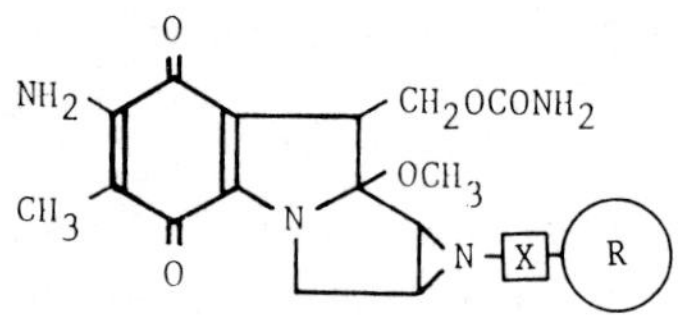

(1) Linkage structure * X *

   a. Chemical stability(stability in dosage form)

   b. Lability: enzymatic or chemical conversion

     (regeneration of mitomycin C)

(2) Carrier moiety * R *

   a. Lipophilicity, lipid and water solubility,

     lipid interaction (entrapment, release rate)

(3) Other aspects

   a. Antitumor activity

   b. Pharmacokinetic fate

Figure 3. Basic consideration for designing lipophilic prodrug of mitomycin C.

the most advantageous with regard to chemical stability and biological lability, i.e., compound VI was more stable than MMC and was readily converted to MMC by rat plasma.

Based on these observations, alkoxycarbonyl-type prodrugs with different pro-moieties (compounds VI–X) were subsequently synthesized and subjected to further examination. As shown in Table 1, these prodrugs showed increased lipophilicities depending on the property of the pro-moieties: in compounds VII, VIII and IX, the partition coefficient between chloroform and water increased from 183 to 29,200 with an increase in the alkyl chain length from three to nine. The possibility of controlling lipophilicity by changing the pro-moieties was thus demonstrated. These compounds (except for X) were converted to MMC by plasma and had significant antitumour activities against P388 leukemia (Sasaki et al., 1983c).

3.2. Incorporation of lipophilic prodrugs of MMC into liposomes and O/W emulsions
The lipophilic derivatives of MMC listed in Table 1 were then used in lipidic dosage forms, such as liposomes and O/W emulsions. Liposomes were prepared by the method of Bangham and Horne (1964) employing egg phosphatidylcholine (PC). Chloroform containing egg PC and the drug was evaporated under vacuum to give a thin lipid film. The dry lipid film was then suspended in a saline solution by vortex shaking, and resulting suspension was disrupted sonically at 0°C for 3 minutes under a nitrogen atmosphere. An electron microscopic observation revealed that the liposomes obtained kept a multilamellar structure, even when lipophilic prodrugs such

TABLE 1

Structures and physicochemical properties of lipophilic prodrugs of mitomycin C

Compound	X	R	Partition coefficient		Solubility at 37°C		
			PC_{CHCl_3}	PC_{oct}	Water (mM)	Sesame oil (mM)	Hexane (µM)
I, mitomycin C (MMC)	-H		0.26	0.41	2.730	0.0180	0.0234
II, benzyl MMC	-CH$_2$-	⬡	231.9	38.55	1.493	4.165	0.726
III, benzoyl MMC	-CO-	⬡	522.9	77.94	0.0096	0.0484	0.0198
IV, benzylcarbonyl MMC	-COCH$_2$-	⬡	163.1	34.48	2.235	0.741	0.209
V, benzoyloxymethyl MMC	-CH$_2$OCO-	⬡	–	–	–	–	0.471
VI, benzyloxycarbonyl MMC	-COOCH$_2$-	⬡	1643	113.0	0.528	3.291	0.415
VII, propyloxycarbonyl MMC	-COO-	-C$_3$H$_7$	183.7	32.73	0.333	0.104	0.02
VIII, pentyloxycarbonyl MMC	-COO-	-C$_5$H$_{11}$	1785	279.2	0.590	3.48	2.02
IX, nonyloxycarbonyl MMC	-COO-	-C$_9$H$_{19}$	29200	3637	0.0003	15.17	0.304
X, cholesteryloxycarbonyl MMC	-COO-	-C$_{27}$H$_{45}$	8216	7606	0.0003	12.10	6.610

as compound IX were incorporated into them. An O/W emulsion was prepared with 4 volumes of sesame oil containing drugs and 6 volumes of aqueous phase containing a dissolved surfactant. Emulsification was carried out by sonication.

In Table 2, the entrapment of five lipophilic prodrugs and the original MMC in the liposomes and oil droplets of the O/W emulsion are summarized. The entrapment efficiency was calculated by determining the drug concentrations in the outer aqueous phase obtained by ultrafiltration. All prodrugs were incorporated in these carrier systems to relatively high extents depending on their physicochemical properties, whereas MMC was scarcely incorporated.

Figure 4 shows the extent of entrapment of prodrugs at different lipid volume fractions. The extent of entrapment is expressed as the apparent distribution ratio of the drugs between lipid and aqueous phases (DR_{app}). As shown in these figures, the plots of DR_{app} against lipid volume fractions give straight lines, suggesting that drug incorporation occurred by simple partition between suspended lipid and aqueous phase. Good correlationship was observed between the slopes of these lines, which correspond approximately to partition coefficients between lipid and aqueous phase, and partition coefficients of these compounds between organic solvents and water. These results suggest that the entrapment efficiencies can be estimated from partition coefficients obtained in the usual way.

In order to determine the release properties of the prodrugs from liposomes or an O/W emulsion, the dosage forms were dialysed against 14 times their volume of phosphate buffer (pH 7.4) and the amount of drug in the outer compartment was determined. The amounts of drug recovered in the outer compartment at 1 hour after the start of experiment are summarized in Table 2. These results indicate that compounds having fairly high lipophilicities (such as IX and X) are incorporated well into these dosage forms. In comparison to these results, compound IX showed relatively rapid release from liposomes and subsequent conversion in a medium containing rat plasma. Therefore, it can be concluded that drugs must have rather higher lipo-

TABLE 2

Entrapment and release of mitomycin C prodrugs in liposomes and an O/W emulsion

Compound	Liposome		O/W emulsion	
	Entrap (%)	Release (% in 1 hour)	Entrap (%)	Release (% in 1 hour)
I	0.1	87.2	1.0	93.2
II	33.6	84.8	97.3	30.7
VI	38.2	72.2	98.3	15.2
VIII	61.9	83.5	98.6	14.1
IX	99.9	0.1	99.1	0.1
X	99.9	0.1	99.1	0.1

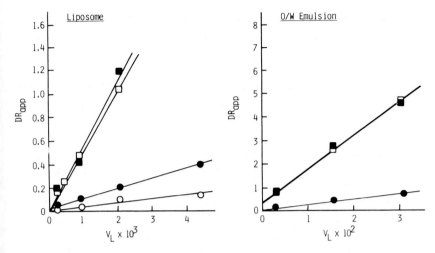

Figure 4. Relation between apparent lipid/water distribution ratio (DR_{app}) of each drug and the volume fraction of the lipid phase in liposomes or an O/W emulsion. ○, Mitomycin C; ●, benzylcarbonyl mitomycin C (IV); ■, benzyloxycarbonyl mitomycin C (VI); □, pentyloxycarbonyl mitomycin C (VIII). Formulations were prepared by changing the lipid content, and the lipid/water distribution ratio was calculated by determining the drug concentrations in the water phase obtained by ultrafiltration.

philicity, probably with chloroform to water partition coefficients of more than 1000, in order to be transported in the body with the carrier. Prodrugs incorporated in both dosage forms exhibited significant antitumour activities against P388 leukemia, except for compound X (Sasaki et al., 1984).

3.3. Specific delivery of MMC incorporated in liposomes and an O/W emulsion in the form of lipophilic prodrug

The potential utility of lipidic dosage forms incorporating MMC in the form of lipophilic prodrugs has been evaluated in rats. Compound IX, nonyloxycarbonyl MMC, was chosen as a representative of a prodrug which is entrapped in these formulations to a high extent. In these experiments, compound IX was assayed by HPLC after extraction by chloroform from biological samples. MMC was determined by a bioassay using *Escherichia coli* B as a test organism. The movements of liposomes and oil droplets were traced using ^{14}C-labeled dipalmitoyl PC or ^{14}C-labeled tripalmitin as a tracer.

Intravenous injection of IX dissolved in DMSO showed rapid conversion of IX to MMC in the body. On the contrary, slow conversion was observed when IX was administered in the form of liposomes and an O/W emulsion. These results indicated that IX was first retained in these carriers and then released gradually, followed by subsequent rapid conversion to MMC in plasma. The wide applicability of these systems for the delivery of MMC to various kinds of target site is thus suggested. In the present discussion, the utility of these combined systems as lymphotropic or local sustained-release delivery systems is demonstrated.

In cancer chemotherapy, a sufficient supply of anticancer agents to the lymphatic system seems to offer a promising means of preventing lymph node metastasis. Therefore, it is vitally necessary to develop a potential drug delivery system which can deliver anticancer agents selectively into the lymphatic system. In previous investigations, various kinds of emulsion formulations were adopted as local drug delivery systems (Hashida et al., 1977a; Sezaki et al., 1982) and an improvement of the lymphatic transfer of anticancer agents, such as 5-fluorouracil (Hashida et al., 1977c) and bleomycin (Hashida et al., 1979; Tanigawa et al., 1980), was successfully achieved. In the same manner, the efficiency of liposomes and O/W emulsions containing the lipophilic prodrug of MMC as a lymphotropic drug delivery system was evaluated, using the thigh muscle of rat as a model injection site.

In Figure 5, the disappearance of IX from the thigh muscle after intramuscular injection in the form of liposomes and an O/W emulsion is shown with that of the lipidic carriers. The absorption profiles of free MMC administered in the form of aqueous solution and lipidic dosage forms are illustrated for comparison. MMC was rapidly absorbed from the injection site, regardless of dosage forms. On the contrary, IX was retained in the injection site for a considerably longer period when administered in the form of liposomes or an O/W emulsion. More retarded absorption was recognized for lipids in carrier systems, as shown in Figure 5. These results suggest the persistent retention of these carrier systems in the muscle and the gradual release of IX from the carrier particles. The use of these formulations as local sustained-release delivery systems is thus demonstrated.

In the same experiment, the transfer of drugs and carrier lipids to the regional lymph nodes was examined and the results are shown in Figure 6. Immediately after injection, free MMC arrived at the regional lymph nodes, but then disappeared rapidly and no active MMC was detected at 15 minutes after injection, regardless

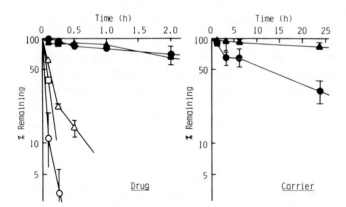

Figure 5. Disappearance of drug and carrier lipid from the thigh muscle after intramuscular injection in rats. Drug: □, mitomycin C with saline solution; ○, mitomycin C with liposome; △, mitomycin C with O/W emulsion; ●, nonyloxycarbonyl mitomycin C (IX) with liposome; ▲, nonyloxycarbonyl mitomycin C with O/W emulsion. Carrier: ●, liposome (^{14}C-labeled dipalmitoylphosphatidylcholine); ▲, O/W emulsion (^{14}C-labeled tripalmitin).

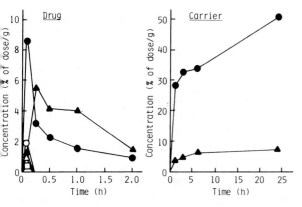

Figure 6. Regional lymph node concentration of drug and lipid carrier after the intramuscular injection of liposomes and an O/W emulsion into rats. Drug: □, mitomycin C with saline solution; ○, mitomycin C with liposome; △, mitomycin C with O/W emulsion; ●, nonyloxycarbonyl mitomycin C (IX) with liposome; ▲, nonyloxycarbonyl mitomycin C with O/W emulsion. Carrier: ●, liposome (^{14}C-labeled dipalmitoylphosphatidylcholine); ▲, O/W emulsion (^{14}C-labeled tripalmitin).

of dosage forms. On the other hand, a remarkable accumulation of liposomal lipid was observed in the lymph nodes, and the O/W emulsion labeled with ^{14}C-labeled tripalmitin gave a similar picture. IX also appeared in the lymph nodes at the early stage after injection and then concentrations decreased gradually, but IX still remained there at 2 hours after injection. It was suggested from these results that liposomes or oil droplets in an O/W emulsion were taken up by the lymphatic vessels and accumulated in the lymph nodes. The lipophilic prodrug IX was liberated from these carriers in the lymph nodes, and probably converted to MMC by enzymes. The usefulness of delivery systems designed by combining lipidic carrier devices with a lipophilic prodrug approach as lymphotropic delivery systems for preventing lymphatic metastasis of cancer was suggested.

4. Other approaches combining physical and chemical modifications

In previous reports (Hashida et al., 1977b, 1978; Kojima et al., 1978), anticancer agents such as MMC and cytosine arabinoside were coupled to agarose beads activated by cyanogen bromide. Both drugs were slowly released from the beads in vitro and in vivo. Significant antitumour activities were obtained by intraperitoneal administration of these conjugates in mice bearing experimental tumours. Based on these findings, it was concluded that antitumour agents-agarose beads conjugates can be used as injectable implants for local cancer chemotherapy.

The stable incorporation of bleomycin into the inner aqueous phase of an O/W emulsion was achieved by using complex formation between bleomycin and the polyanionic macromolecule, dextran sulfate (Muranishi et al., 1979).

5. Summary

In this chapter, we have reviewed our investigations on the development of drug delivery systems of anticancer agents which were designed on the basis of a combined utilization of physical devices and chemical modifications. In Figure 7 the basic concept and mechanism of drug delivery in the present approach are illustrated schematically. In order to improve entrapment efficiency in lipidic carriers, MMC is first derivatized to the highly lipophilic prodrug and then incorporated into these carriers. Following the administation of various dose systems, MMC was delivered to the target site, such as lymph node, according to the property of carrier particle. In the target site, the lipophilic prodrug of MMC is released from the lipidic carriers in accordance with their lipophilicity (rate-limiting step). The released prodrug is promptly converted and the regenerated MMC should exhibit its cytotoxic action. In the release of MMC from microspheres containing the MMC-dextran conjugate, the rate of chemical hydrolysis of the linkage between MMC and the spacer-introduced dextran plays a role as the rate-limiting step and the pro-moiety, i.e., dextran, may be left in the sphere. Thus, chemical modifications can be utilized for designing drug delivery systems.

The integrated approach using both physical and chemical modifications seems to offer a promising future in the optimization of drug delivery. The prodrug manipula-

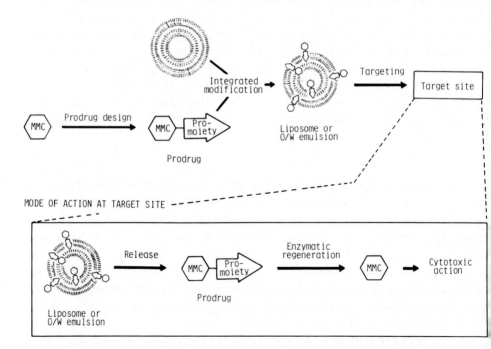

Figure 7. Schematic model showing the basic concept and mechanism of drug-delivery systems designed using a combination of physical device with chemical modification.

tion can be used as another variable in the design of carriers with controlled drug release and may expand the applicability of existing dosage forms.

References

Bangham, A.D. and Horne, R.W. (1964) J. Mol. Biol. 8, 660–668.

Fendler, J.H. (1980) in Liposomes in Biological Systems (Gregoriadis, G. and Allison, A.C., Eds.) pp. 87–100, John Wiley & Sons, New York.

Forssen, E.A. and Tökès, Z.A. (1981) Proc. Natl. Acad. Sci. U.S.A. 78, 1873–1877.

Gregoriadis, G. (1980) Nature 283, 814–815.

Hashida, M., Egawa, M., Muranishi, S. and Sezaki, H. (1977a) J. Pharmacokin. Biopharm. 5, 225–239.

Hashida, M., Kojima, T., Takahashi, Y., Muranishi, S. and Sezaki, H. (1977b) Chem. Pharm. Bull. 25, 225–239.

Hashida, M., Muranishi, S. and Sezaki, H. (1977c) Chem. Pharm. Bull. 25, 2410–2418.

Hashida, M., Kojima, T., Muranishi, S. and Sezaki, H. (1978) Gann 69, 839–843.

Hashida, M., Muranishi, S., Sezaki, H., Tanigawa, N., Satomura, K. and Hikasa, Y. (1979) Int. J. Pharm. 2, 245–256.

Hashida, M., Kato, A., Kojima, T., Muranishi, S., Sezaki, H., Tanigawa, N., Satomura, K. and Hikasa, Y. (1981) Gann 72, 226–234.

Hashida, M., Takakura, Y., Matsumoto, S., Sasaki, H., Kato, A., Kojima, T., Muranishi, S. and Sezaki, H. (1983) Chem. Pharm. Bull. 31, 2055–2063.

Juliano, R.L. and Stamp, D. (1978) Biochem. Pharmacol. 27, 21–27.

Kato, A., Takakura, Y., Hashida, M., Kimura, T. and Sezaki, H. (1982) Chem. Pharm. Bull. 30, 2951–2957.

Kojima, T., Hashida, M., Muranishi, S. and Sezaki, H. (1978) Chem. Pharm. Bull. 26, 1818–1824.

Kojima, T., Hashida, M., Muranishi, S. and Sezaki, H. (1980) J. Pharm. Pharmacol. 32, 30–34.

Kosloski, M.J., Rosen, F., Milholland, R.J. and Papahadjopoulos, D. (1978) Cancer Res. 38, 2848–2853.

Muranishi, S., Takahashi, Y., Hashida, M. and Sezaki, H. (1979) J. Pharm. Dyn. 2, 383–390.

Patel, H.M. and Ryman, B.E. (1981) in Liposomes: From Physical Structure to Therapeutic Applications (Knight, C.G., Ed.), pp. 409–436, Elsevier, Amsterdam.

Rahman, A., More, N. and Schein, P.S. (1982) Cancer Res. 42, 1817–1825.

Sasaki, H., Fukumoto, M., Hashida, M., Kimura, T. and Sezaki, H. (1983a) Chem. Pharm. Bull. 31, 4083–4090.

Sasaki, H., Mukai, E., Hashida, M., Kimura, T. and Sezaki, H. (1983b) Int. J. Pharmaceut. 15, 49–59.

Sasaki, H., Mukai, E., Hashida, M., Kimura, T. and Sezaki, H. (1983c) Int. J. Pharmaceut. 15, 61–71.

Sasaki, H., Takakura, Y., Hashida, M., Kimura, T. and Sezaki, H. (1984) J. Pharm. Dyn. 7, 120–130.

Segal, A.W., Gregoriadis, G. and Black, C.D.V. (1975) Clin. Sci. Mol. Med. 49, 99–106.

Sezaki, H., Hashida, M. and Muranishi, S. (1982) in Optimization of Drug Delivery (Bundgaard, H., Hansen, A.B. and Kofod, H., Eds.), pp. 241–255, Munksgaard, Copenhagen.

Szoka, F.C. and Papahadjopoulos, D. (1978) Proc. Natl. Acad. Sci. U.S.A. 75, 4194–4198.

Tanigawa, N., Satomura, K., Hikasa, Y., Hashida, M., Muranishi, S. and Sezaki, H. (1980) Surgery 87, 147–152.

Yoshioka, T., Hashida, M., Muranishi, A. and Sezaki, H. (1981) Int. J. Pharmaceut. 8, 131–141.

Yoshioka, T., Ikeuchi, K., Hashida, M., Muranishi, S. and Sezaki, H. (1982) Chem. Pharm. Bull. 30, 1408–1415.

Microspheres and Drug Therapy. Pharmaceutical, Immunological and Medical Aspects
edited by S.S. Davis, L. Illum, J.G. McVie and E. Tomlinson
© 1984, Elsevier Science Publishers B.V.

CHAPTER 9

Drug entrapment within native albumin beads

Theodore D. Sokoloski and Garfield P. Royer

1. General objective

The use of cross-linked albumin in systems designed for the parenteral delivery of drugs has been explored along several avenues. The systems can probably be used for oral delivery, but whether or not they would be able to compete economically with other methods is uncertain. In the search for a delivery system for parenteral use it is desirable to be able to engineer a device that has an easily modified and controlled release of drug. Another, and perhaps more challenging, problem is to give the system the capability of delivering a drug to a tissue target to maximize effectiveness and/or minimize side effects. Cross-linked albumin delivery systems have the potential to meet both objectives: controlled release and tissue targeting. Cross-linked albumin delivery systems seem particularly advantageous since they utilize a natural product, albumin, which, if not altered to any significant extent (particularly its surface), should result in a product that is both biocompatible and biodegradable.

2. Cross-linking mechanisms

Intra- and intermolecular cross-linking of albumin molecules can occur via either heat treatment or chemical reaction, or a combination of both. Cross-linking by heat treatment occurs through the formation of lysinoalanine, N-(DL-2 amino-2-carboxy-ethyl)-L-lysine. The heat treatment approach is not discussed in this chapter. The method used by us and some others is the milder chemical cross-linking approach, which involves the ε-amino groups of lysine residues making up a part of the primary structure of albumin. There are in the vicinity of 50 lysines per 100,000 molecular weight of albumin.

2.1. Active esters

Active esters, such as ethyleneglycol-bis-succinimidyl succinate (I) or dithio-bis-succinimidyl succinate (II), were used by Abdella et al., (1979) as cross-linkers. Although their precise mechanism of action is not extensively studied, it is presumed that the active ester on either end of the molecule forms an amide with the amino function of a lysine in a straightforward manner. The assumption that this reaction is straightforward is undoubtedly tenuous in light of what follows. Some active esters, such

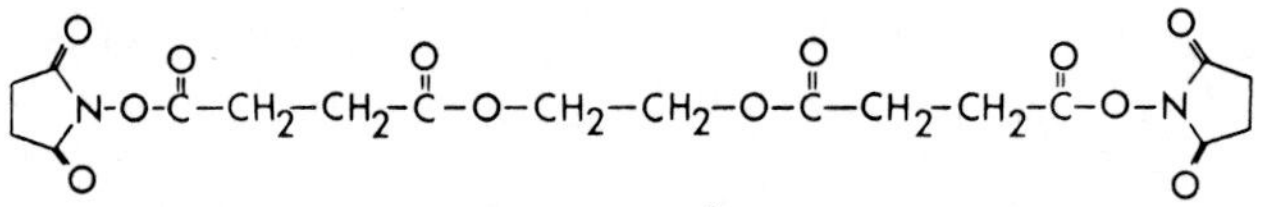

I

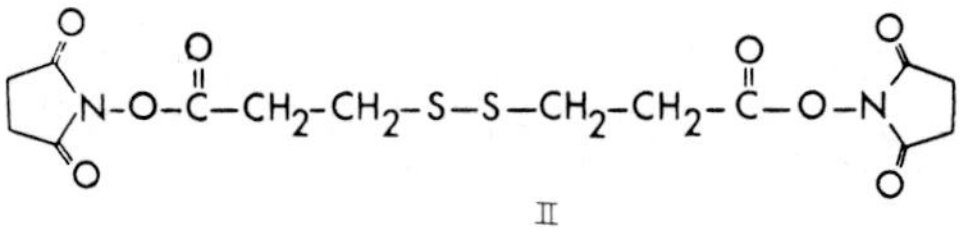

II

as I and II, have amphiphilic properties that make them attractive in the production of certain delivery systems, such as in the capsule type discussed later.

2.2. Glutaraldehyde

The most widely used cross-linking agents for protein are aldehydes, with the five-carbon dialdehyde glutaraldehyde being particularly effective. Aqueous solutions of this dialdehyde are found to contain free glutaraldehyde (III), the cyclic hemiacetal of its hydrate (IV), and oligomers of the hemiacetal (V) (Korn et al. 1972).

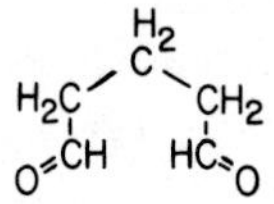

III

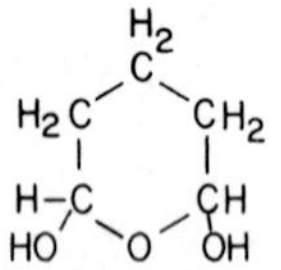

IV 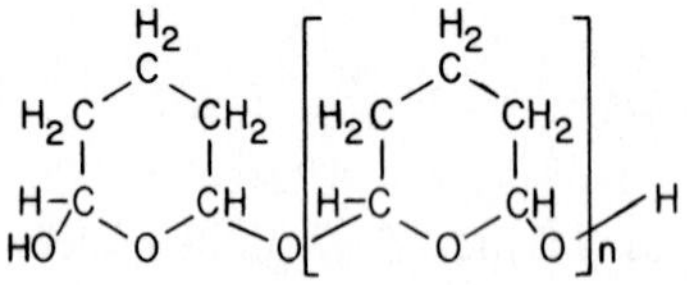   V

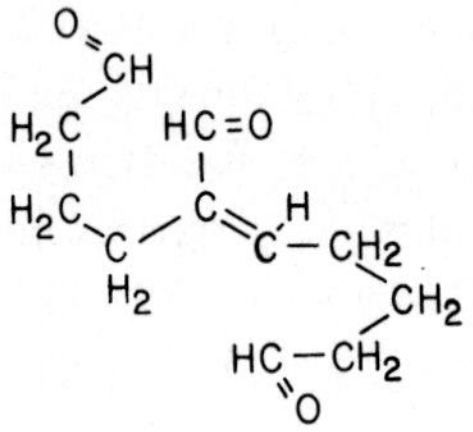

VI

Glutaraldehyde is the most efficient cross-linking agent presently used. Unfortunately, the mechanism of its interaction with protein is quite complex, and as a consequence its reactivity is not yet clearly defined. The interaction of the aldehyde with the amino groups of lysine is not a simple Schiff's base addition because the products formed are extremely stable. One explanation for this unusual stability was offered by Richards and Knowles (1968) who speculated that an α-β unsaturated aldehyde such as VI could exist in aqueous glutaraldehyde solution as a result of condensation. An aldol condensate of this type could react with an amine and then undergo a Michael rearrangement to form a stable product, as depicted in Scheme 1.

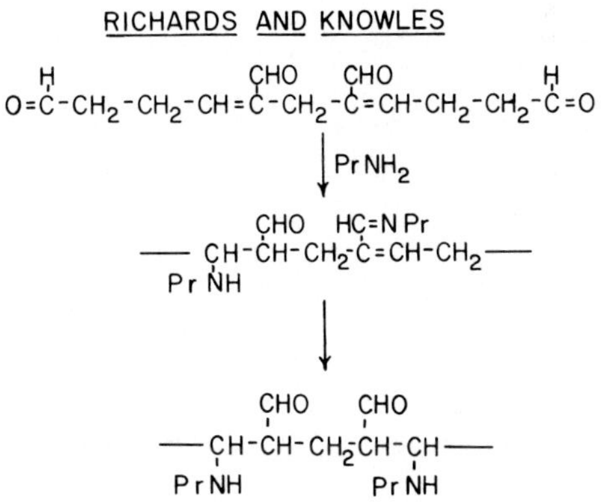

RICHARDS AND KNOWLES

$$O=\overset{H}{\underset{}{C}}-CH_2-CH_2-CH=\overset{CHO}{\underset{}{C}}-CH_2-\overset{CHO}{\underset{}{C}}=CH-CH_2-CH_2-\overset{H}{\underset{}{C}}=O$$

$\downarrow$ Pr NH$_2$

$$\underset{Pr\ NH}{\overset{CHO}{\underset{}{C}}H}-\overset{}{C}H-CH_2\overset{HC=N\,Pr}{\underset{}{C}}=CH-CH_2\underline{}$$

$\downarrow$

$$\underline{}\underset{Pr\,NH}{\overset{CHO}{\underset{}{C}}H}-\overset{}{C}H-CH_2\underset{Pr\,NH}{\overset{CHO}{\underset{}{C}}H}-\overset{}{C}H\underline{}$$

Scheme 1

Hardy et al., (1979) speculated it is not necessary to invoke the formation of an α-β unsaturated aldehyde and that the physical evidence offered by Richards and Knowles supporting its presence could be explained by the formation of a pyridinium compound resulting from oxidative cyclization of a Schiff base adduct.

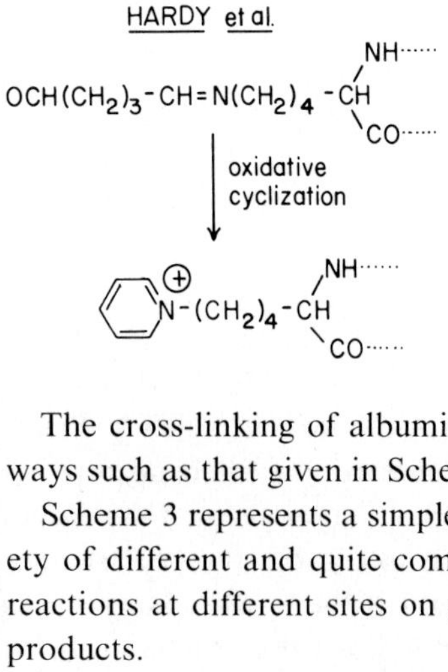

HARDY et al.

$$OCH(CH_2)_3-CH=N(CH_2)_4-\overset{\overset{\displaystyle NH\cdots}{|}}{\underset{\underset{\displaystyle CO\cdots}{|}}{C}H}$$

$\downarrow$ oxidative cyclization

Scheme 2

The cross-linking of albumin by glutaraldehyde might then occur through pathways such as that given in Scheme 3.

Scheme 3 represents a simple pathway and it goes without saying that a wide variety of different and quite complex structures are possible through similar types of reactions at different sites on glutaraldehyde condensates and amino acid addition products.

Lubig et al. (1981) suggest that monomeric glutaraldehyde reacts with protein to give intermediate N-alkyl-2,6-dihydroxypiperidines. Intramolecular dehydration leads to the corresponding N-alkyl-1,4-dihydro-pyridines. The latter can form pyridinium compounds. Condensation of the cyclic monohydrate of glutaraldehyde and N-alkyl-2,6-dihydroxy-piperidines give linear polymeric cross-links containing α-oxo-N-alkylpiperidine salts. These reactions are presented in Scheme 4.

It would appear that the scheme suggested by Lubig et al. would encompass the

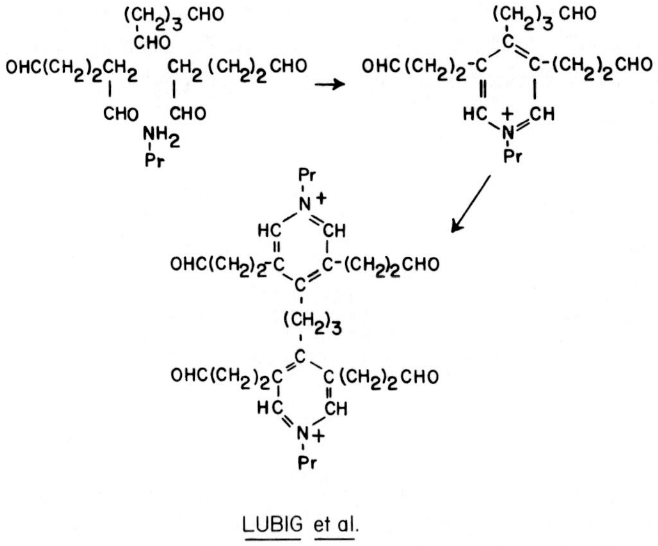

Scheme 3

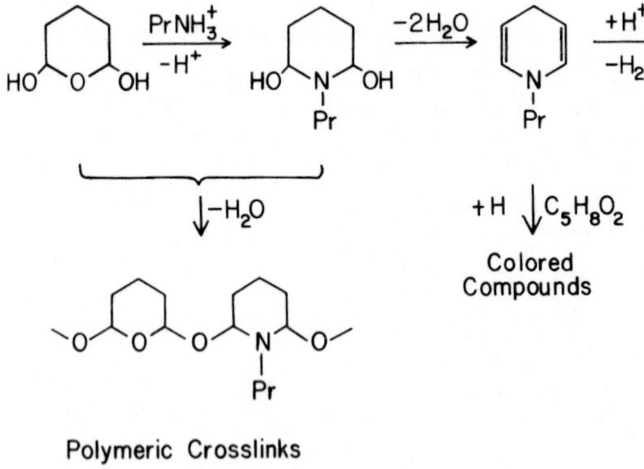

LUBIG et al.

Polymeric Crosslinks

Scheme 4

mechanisms offered by Hardy et al. and by Richards and Knowles. Scheme 4 indicates a pH dependence of the reaction. However complicated, the mechanism of action of cross-linking agents with proteins is well worth studying because, if the nature and extent of the cross-linking can be controlled, it is likely that the performance of the delivery system can be better engineered, since it is the cross-linking that is absolutely essential to the successful formulation and biological usefulness of such delivery systems.

3. Delivery systems

Several different approaches have been used in the design of drug delivery systems where chemical cross-linking is the basic reaction involved. Four of these systems will be described. Those methods that involve preparation of microspheres utilizing heat coagulation (110–165°C) or heat coagulation followed by 'curing' with a chemical cross-linking agent will not be discussed. Examples of the heat coagulation method can be found in the work of Widder et al. (1979, 1981). In the four systems to be described, one results in a hollow and initially empty albumin cross-linked ghost, another results in a capsule with drug inside, and the remaining two result in solid beads in which drug is embedded. The ghost, capsule, and one of the beads (Longo et al., 1982) came about by a cross-linking reaction that occurs primarily at a surface or interface. The other bead system developed in our laboratories (Lee et al., 1981; Royer et al., 1983) comes about through a cross-linking reaction that essentially is homogeneous throughout the solid particle.

3.1. Ghost

In the formation of a ghost (Lee, 1981), albumin is first absorbed on the surface of an inorganic particle (silica or aluminum oxide particles) and then cross-linked. Following this, the core is dissolved away and what remains is a hollow balloon-like structure, which presumably might then be loaded with drug. Typical reaction conditions consist of 1 g of very small silica beads suspended in a 3% serum albumin solution. The beads are separated and dried in a desiccator. These coated beads are then treated with an aqueous glutaraldehyde solution. Excess glutaraldehyde can be removed by successive additions of sodium borohydride. The structures are washed and then the silica core is leached using normal sodium hydroxide solution. Aluminium oxide can also be used as the core. After the cross-linked shell is formed, the aluminium oxide can be removed using dilute acid. One intriguing aspect of this delivery system approach is that it is possible to use not only different sized cores but different shaped ones as well that conceivably could result in systems having different shape-related release patterns. The ghosts behave very much like a semipermeable membrane: they swell in water and shrink in salt solution. Amino acid analysis shows that cross-linking consumes all of the lysines present and three molecules of histidine. In the formation of any cross-linked albumin system it seems axiomatic that the structure of the protein should not be altered to an extent where the delivery system is essentially not recognized and is rejected by the body. The loss of lysine residues and three histidines may not in itself lead to a toxic reaction. It is found, however, that the leaching of the core with sodium hydroxide affects threonine and serine components as well, giving rise to some concern as to whether the protein has been significantly changed. Trypsin has no effect on the ghost and α-chymotrypsin (1 mg/ml) digests the structure in 3 hours, suggesting that the ghost will be biodegradable. Attempts have been made by us to entrap materials such as enzymes and norgestrel by alternatively shrinking and swelling the ghosts or by using organic solvents. All attempts failed. It appears that the membrane may not be stable enough to endure such manipulation, and using active esters as cross-linking agents is no advantage.

3.2. Capsule

In the preparation of a cross-linked serum albumin capsule, use is made of an oil in water emulsion (Lee, 1981). The aqueous phase contains the albumin and the internal oil phase contains the cross-linking agent (active esters in this system) together with drug in solution or suspension. The active ester agents are excellent candidates for the capsular delivery approach since they have some surface-active character. This is important since what happens in these systems is a migration of the cross-linking agent to the interface, where it reacts with serum albumin to form a cohesive membrane. One other attractive feature about serum albumin in the preparation of capsules is that it is compatible with as much as 40% methanol in water. The use of methanol in the external phase decreases the polarity of water and might foster migration of the cross-linking agent to the interface. A typical formulation uses chloroform as the internal phase containing cross-linking agent (0.1%) and drug. In one system norgestrel was the drug used and it, of course, is chloroform-soluble. The external phase consists of 5% serum albumin in a 40% methanol solution. The capsules form spontaneously. Their size is determined by the size of the emulsified particle. The capsules are easily separated and the chloroform can be removed, leaving drug crystals inside the capsule.

It is apparently necessary to use a high molar ratio of amino groups to cross-linking agent (8:1) in order to minimise linkage between capsules to form aggregated structures. The use of such a high ratio results in a relatively thin membrane that may not withstand syringing. However, because of the fewer amino groups that would be modified, the resulting capsule would probably be quite biocompatible and biodegradable. The capsule may also offer an added advantage of providing a zero-order release, and appears to warrant further investigation.

3.3. Beads via surface linking

Longo et al. (1982) have prepared bead-like albumin microspheres using polymeric dispersing agents. The resulting structures are apparently solid spheres, even though the cross-linking reaction is concentrated at an interface. In the preparation of their microspheres, aqueous serum albumin is dispersed in a 25–30% solution of poly-methylmethacrylate or polyoxyethylene-polyoxypropylene copolymer in a non-polar solvent or solvent mixture (chloroform or chloroform/toluene). A solution of glutaraldehyde in toluene or chloroform is added to the dispersion to effect cross-linking (5–6 hours). After cross-linking is completed, 2-aminoethanol or amino acetic acid is added to cap free aldehyde groups on the surface, and the microspheres are then washed. Longo et al. visualized several advantages in their method. A major one is that the microspheres are hydrophilic in nature, and thus would have a lowered propensity for aggregation. Another advantage they see is that there is a relatively high concentration of aldehyde functionality on the surface (Fig. 1a), which they feel facilitates a variety of chemical modifications, including further enhancing hydrophilicity and antibody or enzyme attachment. It remains to be seen if microspheres with such a high concentration of surface modification will remain biocompatible and biodegradable.

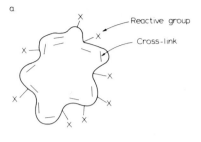

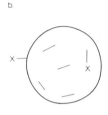

Figure 1. Representation of the nature of albumin beads resulting from interfacial cross-linking (a) and by internal cross-linking (b). From Royer et al. (1983).

3.4. Beads via internally homogeneous linking

The formulation of a cross-linked albumin bead delivery system has given us our greatest success in comparison with the ghosts and capsules discussed earlier. In our method of forming a bead, cross-linking is not concentrated on the surface of the particle and the procedures used are remarkably simple (Lee et al., 1981; Royer et al., 1983). In addition, there is close to a quantitative entrapment of added drug. A water in oil emulsion is used in this system, with the size of the dispersed internal phase dictating the size of the finished bead.

Figure 2 is a simple representation of the procedure. The internal phase consists of a cooled (4°C) albumin solution with drug (in solution or suspension) and glutaraldehyde. The ingredients are rapidly mixed. The low temperature slows the reaction between aldehyde and protein. This aqueous phase is rapidly added to the oil phase, which is at room temperature. Spontaneous emulsification results and analysis shows that cross-linking is essentially completed in 10 minutes. The dispersion is allowed to cure for 1 hour. The resulting bead is visualised as having linkages occurring homogeneously throughout the bead (Fig. 1b), as opposed to those resulting from the procedure of Longo et al. (1982) (Fig. 1a). A typical formulation where no surfactants are used consists of drug and 200 mg of albumin in 0.8 ml. of pH 7 buffer at 4°C. To this is added 0.2 ml of a chilled 5% glutaraldehyde solution. The resultant solution gives a 1:1 ratio of cross-linker to amino groups. The aqueous solution is pipetted into a rapidly stirred 100 ml of a 1:4 corn oil/petroleum ether mixture at room temperature. After 1 hour the oil is decanted and the beads are washed with

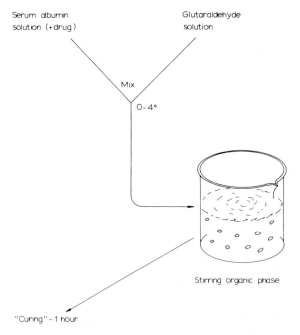

Figure 2. Method of preparation of cross-linked albumin beads under non-denaturing conditions. From Royer et al. (1983).

petroleum ether and/or alcohol. The beads are easily collected and dried in a vacuum desiccator or freeze drier. The active ester cross-linkers and dimethyl adipimate can also be used with this approach. Using a system containing no emulsifier results in beads having a size of 100–200 μm in diameter. When a water-insoluble drug is used it may be necessary to add a wetting agent to facilitate dispersement of the drug in water – 0.1% sodium dodecyl sulphate is suitable.

A water-soluble material, methyl orange, was entrapped in such beads and its in vitro release into phosphate buffer and into buffers containing α-chymotrypsin was measured. Compared to a 100% availability of non-entrapped drug in 4 minutes, about 12% of dye was released from the bead into buffer in 9 minutes and about 20% delivered in the same time into the α-chymotrypsin solution. It seems obvious that digestion of the bead would contribute to the rate of release. Beads containing entrapped methyl orange having an average particle size of 75 μm were themselves entrapped in a bead using these core 75-μm beads as particles suspended in the internal aqueous phase containing albumin and glutaraldehyde. In vitro release studies showed a considerable prolongation of dye availability from the bead within a bead system (Fig. 3). The linear relationship between percent released and the square root of time suggests that the release may be a matrix diffusion-controlled process.

10 mg of a water-insoluble material, norgestrel, were incorporated into beads having a final size of 50–200 μm. Release of the drug into a 40% poly(ethylene glycol) 300 (PEG 300) aqueous solution was measured. The solvent used gave rates that were

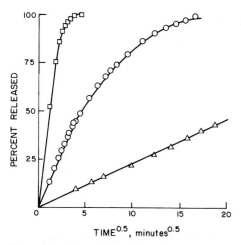

Figure 3. Percent of a water-soluble material (methyl orange) released from cross-linked albumin beads as a function of square root of time. Symbols: □, non-entrapped methyl orange; ○, core beads; △, core beads embedded in beads.

slow but measurable, and certainly fast in comparison with what would be expected into buffer alone (Fig. 4). The linear relationship found between amount released and square root of time again suggests a diffusion-controlled mechanism. As expected, the extent of cross-linking affects the rate of release. In a study of release from beads made using 1, 2, 3 and 4% glutaraldehyde (Fig. 4) it was found that cumulative

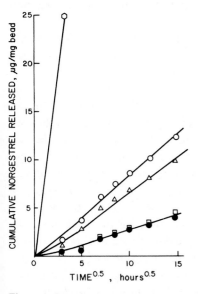

Figure 4. Cumulative amount of a water-insoluble drug (norgestrel) released from cross-linked albumin beads into 40% poly(ethylene glycol) in water as a function of the square root of time. Different amounts of glutaraldehyde were used to prepare the beads: ○, 1%; △, 2%; □, 3%; ●, 4%. Non-entrapped drug is represented by ○ for reference. From Royer et al. (1983).

TABLE 1

Lysine content of serum albumin beads using various glutaraldehyde concentrations

	Bovine serum albumin	Glutaraldehyde concentration (%)			
		1	2	3	4
Lysine residues/mol	53	32	20	9	6
Lysine residues modified, No. (%)	—	21 (40)	33 (62)	44 (83)	47 (89)

amounts released into PEG 300/water were linear with square root of time, with rates decreasing as amounts of glutaraldehyde used increased. Amino acid analysis of the beads that were produced gave the results shown in Table 1. Those systems resulting from the use of glutaraldehyde concentrations greater than 1% (where more than 40% of the lysines were modified) resulted in beads that were not digested by 1 mg/ml of α-chymotrypsin. The implication of this is that there are very close constraints with respect to how much cross-linking can be introduced and still result in a biologically useful product.

The effect of drug loading on release was also studied using norgestrel-embedded beads. As expected, it was found that there are differences in release rates, with the greater the loading (a range of 5–33% was used), the greater and faster the amount released.

To test the in vivo performance of albumin beads, progesterone embedded in rabbit serum albumin beads has been studied. The steroid made up 20% of the bead weight. Male rabbits were injected intramuscularly and subcutaneously with beads as suspensions in corn oil. Release following subcutaneous injection is depicted in Figure 5. There is an initial burst of drug release followed by an almost zero-order release for 20 days. In control experiments, equivalent doses of unentrapped progesterone were made available within 1 day. Body weight and temperature of the animals were monitored over the course of the study. No significant change was found, nor was there any inflammation or necrosis at the injection site. Surgery in an animal after 6 days showed a pellet-like repository of intact beads from which progesterone could be extracted. Examination of a 2-month injection site confirmed that the beads were biodegradable and well tolerated. The biocompatibility of the beads was confirmed in studies where unloaded beads were repeatedly injected into calves and in studies where tetanus toxoid was entrapped and injected into rabbits.

Providing sustained release of polypeptide hormones and antigens is an important challenge being addressed by many. The cross-linked albumin system might be used for such compounds if the amino groups of the polypeptides could be reversibly blocked. Prior to embedding, polypeptides were maleylated or citraconylated as shown in Scheme 5. Acylation is carried out at pH 8–10 and deprotection can be

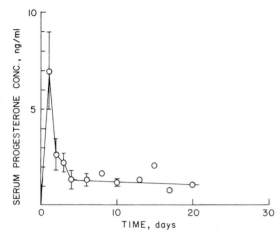

Figure 5. Serum progesterone levels in rabbits as a function of time following subcutaneous injection of cross-linked albumin beads into which drug was embedded. Rabbit serum albumin was used. Serum levels of drug were determined by RIA. From Royer et al. (1983).

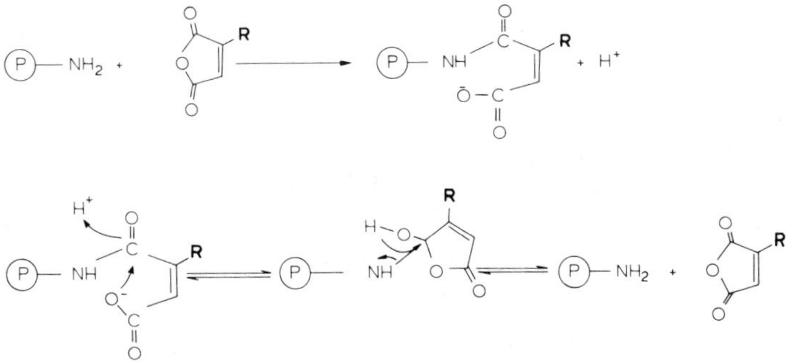

Scheme 5

accomplished by soaking the beads in an acid solution which will not dissolve the protein (salt, ethanol/water, etc.). Insulin was citraconylated and then embedded. 60% of the polypeptide was released in 5 minutes, followed by a second phase lasting 9 hours.

Tetanus toxoid is a single polypeptide with a molecular weight of about 140,000. 90% of the amino groups were maleylated prior to embedding. These toxoid laden beads were injected into rabbits. Two injections, 3 weeks apart, failed to raise antibodies, although untreated and unembedded tetanus toxoid gave an expected antibody titre. Even though no antibodies were produced with the citraconylated toxoid, the beads were found to be biocompatible and biodegradable.

Using the bead system developed by us, Goosen et al. (1982, 1983) embedded insulin crystals in systems of different size and cross-link density. These studies are different from our own, which used a citraconylated product. The studies of Goosen et al. give excellent examples of the advantages of the device, its potential, and future directions for investigation. In their most recent work, microspheres were made using

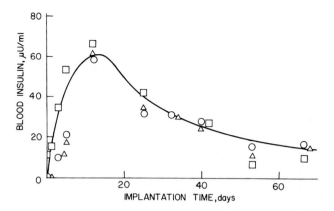

Figure 6. Blood insulin levels of diabetic rats implanted with varying doses of insulin-albumin microbeads. Bovine serum albumin was used with 1% glutaraldehyde as cross-linking agent. Insulin levels were determined by radioimmunoassay. Bead loading was 200 mg insulin per gram of beads. Symbols: ○, 10 mg dose; △, 20 mg dose; □, 40 mg dose (on day 28, a sample of microbeads and surrounding tissue was recovered from the animal which received the 40 mg dose). Redrawn from Goosen et al. (1982).

0.5% glutaraldehyde. Subcutaneous implantation of a single dose in diabetic rats provided sustained insulin blood levels over a period of 2 weeks. The beads were well tolerated, and biodegraded with time. This result is particularly interesting since the beads were made using bovine serum albumin. It is apparent that drug release is a function of bead size: smaller beads (200 μm) disappeared in 4 weeks whereas large microspheres (600 μm) took up to 8 weeks. In their earlier study where 1% glutaraldehyde was used (Goosen et al., 1982) up to 2 months of sustained release of insulin was observed (Fig. 6). This dramatically illustrates the marked affect that density of cross-links has on bead performance. The actual mechanism of release of bioactive macromolecules such as insulin (or that of small molecules as well) has yet to be determined. Diffusion through the albumin matrix as well as bioerosion of the sphere are most likely involved. Figure 6 shows that insulin blood levels are independent of dose administered. The dose-independent release could be the consequence of an effect such as the formation of a cyst-like capsule surrounding the implant. This was observed in the rat studies.

4. Future studies

A tailored, controlled release of drugs embedded in albumin microspheres is the prime objective of future studies. Size effects, density of cross-links, and biological system effects must be characterised and then orchestrated into a truely engineered delivery. None of these parameters that affect performance are easily characterised. Indeed, trying to sort out the mechanism of release is in itself a formidable problem.

References

Abdella, P.M., Smith, P.K. and Royer, G.P. (1979) Biochem. Biophys. Res. Commun. 87, 734–742.

Goosen, M.F.A., Leung, Y.F., Chou, S. and Sun, A.M. (1982) Biomat. Med. Devices Artif. Organs 10, 205–212.

Goosen, M.F.A., Leung, Y.F., O'Shea, G.M., Chou, S. and Sun, A.M. (1983) Diabetes 32, 478–481.

Hardy, P.M., Hughes, G.J. and Rydon, H.N. (1979) J.C.S. Perkin I, 2282–2288.

Korn, A.H., Feairheiler, S.H. and Filachione, E.M. (1972) J. Mol. Biol. 65, 525–529.

Lee, T.K. (1981) Ph.D. Thesis: I. The Development of a Sustained Release Device for Biologically Active Compounds, Ohio State University, Columbus.

Lee, T.K., Sokoloski, T.D. and Royer, G.P. (1981) Science 213, 233–235.

Longo, W.E., Iwata, H., Lindheimer, T.A. and Goldberg, E.P. (1982) J. Pharm. Sci. 71, 1323–1328.

Lubig, R., Kusch, P., Roper, K. and Zahn, H. (1981) Monatsh. Chem. 112, 1313–1323.

Richards, F.M. and Knowles, J.R. (1968) J. Mol. Biol. 37, 231–233.

Royer, G.P., Lee, T.K. and Sokoloski, T.D. (1983) J. Parenteral Sci. Techn. 37, 34–37.

Widder, K., Flouret, G. and Senyei, A. (1979) J. Pharm. Sci. 68, 79–82.

Widder, K.J., Senyei, A.E., Ovadia, H. and Paterson, P.Y. (1981) J. Pharm. Sci. 70, 387–389.

Microspheres and Drug Therapy. Pharmaceutical, Immunological and Medical Aspects
edited by S.S. Davis, L. Illum, J.G. McVie and E. Tomlinson
© *1984, Elsevier Science Publishers B.V.*

CHAPTER 10

Hydrophilic albumin and dextran ion-exchange microspheres for localized chemotherapy

E.P. Goldberg, H. Iwata and W. Longo

1. Introduction

A major goal of drug research today is the control of pharmacokinetics and the localisation of activity, especially for highly toxic drugs. In particular, the safety and efficacy of cancer chemotherapy could be improved significantly by confining antitumour drugs to neoplastic tissue (Nicolson, 1976; Gregoriadis, 1981; Goldberg et al., 1983). There are many studies in progress aimed at achieving this goal using tumour-specific polyclonal and monoclonal antibodies (Ghose and Blair, 1978; Ghose et al., 1983), liposomes (Fendler and Romero, 1977), microspheres (Mosbach and Schroder, 1979) and polymeric drug carriers (Bernstein et al., 1979). However, only limited success has been achieved to date in vivo. Although surface cytochemical differences between normal and malignant tissue will surely be exploited for targeting chemo- or immunotherapy, many other types of drug localization will continue to be explored (Goldberg 1983).

One approach to drug localisation, studied in this laboratory, is the direct injection of cytotoxic agents and immunostimulants into tumour tissue, i.e., intratumour therapy. This has been one of the few drug targeting methods that has shown significant promise for the complete cure of some animal tumours (Likkite and Halpern, 1974; Scott 1974; Takahashi et al., 1976; McLaughlin et al., 1978). It should be noted that in many animal studies, not only the injected primary tumour but also distant metastases were irradiated. Cured animals also often exhibited specific immune resistance to new tumour challenges. In guinea pig hepatoma studies, no cures occurred when drug was given by the intravenous route. Because of the systemic immune responses, such local chemotherapy may therefore be considered to be a type of immunotherapy (McLaughlin and Goldberg, 1983).

The diffusion of drugs away from local intratumour injections has been studied (Takahashi et al., 1976; McLaughlin and Goldberg, 1983). It was found that low-molecular-weight compounds such as bleomycin (BLM) and adriamycin (AD) tend to leave the tumour injection site very rapidly (Fig. 1). These experiments have also shown that multiple intratumour injections or drug-water/oil emulsions increase drug retention time, with resulting higher cure rates. Such studies point to a correla-

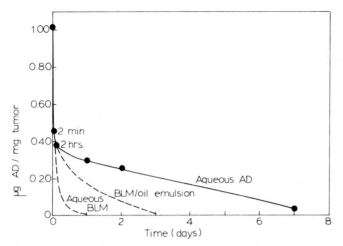

Figure 1. Concentration of adriamycin (AD) and bleomycin (BLM) in tumour tissue vs time.

tion between drug retention time and the effectiveness of intratumour chemotherapy. To circumvent this problem of rapid drug diffusion, we have become interested in the use of soluble or insoluble macromolecular drug carriers which would be fixed at the injection site (chemically or physically) and thereby provide sustained localised drug activity (Goldberg et al., 1981, 1983; Iwata et al., 1982; Longo et al., 1983).

Reported here are recent studies aimed at producing insoluble microsphere (MS) carrier systems for local or intratumour therapy. Although originally intended primarily for tissue immobilization, we now regard the opportunities for using submicron MS for intravenous drug delivery as also promising. MS preparations were aimed at satisfying the following criteria: (1) ability to bind and release high concentrations of drugs, (2) stability after synthesis with a clinically acceptable shelf life, (3) controllable particle size and dispersibility in aqueous media for easy injection, (4) release of active drug with a good control over a wide time scale, (5) biocompatibility with a controllable biodegradability, (6) easy chemical modification and (7) controllable particle size and porosity or cross-link density.

MS systems considered most readily applicable were based on albumin and dextran. These two polymers are biocompatible and are degraded in vivo. Human serum albumin (HSA) is of course the major blood plasma protein. It has been recognized as a natural circulatory drug carrier (Koch-Weser and Sellers, 1976a,b). Equilibrium binding to various therapeutic agents depends primarily on hydrophobic and electrostatic interactions (Sjöholm et al., 1979). This type of binding avoids the need for covalent attachment between drug and albumin and facilitates drug release. Dextran is also an excellent candidate for a drug carrier. This polysaccharide and its derivatives have been used extensively in medicine and biochemistry (Gronwall, 1957; Fischer, 1980). Its chemistry and interactions with biological compounds have been studied in detail, and cross-linked dextran is widely used for gel, ion-exchange and affinity chromatography. The extensive literature for both HSA and dextran affords a good background in studies for use as antitumour drug carriers in the form of cross-linked MS.

Important deficiencies of HSA/MS preparations made by the usual vegetable oil dispersion method include hydrophobicity and limitations in drug loading. Therefore, a significantly improved method, based on steric stabilization of HSA dispersions in polymer solutions, was developed. This method yields hydrophilic HSA/MS which may be loaded with high drug concentrations or readily modified chemically to achieve special surface properties (Longo et al., 1982). However, although drug containing MS based on the physical association of drugs to HSA and dextran are of considerable interest, it has also been found that application of ion-exchange principles can yield compositions with even higher drug loadings and more versatile release properties. Thus, for example, anionic modifications of HSA and dextran facilitate binding and controlled release of basic drugs. Therefore, this chapter will concentrate on such modified ion-exchange MS.

2. Albumin microspheres

The unique properties of HSA have led to the development of HSA/MS as drug carriers, and studies by a number of investigators have been reported (Yapel, 1978; Royer, 1982; Senyei and Widder, 1982). The biodegradability of HSA/MS is also important and is a function of the degree of albumin cross-linking, porosity and accessibility of HSA/MS to enzymatic and phagocytic processes in the body (Widder et al., 1980).

We became interested in HSA/MS because they seem to be uniquely suitable for intratumour or intravenous injection. However, it was considered important to improve upon current methods for synthesis because of hydrophobicity and the relatively low drug concentrations achieved (Kramer, 1976; Widder et al., 1979; Ishizaka et al., 1981; Lee et al., 1982). These methods are essentially all modifications of a process developed in 1969 by Rhodes et al. involving either denaturation of albumin at elevated temperatures (Kramer, 1976) or chemical cross-linking (Senyei et al., 1981) in vegetable oil emulsions. Surfactants are needed to disperse such HSA/MS in water. They appear to be somewhat hydrophobic because of the method of formation.

Therefore, a new method was sought to produce hydrophilic HSA/MS that could be made with high concentrations of drugs and which would satisfy the other criteria set forth earlier for improved drug carriers. Hydrophilicity was regarded as important because water-soluble drugs could then, for the first time, be incorporated into the HSA/MS after synthesis. Additionally, wet chemistry for surface and bulk modification would be more readily accomplished. Such MS would also be dispersed easily for injection use without the need for surfactants which might affect the drugs and the release properties of drugs from HSA/MS.

Described here is a method for the synthesis of such hydrophilic HSA/MS as well as HSA/MS containing the clinically important anti-tumour agent, adriamycin (AD).

312

This method offers excellent control of particle size and surface and bulk chemistry and yields AD-HSA/MS which are readily dispersed for injection. Ion-exchange polyglutamic acid (PGA) containing HSA/MS were also prepared with up to 45 wt.% of AD. These preparations are based upon our earlier studies wherein poly(L-glutamic acid) (molecular weight, 40,000) was shown to form a stable stoichiometric polymer-drug salt with basic antitumour agents such as AD (Goldberg et al., 1981). Such polymer-drug complexes could be prepared containing up to 80 wt.% of AD. Although insoluble and stable in water, the salt readily dissociates in physiological saline to release free drug. Therefore, incorporation of PGA into HSA/MS was studied; it was readily achieved for the preparation of ion-exchange MS containing high drug concentrations.

In vitro studies showed that AD was released from AD-PGA-HSA/MS in a controllable manner as a function of the ionic strength of the eluting medium and the MS surface and bulk properties. AD-PGA-HSA/MS showed much lower toxicity than free drug (Fig. 2). Also important was the elimination of necrotic reactions at the injection site for AD-PGA-HSA/MS, as compared with AD (Figs. 3 and 4). This is frequently a significant clinical problem accompanying injections of AD.

2.1. Synthesis of hydrophilic HSA/MS and PGA-HSA/MS
The synthesis of hydrophilic HSA/MS is described in detail elsewhere (Longo et al., 1982). For a typical AD-PGA-HSA composition, 150 mg of HSA (or HSA with 10–20 wt.% PGA, molecular weight, 60,000) was dissolved in 0.5 ml of distilled H_2O and added dropwise to 4.0 ml of a 25 wt.% solution of polymethylmethacrylate

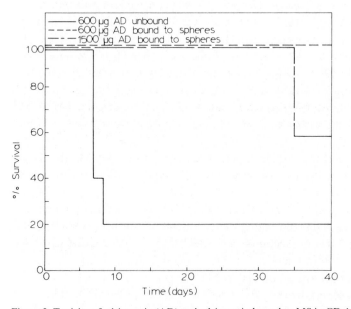

Figure 2. Toxicity of adriamycin (AD) and adriamycin bound to MS in CD-1 mice.

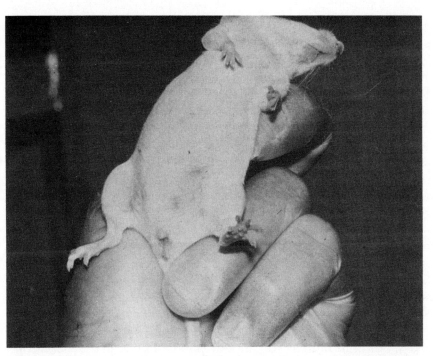

Figure 3. CD-1 mouse injected intraperitoneally with adriamycin (600 μg) bound to MS; no ulcer formation.

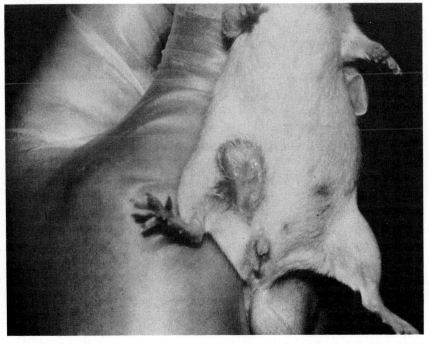

Figure 4. CD-1 mouse showing ulceration from intraperitoneal injection of free adriamycin (600 μg).

314

(PMMA) in an equal mixture of chloroform and toluene. After dispersion of the aqueous phase to a desired particle size, cross-linking of the HSA was initiated by the addition of 1.0 ml of glutaraldehyde-saturated toluene. Free reactive aldehyde groups were quenched, if desired, with glycine. MS were washed with acetone to remove the PMMA completely and were either dehydrated under vacuum or suspended in water and frozen or lyophilized. This procedure typically produces MS that are very uniform, show good spherical geometry and have a solid porous interior, as shown in Figures 5 and 6. The average size of the HSA/MS in Figure 5 is 10 μm. Smaller or larger HSA/MS were produced by adjusting the dispersion time and the mixing energy. The high concentration of PMMA used in this process facilitates good dispersion and stabilization in the organic phase and is based on steric stabilization concepts (Heller, 1966).

For in vitro and in vivo drug studies, HSA/MS and PGA-HSA/MS of 30 μm average diameter (with either free residual aldehyde groups or quenched with glycine) were synthesized as described. To prepare AD containing HSA/MS or PGA-HSA/MS, MS were added to a known weight of AD in aqueous solution and mixed for 16 hours at 4°C. MS were then separated from the drug solution by centrifugation and washed repeatedly with distilled water. The concentration of unbound AD in the wash was determined spectrophotometrically (DiMarco and Arcamone, 1975). Bound AD varied from 18 to 45 wt.% (Table 1) as a function of PGA in the MS and quenching of reactive aldehyde groups (unquenched HSA/MS yield some covalent binding of AD).

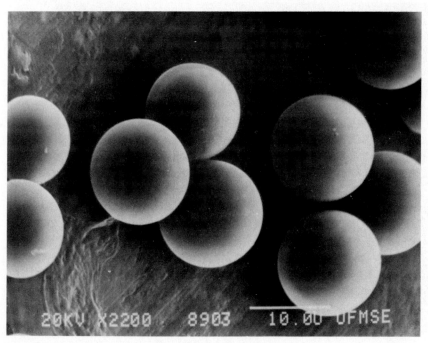

Figure 5. Scanning electron micrograph of HSA/MS, 10 μm average diameter.

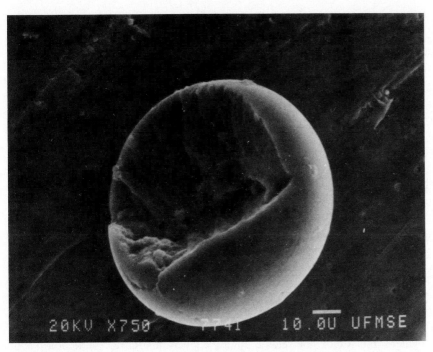

Figure 6. Scanning electron micrograph of 100 μm HSA/MS showing internal structure.

2.2. In vitro drug release from HSA/MS

In vitro AD release rates from AD-HSA/MS and AD-PGA-HSA/MS were evaluated using a dynamic column flow method. Release rates were found to be readily controlled by utilizing three binding mechanisms: (1) slow release: hydrolytic degradation of covalent bonds, (2) medium release: dissociation of drug-salt complex, and

TABLE 1

Adriamycin binding to HSA/MS and PGA-HSA/MS

% PGA in MS	Weight % bound AD
Unquenched	
0	18
12	33
16	39
22	46
Quenched	
0	18
11	21
15	25
19	33

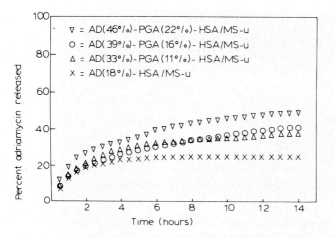

Figure 7. In vitro release of adriamycin from HSA/MS-U and PGA-HSA/MS-U, average diameter 30 μm.

(3) fast release: desorption of physically associated drug.

For the unquenched (U) MS (HSA/MS-U and PGA-HSA/MS-U), drug binding is both covalent and ionic. The release data are given in Figure 7. The amount of AD released using saline as the elution medium in 15 hours varied from 23% for AD-HSA/MS-U to 50% for AD-PGA(22%)-HSA/MS-U. Increasing the concentration of PGA in HSA/MS increased the release rate of AD. This is due to the faster dissociation of PGA-AD salt complex compared to the hydrolytic release of covalently bound AD. The release curves shown in Figure 8 are representative for glycine quenched (Q) MS (HSA/MS-Q and PGA-HSA/MS-Q) with physically adsorbed and ionic bound AD. Unlike the results shown in Figure 7, the physically associated AD

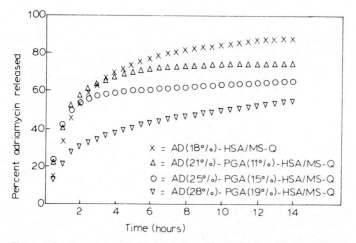

Figure 8. In vitro release of adriamycin from HSA/MS-Q and PGA-HSA/MS-Q, average diameter 26 μm.

is released faster than by salt dissociation. As the amount of the PGA is increased in the MS-Q, a higher percentage of the bound AD is associated with the salt complex. This causes a relatively larger concentration of AD to be released by salt dissociation, which then reduces the overall release rate.

The ion-exchange properties of the AD-PGA salt complex are shown in Figure 9, which depicts dynamic flow release for AD from AD-HSA/MS-Q(OH), AD-HSA/MS-Q(COOH) and AD-PGA-HSA/MS-Q(COOH). (OH) indicates that the MS were quenched with aminoethanol while (COOH) indicates glycine quenching of aldehyde groups. Glycine adds additional anionic carboxyl groups as compared with aminoalcohol quenching. Increasing carboxyl group concentration increases AD binding by salt formation. Because the salt complex is stable in water, the MS with the highest concentration of carboxyl groups, AD-PGA-HSA/MS-Q(COOH), released the least AD (4%) with water as the mobile phase. AD-HSA/MS-Q(OH), which contains minimal carboxyl groups (from albumin itself), releases the greatest amount of AD (35%) to water elution. When the water mobile phase is replaced with saline, the AD-COOH salt dissociates releasing AD, as shown in Figure 9.

Dynamic flow drug release in vitro may not adequately represent the kinetic behaviour in vivo. However, in vitro comparisons between drug carriers are useful to guide animal testing. The dynamic column elution system is, at best, a model for drug delivery in a circulatory blood system with fast continuous flow. In contrast, MS immobilized in solid tumours or tissue would not be subjected to a rapid turnover of fluid. The much slower fluid turnover in tissue can be better represented by a semistatic in vitro release model. In a static fixed-volume system, drug release from AD-HSA/MS would be regulated by diffusional dependence on the concentration of drug released into a relatively closed system (e.g., a tumour). A tissue concentration level would be reached where further drug release would be inhibited by a drug-MS equilibrium. Drug diffusion away from the tumour area would then reduce the con-

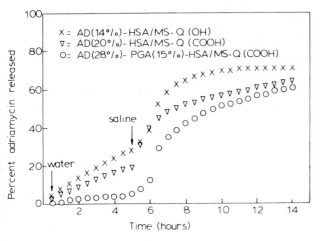

Figure 9. Ion-exchange release of adriamycin from HSA/MS-Q (glycine or aminoethanol) and PGA-HSA/MS-Q (glycine).

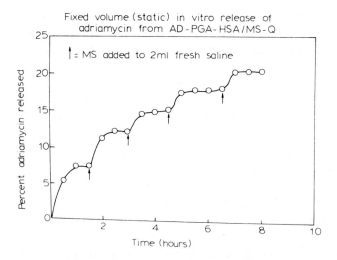

Figure 10. Fixed volume (static) in vitro release of adriamycin from PGA-HSA/MS-Q.

centration to a point where more drug would be released. Figure 10 demonstrates this point. It shows the release of AD from AD-PGA-HSA/MS, containing 2.6 mg of AD, suspended in 2.0 ml of saline. This may be regarded as equivalent to approximately 1 mg AD per ml of a porous tumour volume. Figure 10 shows that AD-PGA-HSA/MS released AD until a concentration equilibrium was reached and further AD release then stopped. When the AD-PGA-HSA/MS was added to a fresh 2 ml volume of saline, AD release again occurred. HSA/MS, containing therapeutic agents such as AD, injected into areas that have a low fluid turnover would thereby maintain high concentrations of drug in the target area for extended periods.

2.3. In vivo properties of AD-PGA-HSA/MS

AD is an extremely toxic antitumour drug and can be administered clinically only in low doses (Carter, 1975). The toxicity of the drug was reduced significantly by MS binding. This was demonstrated using CD-1 mice injected intraperitoneally, with AD, AD-PGA-HSA/MS and PGA-HSA/MS (containing no drug). Figure 2 shows the percent survival for the treated animals. A dose of 600 μg of AD killed 80% of animals within 10 days. The same amount of AD bound to PGA-HSA/MS was not toxic to 40 days. Thus, for intratumour or intravenous injections, much higher concentrations of AD might be used clinically when bound to MS.

Another clinical problem often encountered with AD is the severe necrotic lesion that develops at the site of injection, especially when there is drug leakage around the needle (Rudolph et al., 1976). These ulcers resist healing. It was found that when AD (600 μg) was administered intraperitoneally to mice, ulcer formation occurred at the site of injections, as shown in Figure 4. All animals treated with AD developed these ulcers. Figure 3 shows a mouse injected with the same dose of AD bound to HSA/MS. No ulcer formation occurred with any of the test animals injected with

MS preparations. Control groups of PGA-HSA/MS also showed no toxic effects.

The binding of AD to HSA/MS clearly reduced the toxicity of AD. Other investigators (Bernstein et al., 1979) have also found reduced toxicity for AD bound to large macromolecules such as dextran. The significant reduction in toxicity for AD-PGA-HSA/MS suggests that MS may be more effective carriers, even for intravenous administration of AD (using submicron MS) as well as for localized tissue injection therapy.

3. Dextran microspheres

Unlike albumin, hydrophilic cross-linked dextran microspheres (DEX/MS) are well known and widely used for chromatography. DEX/MS are suitable for intratumour injection and are commercially available in several particle sizes and cross-link densities (e.g., Sephadex). They are relatively biocompatible and can degrade in vivo. Chemical modification of dextran to produce carboxylated or sulphonated polymer was easily carried out by carboxymethylation or sulphopropylation. Thus, addition of functional groups for drug-salt complex formation was readily accomplished. The ion-exchange capability was very similar to the PGA-HSA/MS system that has already been discussed. Additionally, by oxidation of DEX/MS with periodate, it was possible to add an aldehyde group for covalent (imine) binding of amino-functional drugs such as AD. One interesting and very significant aspect of such oxidation was the greatly increased hydrolytic instability of oxidized DEX/MS, which permits the tailoring of very rapidly degradable MS. Although not discussed further in this chapter, periodate-oxidized DEX/MS have been prepared which are readily degradable in saline. Degradation was related to the degree of oxidation. The oxidized DEX/MS shown in Figure 11 degraded in saline in only 2 hours. With bound drug (mitomycin C in this case), degradation was somewhat slower.

3.1. Carboxymethyl-dextran microspheres (CMDEX/MS)
Cross-linked dextran gels (Sephadex G-10 and G-40-50) were used to prepare carboxymethyldextran (CMDEX) ion-exchange MS drug carriers. In a typical preparation, 3 g of dextran gel were suspended in 50 ml of 40 wt.% sodium hydroxide solution and 16 g of chloroacetic acid were then added to this suspension. The reaction mixture was gently agitated for 12 hours at room temperature. The reaction product was washed extensively with distilled water and then with acetone. It was dehydrated under vacuum. DEX/MS of low cross-link density (LCD, from Sephadex G-10) and high cross-link density (HCD, from Sephadex G-50-40) were prepared.

3.2. AD-CMDEX microspheres
AD-loaded CMDEX/MS were made by mixing aqueous AD solutions with dehydrated CMDEX/MS. In a typical preparation, 80 mg of AD were dissolved in 10 ml of water and 158 mg of CMDEX/MS(LCD) were added. A pH of 7.0 was main-

320

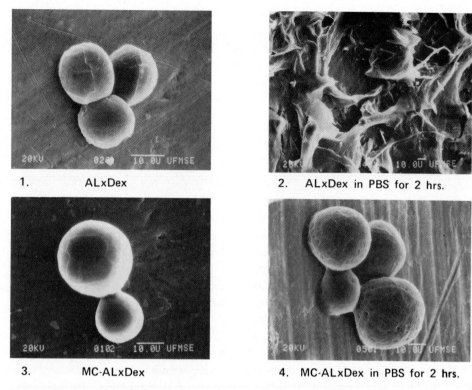

1.   ALxDex   2.   ALxDex in PBS for 2 hrs.

3.   MC-ALxDex   4.   MC-ALxDex in PBS for 2 hrs.

Figure 11. Scanning electron micrographs of oxidized DEX/MS and mitomycin C (MC) containing MS: 1, ALXDEX/MS; 2, ALXDEX/MS exposed to phosphate-buffered saline for 2 hours; 3, MC-ALXDEX/ MS and 4, MC-ALXDEX/MS exposed to phosphate-buffered saline for 2 hours.

tained. After 30 minutes, it was centrifuged and the supernatant removed. The AD-CMDEX/MS(LCD) preparation was washed with distilled water and lyophilized. Uncomplexed AD in the wash was determined by UV/VIS spectroscopy (DiMarco and Arcamone, 1975).

Cross-linked carboxylated or sulphonated dextran microspheres act as cation-exchange drug carriers. Basic drugs such as adriamycin (amino functional) readily form ionic salts. The resulting polymer-drug stoichiometric salts exchange free drug for other cations. Preparative conditions and drug concentrations in various DEX/MS preparations are given in Table 2. Salt formation was quantitative.

The main driving force for formation of ionic salt complexes should be the electrostatic interaction between the anionic acidic DEX/MS derivatives and the basic primary sugar amino group of the drug, AD. However, the relative stability and extremely high yields for these polymeric salts seem not entirely explained by simple ionic group interactions. Secondary interactions may help explain this behaviour. AD can form molecular aggregates by association of the anthracycline chromophore (Chambers et al., 1974). AD molecules may thereby form both an ionic salt and a stacked complex by interactions between the AD chromophores. This secondary

TABLE 2

Adriamycin-containing ion-exchange dextran microspheres

	Dextran microspheres (mg)	Adriamycin (mg)	Volume H_2O (ml)	% yield (on AD)	Microsphere drug content (mg adria-mycin/100 mg)	Average diameter (μm)
CMDEX/MS-LCD	158.47	80.26	10.0	99.9	33.6	128
CMDEX/MS-LCD	3.29	4.13	1.25	82.3	55.6	N.D.[b]
CMDEX/MS-HCD	87.75	11.10	3.0	97.3	11.0	79
SPDEX/MS[a]	4.62	1.18	1.0	99.3	20.2	97

[a] Sulphopropyldextran.
[b] Not determined.

complex interaction would promote formation and enhance stability of the AD polymeric salts.

3.3. In vitro drug release from AD-CMDEX/MS

Figure 12 presents the drug release curves for adriamycin from AD-CMDEX/MS(LCD) under dynamic flow conditions. The drug salt is relatively stable in distilled water. However, upon changing to physiological saline, adriamycin was released almost quantitatively in a few hours.

Figure 13 shows the release profile in saline under closed static conditions. This is a drug release experiment with a fixed volume, similar to that discussed for PGA-HSA/MS. In contrast to the results under flow conditions, only 15% AD was released

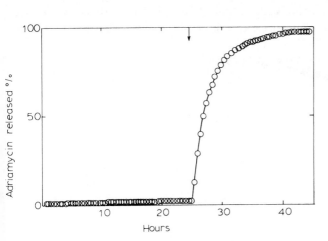

Figure 12. In vitro release of adriamycin from CMDEX/MS-LCD. Arrow indicates the change of mobile phase from distilled water to saline.

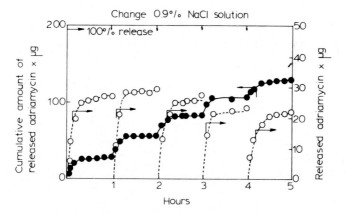

Figure 13. In vitro release of adriamycin from CMDEX/MS-LCD. Arrow indicates the change to fresh saline. ○, amount of adriamycin in each experiment; ●, cumulative amount of released adriamycin.

in the first step. In this closed system, an equilibrium concentration of released drug was established within 30 minutes. Upon changing to a fresh volume of saline, AD was again released immediately and a new equilibrium was rapidly reestablished. This release was repeated several times, as shown in Figure 13.

The release rate may also be governed by many properties of the polymer matrix, such as porosity or cross-link density, number of ionic groups and ionic group strength. Figure 14 shows AD release at a slow flow rate for LCD and HCD CMDEX/MS. Although there are differences in cross-linked density and total functional groups, the release curves show only slight dependence on these parameters at slow flow rates.

Figure 15 shows the dependence of drug release rate on the cross-link density at a higher flow rate. Here, some influence of the cross-link density was observed, i.e., a slower drug release for the higher cross-link density. With a slow flow rate, 50%

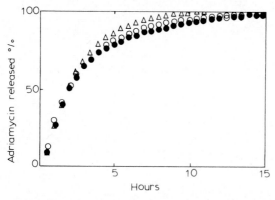

Figure 14. In vitro release of adriamycin from CMDEX/MS and SPDEX/MS using slow flow rate. ○, CMDEX/MS-LCD; ●, CMDEX/MS-HCD; △, SPDEX/MS.

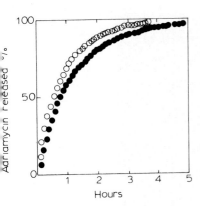

Figure 15. In vitro release of adriamycin from CMDEX/MS using a fast flow rate. ○, CMDEX/MS-LCD; ●, CMDEX/MS-HCD.

AD release occurred in 2 hours, as compared to 40 minutes at a high flow rate (Figs. 14 and 15).

The retention of drug activity for released AD was also measured by DNA complexing. Anti-tumour activity has been related to the formation of a molecular complex with DNA and inhibition of nucleic acid synthesis. Therefore, retention of AD activity may be assessed by measuring the formation of the DNA complex in vitro (DiMarco and Arcamone, 1975). The decrease in absorbance of AD at 480 nm upon addition of DNA was measured. AD released from MS behaves similarly to AD. There appears to be no effect upon biological activity as a result of AD binding and release from the MS, as judged by DNA complexing.

4. Summary

The emphasis of this research has been upon the synthesis and properties of chemically modified albumin and dextran microspheres for use as drug carriers in localized therapy. A novel method was developed for the preparation of hydrophilic HSA/MS. These were readily modified with an anionic polypeptide, polyglutamic acid, to afford ion-exchange drug carriers capable of 40–50% adriamycin loading and relatively rapid drug release. Similar anionic dextran microspheres carriers were prepared by carboxymethylation of epichlorohydrin cross-linked dextran. Although the HSA/MS and DEX/MS systems were slowly biodegradable in vivo (weeks to months, depending upon the cross-link density), more rapidly degradable DEX/MS (hours to days) were achieved by periodate oxidation of DEX/MS.

Drug-containing MS exhibited a significantly reduced toxicity and much less tissue necrosis, encouraging consideration of submicron MS-drug compositions for intravenous administration. The protective environment of the MS may also reduce metabolic degradation of antitumour drugs and further enhance efficacy. Prolonged local

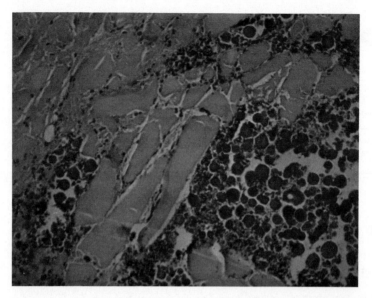

Figure 16. Optical photomicrograph (× 100) of HSA/MS immobilized in rabbit muscle tissue 1 week after injection.

immobilization of 30–50-μm HSA/MS in rabbit muscle tissue for at least 4–6 weeks was demonstrated (Figure 16). The potential for use of HSA/MS or DEX/MS in intratumour chemo- or immunotherapy appears encouraging. Additionally, these MS carriers offer considerable promise for localised delivery of hormones and antibiotics as well as for improved adjuvant compositions with prolonged activity and minimal adverse behaviour. These various applications are under investigation.

Acknowledgments

The studies reported here were supported in part by the State of Florida Biomedical Engineering Center. We wish to thank Dr. Arcamone of Farmitalia for generous samples of adriamycin and M. Smith for her help with this manuscript.

References

Bernstein, A., Hurwitz, E., Maron, R., Arnon R., Sela, M. and Wilchek, M. (1979) J. Natl. Cancer Inst. 60, 379–384.
Carter, S.K. (1975) Cancer Chemotherapy 6, 389–397.
Chambers, R.W., Kajiwara, T. and Kearns, R.D. (1974) J. Phys. Chem, 78, 380–387.
DiMarco, F.L. and Arcamone, F. (1975) Arzneim-Forsch. 25, 3681–3760.
Fendler, J.H. and Romero, A. (1977) Life Sci. 20, 1109–1120.

Fischer, L. (1980) in Laboratory Techniques in Biochemistry and Molecular Biology (Work, T.S. and Burdon, R.H., Eds.), Elsevier/North-Holland, Amsterdam.

Ghose, T. and Blair, A.H. (1978) J. Natl. Cancer Inst. 61, 657–676.

Ghose, T., Blair, A.H., Vaughan, K. and Kulkaru, P. (1983) in Drug Targeting (Goldberg, E.P., Ed.), pp. 1–22, Wiley Interscience, New York.

Goldberg, E.P., Terry, R.N. and Levy, M. (1981) ACS Div. Organ. Coatings Plastic Chem. 44, 132–136.

Goldberg, E.P., Iwata, H., Terry, R.N., Longo, W.E., Levy, M. and Cantrell, J.I. (1983) in Affinity Chromatography and Related Techniques (Gribnau, T.C., Visser, J. and Nivard, R.J., Eds.), pp. 375–386, Elsevier, Amsterdam.

Goldberg, E.P. (Ed.) (1983) Targeted Drugs, Wiley Interscience, New York.

Gregoriadis, G. (1981) Lancet 8, 241–247.

Gronwall, A. (1957) Dextran and its Use in Clinical Infusion Solution, Academic Press, New York.

Heller, W. (1966) Pure Appl. Chem. 12, 249–274.

Ishizaka, T., Eudo, K. and Koish, M. (1981) J. Pharm. Sci. 70, 358–363.

Iwata, H., Longo, W.E., Lindheimer, T.A. and Goldberg, E.P. (1982) Trans. Soc. Biomat. 8, 61–62.

Koch-Weser, J. and Sellers, E.M. (1976a) N. Engl. J. Med. 294, 311–316.

Koch-Weser, J. and Sellers, E.M. (1976b) N. Engl. J. Med. 294, 526–531.

Kramer, P.A. (1976) J. Pharm. Sci. 63, 1646–1647.

Lee, T.K., Sokoloski, T.D. and Royer, G.P. (1982) Science 213, 233–235.

Likkite, V.V. and Halpern, B.N. (1974) Cancer Res. 34, 341–344.

Longo, W.E., Iwata, H., Lindheimer, T.A. and Goldberg, E.P. (1982) J. Pharm. Sci. 71, 1323–1328.

Longo, W.E., Iwata, H., Lindheimer, T.A. and Goldberg, E.P. (1983) Am. Chem. Soc., ACS Div. Polymer Chem. 24, 56–57.

McLaughlin, C.A., Cantrell, J.L., Ribi, E. and Goldberg, E.P. (1978) Cancer Res. 38, 1311–1316.

McLaughlin, C.A. and Goldberg, E.P. (1983) in Targeted Drugs (Goldberg, E.P., Ed.), pp. 254–268, Wiley Interscience, New York.

Morimoto, Y., Sugibayashi, K. and Yoshio, K. (1981) Chem. Pharm. Bull. 29, 1433–1438.

Mosbach, K. and Schroder, U. (1979) FEBS Lett. 102, 112–116.

Nicolson, G.L. (1976) Biochim. Biophys. Acta 458, 1–72.

Rhodes, B.A., Zolle, I., Buchanan, J.W. and Wagner, H.W. (1969) Radiology 92, 1453–1459.

Royer, G.P. (1982) U.S. Patent, 4,349,530.

Rudolph, R., Steins, S. and Pattillo, R.A. (1976) Cancer 38, 1087–1094.

Scott, M.T. (1974) J. Natl. Cancer Inst. 53, 855–859.

Senyei, A.E. and Widder, K.J. (1982) U.S. Patent, 4,357,259.

Senyei, A.E., Reich, S.D., Gonczy, C. and Widder, K.J. (1981) J. Pharm. Sci. 70, 389–391.

Sjöholm, I., Ekman, B., Kober, A., Tjungstedt-Påhlman, I., Seiving, B. and Sjödin, T. (1979) Mol. Pharm. 16, 767–777.

Takahashi, T., Ueda, S., Kono, K. and Majima, S. (1976) Cancer 38, 1507–1514.

Widder, K.J., Flouret, G. and Senyei, A.E. (1979) J. Pharm. Sci. 68, 79–82.

Widder, K.J., Senyei, A.E. and Ranney, D.F. (1980) Cancer Res. 40, 3512–3517.

Yapel, A.F. (1978) U.S. Patent, 4,147,767.

Microspheres and Drug Therapy. Pharmaceutical, Immunological and Medical Aspects
edited by S.S. Davis, L. Illum, J.G. McVie and E. Tomlinson
© 1984, Elsevier Science Publishers B.V.

Biodegradable microspheres for prolonged local anesthesia

Masahiro Nakano, Naoki Wakiyama, Tsuyoshi Kojima, Kazuhiko Juni, Reiko Iwaoku, Shohei Inoue and Yasuhiko Yoshida

1. Introduction

Although long-acting local anesthetics such as bupivacaine and etidocaine have been developed, the duration of action is not long enough to control intractable pain caused by advanced cancer and trigeminal neuralgia.

In order to increase the duration of action of local anesthetics, delivery of the drug to the site of action has to be prolonged, by either slow dissolution or slow release. In order to slow down a dissolution process, Nakano et al. (1978) synthesized poorly soluble salts of lidocaine, mepivacaine and bupivacaine and examined their dissolution characteristics.

In the present work, the authors examined if the delivery of local anesthetics could be sustained by enclosing the drugs in microspheres. For preparation of microspheres, biodegradable polymers were employed since it is desirable for the rate-controlling materials to disappear after the mission has been completed. Since polylactic acid has been reported to be biodegradable (Miller et al., 1977), it was used for preparation of microspheres. Polycarbonates were also examined since biodegradability of poly(ethylene carbonate) has been demonstrated in rats (Kawaguchi et al., 1983) and sustained release of antimetabolites from polycarbonate matrices has been demonstrated in vitro (Kawaguchi et al., 1982).

2. Polylactic acid microspheres

Two lots of poly((±)-lactic acid) were synthesized from (±)-lactic acid, and their molecular weights were estimated to be 9.1×10^3 and 1.7×10^4 by measuring the intrinsic viscosity (Wakiyama et al., 1982b). The former was used in butamben microspheres and the latter was employed in tetracaine microspheres (Wakiyama et al., 1981) and dibucaine microspheres (Wakiyama et al., 1982c).

2.1. Preparation of microspheres

Microspheres were prepared by a solvent-evaporation process using poly((±)-lactic

TABLE 1

Effect of nonsolvents and methods of evaporation on the size of butamben microspheres

Nonsolvent	Stirring rate (rpm)	Method of evaporation	Diameter (μm)
1% Gelatin	800	In vacuo	50.6 ± 3.4
1% Gelatin	800	Warming at 40°C	84.7 ± 6.0
1% Sodium alginate	1000	In vacuo	10.5 ± 0.9
1% Sodium alginate	1000	Warming at 40°C	12.3 ± 1.0

Prepared with an initial butamben/polylactic acid ratio of 10:90 using methylene chloride as a polymer solvent.

acid) as a polymer, methylene chloride as a polymer solvent, and 1–2% gelatin or 1% sodium alginate as nonsolvents of the polymer.

Table 1 shows the effects of nonsolvents and methods of evaporation of the solvent on the size of butamben microspheres obtained. Smaller microspheres were obtained when 1% sodium alginate was used as a nonsolvent, probably due to greater viscosity of the sodium alginate solution than that of the gelatin solution. Microspheres obtained by evaporation of the solvent by heat tended to be larger than those obtained by evaporation of the solvent in vacuo. This is probably due to the reduced viscosity of the aqueous phase at higher temperatures.

Drug contents increased with an increase in the initial drug/polymer ratio, as shown in dibucaine microspheres (Table 2). Because of some loss of the drug due to partitioning into the aqueous phase, amounts of the drug enclosed in the microspheres tended to be smaller than the amounts of the drug added.

2.2. Release rates

The effects of the size of microspheres on the release patterns of butamben are shown in Figure 1. As the size decreased from 85 to 10 μm, the initial rate of release

TABLE 2

Effect of drug/polymer ratio on dibucaine contents in polylactic acid microspheres

Initial drug:polymer ratio	Drug content (%)
20:80	13.4
30:70	20.3
35:65	29.9
40:60	35.9
45:55	39.8
50:50	44.7

Prepared by evaporation in vacuo employing methylene chloride as a polymer solvent and 2% gelatin as a nonsolvent.

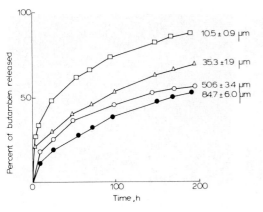

Figure 1. Effect of size on release patterns from polylactic acid microspheres.

increased, due to an increase in surface areas.

The effects of drug contents on release patterns of dibucaine are shown in Figure 2. When the drug contents were small, a nearly constant release rate was obtained. When the drug contents were between 20 and 40%, sigmoidal release patterns were obtained. When the drug contents exceeded 40%, an extremely fast initial release was observed. The sigmoidal release patterns may be attributable to extensive disintegration of the microspheres after about 150 hours, as observed in a morphological study (Fig. 3).

2.3. Duration of local anesthetic effects

The guinea pig skin technique of Quevauviller (1977) was employed for measurement of the local anesthetic activity following dorsal subcutaneous injections of the drugs in solution or dorsal subcutaneous implantations of the drugs in microspheres (Wakiyama et al., 1982a).

When tetracaine was injected in the form of a solution, the pharmacological activity decreased rapidly because of a rapid elimination of the drug from the injected site

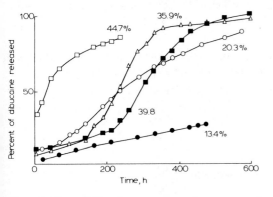

Figure 2. Effect of dibucaine content on release patterns from polylactic acid microspheres, $n = 3$.

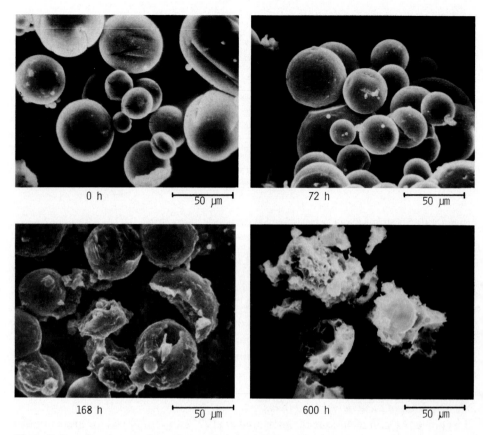

Figure 3. Scanning electron photomicrographs of polylactic acid microspheres containing 35.9% dibucaine.

(Fig. 4). When 15 mg tetracaine were administered in the form of microspheres, the pharmacological activity decreased gradually because of the sustained release of the drug from microspheres in vivo (Fig. 5). When a 5% tetracaine hydrochloride solution containing 15 mg tetracaine was injected subcutaneously to a guinea pig, the guinea pig died of the overdose.

When 20 mg dibucaine were administered in the form of microspheres, the local anesthetic effect lasted for more than 400 hours (Fig. 6). When drug-free microspheres were implanted subcutaneously, some degree of apparent local anesthetic activity was observed (Figs. 5 and 6), possibly due to cutaneous necrosis as a result of surgery.

3. Polycarbonate microspheres of dibucaine

Poly(ethylene carbonate), poly(propylene carbonate) and poly(ethylene propylene

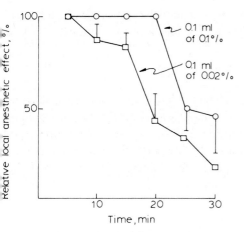

Figure 4. Duration of anesthetic effects following subcutaneous injection of tetracaine hydrochloride solution, $n = 4$.

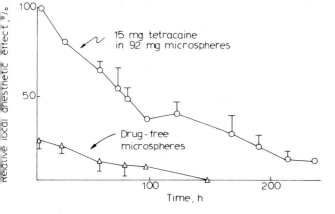

Figure 5. Duration of anesthetic effects following subcutaneous administration of polylactic acid microspheres, $n = 3$.

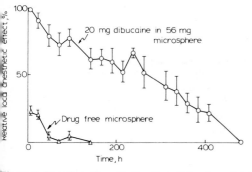

Figure 6. Duration of anesthetic effects following subcutaneous administration of polylactic acid microspheres, $n = 6$.

carbonate) were synthesized from carbon dioxide and the respective alkylene oxide (Inoue et al., 1975), and their intrinsic viscosity values at $25°C$ were 0.37, 0.58 and 0.51 dl/g, respectively.

3.1. Biodegradability of polycarbonates

The biodegradability of poly(ethylene carbonate) has been demonstrated in rats (Kawaguchi et al., 1983). Poly(ethylene carbonate) was shown to be biodegradable in guinea pigs also, whereas little poly(propylene carbonate) degraded during experimental periods of 28–84 days (Fig. 7). Poly(ethylene carbonate) degraded faster in the peritoneal cavity than in the subcutaneous tissue. Biodegradability of poly(ethylene propylene carbonate) has not yet been examined.

3.2. Characteristics of polycarbonate microspheres

Effects of initial dibucaine/polymer ratios on drug contents in poly(ethylene carbonate) microspheres are shown in Table 3. In polycarbonate microspheres also, drug contents increased with an increase in the initial drug/polymer ratio.

In Table 4 are given the sizes and drug contents of microspheres prepared from three different polycarbonates with an initial dibucaine/polymer ratio of 30:70. Diameters and drug contents were not very different from each other.

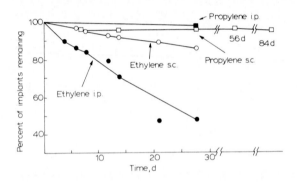

Figure 7. Biodegradation profiles of polycarbonates in guinea pigs, $n = 2$.

TABLE 3

Effect of drug/polymer ratio on dibucaine content in poly(ethylene carbonate) microspheres

Initial drug:polymer ratio	Drug content (%)
20:80	18.0
30:70	29.0
40:60	41.0

Prepared by evaporation in vacuo employing methylene chloride as a polymer solvent and 2% gelatin a a nonsolvent.

TABLE 4

Characteristics of dibucaine-polycarbonate microspheres

Polycarbonate	Diameter (μm)	Drug content (%)
Ethylene	57.2±3.0	29.0
Propylene	48.7±3.6	26.3
Ethylene-propylene	55.1±3.0	27.4

Prepared by evaporation in vacuo employing methylene chloride as a polymer solvent and 2% gelatin as a nonsolvent with an initial drug:polymer ratio of 30:70.

3.3. Release profiles

The release patterns of dibucaine from poly(ethylene carbonate) microspheres containing 29 and 41% dibucaine are shown in Figure 8. Gradual release was obtained from the microspheres with the lower drug content, while an initial burst release was noted in the microspheres with the higher drug content. This difference may be explained by the difference in the surface morphology of the two kinds of microspheres, shown in Figure 9.

The sigmoidal release patterns observed in the polylactic acid microspheres (Fig. 2) were not observed in the poly(ethylene carbonate) microspheres. This difference may be attributed to an extensive disintegration of the polylactic acid microspheres (Fig.3) and little disintegration of the poly(ethylene carbonate) microspheres even after the release of the drug (Fig. 10).

Effects of different polymers on the release rate of dibucaine are shown in Figure 11. Dibucaine was released fastest from poly(ethylene propylene carbonate) microspheres and slowest from poly(propylene carbonate) microspheres.

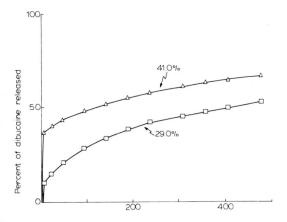

Figure 8. Effect of dibucaine content on release patterns from poly(ethylene carbonate) microspheres, $n = 2$ and 3.

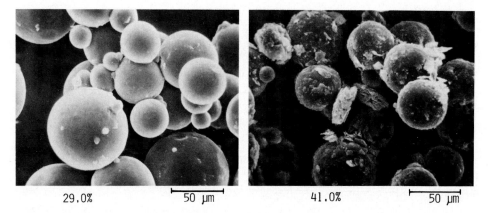

29.0% 50 μm   41.0% 50 μm

Figure 9. Scanning electron photomicrographs of poly(ethylene carbonate) microspheres containing dibucaine.

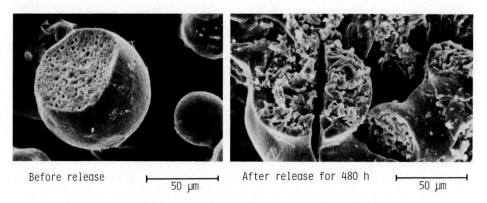

Before release   50 μm   After release for 480 h   50 μm

Figure 10. Scanning electron photomicrographs of cross-sections of poly(ethylene carbonate) microspheres containing 29.0% dibucaine.

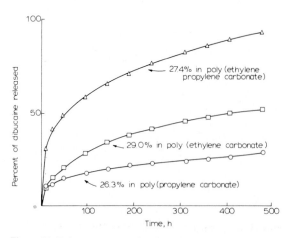

Figure 11. Release patterns of dibucaine from microspheres, n = 3, 3 and 2.

3.4. Duration of local anesthetic effects

Although local anesthetic effects which extended to more than 200 hours were observed following subcutaneous administration of 20 mg dibucaine in 73 mg poly(ethylene propylene carbonate) microspheres to guinea pigs, data are still preliminary, and therefore not presented here in the form of a figure.

4. Concluding remarks

Release rates of drugs from microspheres were shown to be dependent on size and drug content of the microspheres. Prolonged pharmacological effects were observed following administration of the drug in the form of microspheres to an experimental animal.

Although the usefulness of biodegradable polymers such as polylactic acid and poly(ethylene carbonate) as rate-controlling materials for injectable formulations has been demonstrated, the dependency of release rates of drugs and biodegradation rates on molecular weights of polymers have yet to be clarified. Furthermore, since a variety of polymers can be synthesized in the form of copolymers from lactic acid and glycolic acid and from ethylene oxide and propylene oxide, further studies are required to examine the usefulness of these copolymers as biomedical materials from the standpoint of biodegradability and release control.

References

Inoue, S., Tsuruta, T., Takada, T., Miyazaki, N., Kambe, M. and Takaoka, T. (1975) Appl. Polymer Symp. No. 26, 257–267.

Kawaguchi, T., Nakano, M., Juni, K., Inoue, S. and Yoshida, Y. (1982) Chem. Pharm. Bull. 30, 1517–1520.

Kawaguchi, T., Nakano, M., Juni, K., Inoue, S. and Yoshida, Y. (1983) Chem. Pharm. Bull. 31, 1400–1403.

Miller, R.A., Brady, J.M. and Cutright, D.E. (1977) J. Biomed. Mat. Res. 11, 711–719.

Nakano, N.I., Kawahara, N., Amiya, T., Gotoh, Y. and Furukawa, K. (1978) Chem. Pharm. Bull. 26, 936–941.

Quevauviller, A. (1977) in Local Anesthetics (Jong, R.H., Ed.), 2nd edn., pp. 291–318, C.C. Thomas, Springfield.

Wakiyama, N., Juni, K. and Nakano, M. (1981) Chem. Pharm. Bull. 29, 3363–3368.

Wakiyama, N., Juni, K. and Nakano, M. (1982a) J. Pharm. Dyn. 5, 13–17.

Wakiyama, N., Juni, K. and Nakano, M. (1982b) Chem. Pharm. Bull. 30, 2621–2628.

Wakiyama, N., Juni, K. and Nakano, M. (1982c) Chem. Pharm. Bull. 30, 3719–3727.

Microspheres and Drug Therapy. Pharmaceutical, Immunological and Medical Aspects
edited by S.S. Davis, L. Illum, J.G. McVie and E. Tomlinson
© *1984, Elsevier Science Publishers B.V.*
337

Nanoparticles: possible carriers for vaccines and cytostatics

J. Kreuter

Nanoparticles are solid colloidal particles ranging in size from 10 to 1000 nm (1 μm). They consist of macromolecular materials in which the active principle (drug or biologically active material) is dissolved, entrapped, encapsulated, and/or to which the active material is adsorbed or attached. They have been shown to be good adjuvants for vaccines and to exhibit good payload capacities for a variety of drugs.

The distribution pattern of nanoparticles after intravenous injection is very similar to that of other colloidal materials: after 30 minutes about 85% can be found in the liver, 4% in the spleen, and 4% in the lungs. While the coating of the nanoparticles with albumin does not change this distribution pattern, coating with Pluronic® F68 keeps the particles in the blood circulation for a prolonged time period and reduces the liver uptake to about 40% after 30 minutes and 50% after 1 week.

Nanoparticles hold promise as carriers for anti-tumoral drugs. They increased the efficacy of a number of cytostatics. However, the toxicity of some of these compounds, such as 5-fluorouracil, was also increased by binding to nanoparticles.

Microspheres and Drug Therapy. Pharmaceutical, Immunological and Medical Aspects
edited by S.S. Davis, L. Illum, J.G. McVie and E. Tomlinson
© *1984, Elsevier Science Publishers B.V.*

Microspheres and intestinal persorption

P.P. Speiser

Drugs are enterally absorbed by either passive diffusion or active transport mechanisms through the gut wall. Both phenomena take place in the dissolved, molecular or ionic state, but lipophilic droplets and particles such as fat, coal, xenobiotics and others can also be transferred in the solid state. This latter process has been known for quite a long time (Volkheimer); it is called (micro)pynocytosis, citopempsis or persorption, a process very similar to endocytosis and phagocytosis.

It can be shown that drugs bound to or incorporated into ultrafine solid lipophilic resin microspheres as carriers undergo similar persorption processes. The first preliminary results with radioactive tracered polyacrylate microspheres of a particle size between 150 and 350 nm show qualitatively this enteral passage phenomenon in the rat. Quantitatively, the persorption varies between 10 and 48%, depending on the drug, the lipophilicity, and other factors in the microspheres.

The classical opinion that drug can only be absorbed through biologic membranes in the dissolved state will probably be corrected in the near future, by the admission that an intestinal permeation of ultrafine particles as lipophilic microspheres loaded with drugs occurs.

Microspheres and Drug Therapy. Pharmaceutical, Immunological and Medical Aspects
edited by S.S. Davis, L. Illum, J.G. McVie and E. Tomlinson
© *1984, Elsevier Science Publishers B.V.*

Polymeric microspheres for controlled drug delivery

M.A. Wheatley and R. Langer

Previous studies in our laboratory have reported polymer systems that have been developed for the controlled release of macromolecular ($M_r > 1000$) drugs. These polymer systems have been shown to be capable of releasing for up to 100 days and over 50 different releasing substances have been used. These systems are based on ethylene vinyl acetate copolymer and other inert polymers. We now report the development of an injectable drug delivery system. A prototype system composed of sodium alginate and polyamino acids has proved to be a very effective system for the encapsulation of pancreatic islet cells and the growth of hybridoma cells. This report will discuss a modification of this microencapsulation method for use as a drug delivery system.

The capsules are made in three steps: Initial capsule formation: The encapsulation species is mixed with a solution of sodium alginate in saline, with a final alginate concentration of around 1.0%. This mixture is added dropwise into a 1.5% solution of $CaCl_2$ through a 22G syringe needle around which flows a coaxial air stream to detach the alginate drops. The alginate gels into spherical droplets immediately on contact with the $CaCl_2$ solution. Capsule coating: The washed alginate beads are coated by contact with a solution of polyamino acid in saline buffer. Liquefaction of the capsule interior: The alginate inside the polyamino acid-coated capsule is liquefied by sequestering the cross-linking Ca^{2+} with citrate during a sodium citrate wash step.

The release characteristics of the capsules can be modified by varying such parameters as the capsule size, the contact time during the polyamino acid step, or by post-encapsulation modification of the microspheres with bi- or multifunctional reagents. All these factors affect the release rate of different molecular weight substances differently, changing the molecular weight cut-off point for diffusion from the capsule.

Initial studies have been conducted to compare the in vivo release kinetics from this system to the in vitro kinetics. In this case we used a method previously developed in our laboratory which involves the release of radioactively labeled inulin, a substance that is not metabolized by the body, but which is excreted through the kidneys.

This work was supported by a grant from Damon Biotech Corporation.

Microspheres and Drug Therapy. Pharmaceutical, Immunological and Medical Aspects
edited by S.S. Davis, L. Illum, J.G. McVie and E. Tomlinson
© *1984, Elsevier Science Publishers B.V.*

Biodegradable microspheres for injection or inhalation

Patrick P. DeLuca, Motoko Kanke and Toyomi Sato

Microspheres in the 1–100 μm range have been prepared in our laboratories from poly(glycolic acid) and copolymers of glycolide and L-(−)-lactide. By controlling processing conditions, uniform microspheres were prepared by three methods — (a) freeze drying, (b) evaporation and (c) dilution-precipitation. Smaller, more porous spheres were obtained by the precipitation method; the freeze-dry method yielded spheres with the lowest porosity. The addition of a protective colloid before removal of the continuous phase increased the yields, reduced the size of spheres significantly and improved the porosity, as well as the release rates. The three methods enable the preparation of a very porous spherical matrix in which essentially all of the incorporated agent is accessible for leaching from a macroreticular network of interconnecting channels. The release, therefore, can be designed to depend predominantly on dissolution of the drug and diffusion through the fluid-filled pores and not on erosion of the polymer.

Polymer concentration in the dispersed phase was critical in producing spherical particles. 5–10% polymer produced spherical particles at 90% yields. Polymer concentration above 10% resulted in larger particles and lower yields. Controlling the dispersion temperature at 15°C and then increasing the temperature rapidly to 50°C to stabilize the emulsion droplets resulted in small spheres. 50% loading was found to be possible.

The very water-soluble FD&C Blue No. 1 released within 1–3 days, depending on the concentration of dye and polymer concentration. Release was complete before any discernible degradation or erosion of the polymer matrix. About 90% of the less-soluble prednisolone acetate released in 7 days, at which time degradation of the matrix was evident.

Porosity of the matrix and solubility of the drug will govern the release rate. Therefore, the release of a given drug can be controlled by controlling the porosity of the matrix. Erosion of the polymer matrix following release will be a function of the copolymer composition, molecular weight, cross-linking, and degree of hydrophobicity.

In a study of the interaction of 1-, 3- and 12-μm microspheres with blood constituents, 1- and 3-μm spheres were found in the lysosomes inside the cytoplasm of monocytes and granulocytes, with a residence time of up to at least 24 hours. The

12-μm spheres were observed outside the monocytes and granulocytes. There was no evidence of any damage to the lysosomes or other cellular organelles and normal enzymatic function of the monocytes and granulocytes was maintained, as evidenced by normal distribution of α-naphthyl esterase in the monocytes and naphthol AS-D chloroacetate esterase in the granulocytes. The response of T and B lymphocytes to pokeweed, phytohemagglutinin and concanavalin A mitogens showed no change 7 days after microsphere administration, in comparison to the response of lymphocytes obtained prior to administration, and the serum protein levels, including γ-globulin, were unchanged from control values, indicating that the spheres did not stimulate the immune response antigenically.

Microspheres and Drug Therapy. Pharmaceutical, Immunological and Medical Aspects
edited by S.S. Davis, L. Illum, J.G. McVie and E. Tomlinson
© 1984, Elsevier Science Publishers B.V.

Microsphere systems for intraarticular drug administration

J.H. Ratcliffe, I.M. Hunneyball, C.G. Wilson, A. Smith and S.S. Davis

The administration of steroids or cytotoxic drugs into the intra-articular cavity in patients with chronic inflammatory disease is complicated by two factors. Firstly, the release of drug into the systemic circulation and, secondly, the short duration of effect.

The principle requirements for an 'ideal' drug delivery system are as follows: 1. Delivery of the active principle over a sustained period (1 month). 2. The carrier system must be retained in the joint, uniformly distributed, and taken up by the phagocytic cells within the synovium. 3. The preparation and its degradation products must be non-irritant.

Biodegradable polymers have been evaluated as potential carriers for intra-articular steroids. Microparticles of polylactic acid (PLA) and polybutylcyanoacrylate (PBCA) and microspheres of gelatin (PG) (Yoshioka et al., 1981) and albumin (PA) (Tomlinson et al., 1982) have been prepared within the size range 1–10 μm. New Zealand White rabbits ($n = 6$ per group) received, by intra-articular administration, 2.5 mg (10 mg/ml) of each preparation. At 3 and 7 days, the animals were killed and the synovia removed for histological examination.

The PCBA and PLA particulates were found to cause joint inflammation. PBCA particulates caused severe localised hyperplasia of the synovial membrane due to the hydrophobic nature of the polymer and the toxicity of its major degradation product, formaldehyde. Underlying tissues were shown to be normal. PLA particulates caused a more general, less severe hyperplasia but with more extensive involvement of the subsynovial tissues. PG and PA were well tolerated, PG causing more inflammation than PA, with a diffuse cellular infiltration.

On the basis of its biocompatibility, and the observed uptake and retention into synovial cells, albumin microspheres have been chosen for further study. The retention of the radioactively labelled microspheres within the normal and arthritic joint is being evaluated by gamma scintigraphy.

346

References

Tomlinson, E., Burger, J.J., Schoonderwoerd, E.M.A., Kuik, J., Schlötz, F.C., McVie, J.G. and Mills, S.N. (1982) J. Pharm. Pharmacol. 34, 88P.
Yoshioka, T., Hashida, M., Muranishi and Sezaki, H. (1981) Int. J. Pharmaceut. 8, 131–142.

Microspheres and Drug Therapy. Pharmaceutical, Immunological and Medical Aspects
edited by S.S. Davis, L. Illum, J.G. McVie and E. Tomlinson
© *1984, Elsevier Science Publishers B.V.*

CHAPTER 17

The use of polyphthalamide microcapsules for obtaining extended periods of therapy in the eye

M. Beal, N.E. Richardson, B.J. Meakin and D.J.G. Davies

The treatment of chronic eye disease, such as glaucoma, is made difficult because the anatomy and physiology of the eye ensure that the majority of the volume of eye drops instilled on the corneal surface is rapidly removed by drainage and washout by lachrymal secretions. Any method that would extend the period during which the active drug remains in contact with the cornea would increase the period of activity of the drug. Methods so far used have included the use of viscolysers in eye drops, the use of polymeric devices, such as hydrogels, containing absorbed drug and polymeric membranes enclosing the drug, such as the Ocusert.

Our approach has been to prepare a suspension of polymeric microcapsules, of a sufficiently small size to be undetectable as particles by the eye. Of the different microcapsules used in preliminary studies the one chosen for assessment consisted of polyphthalamide prepared by an interfacial polymerisation technique. By careful application of standard procedures it proved possible to produce spherical hollow microcapsules with a mean diameter below 30 μm. These could be handled experimentally, dried, stored and resuspended in water without affecting their integrity.

In vivo studies were carried out whereby the dwell time in the rabbit eye of polyphthalamide microcapsules containing ^{99}Tc-labelled albumin was compared to an aqueous solution of ^{99}Tc-labelled albumin by means of gamma scintigraphy. These measurements showed that the aqueous albumin was rapidly cleared, only 10% of the instilled mass being present after 10 minutes. The microcapsules, however, remained longer and 60% of the instilled mass was still present after 90 minutes. Consequently, the techniques of instilling microencapsulation drugs in the eye for extended activity appears to be hopeful.

Pilocarpine nitrate was then incorporated into these microcapsules and in vitro studies were performed to measure the rate of release of pilocarpine from the microcapsules. The results of these experiments suggested that the walls of the polyphthalamide microcapsules do not significantly control the release of pilocarpine nitrate from the microcapsule core. Parallel studies, whereby the diffusion of pilocarpine nitrate through thin polyphthalamide films was measured, showed that this problem was due to the presence of pores in the microcapsule wall.

Further studies are at present being undertaken to modify the structure of the capsule wall to prepare a material that will control the rate of release of the contained pilocarpine.

Microspheres and Drug Therapy. Pharmaceutical, Immunological and Medical Aspects
edited by S.S. Davis, L. Illum, J.G. McVie and E. Tomlinson
© 1984, Elsevier Science Publishers B.V.

Stability of ^{99m}Tc-labelled liposomes in plasma. Potential use in lymphoscintigraphy

S. Frøkjaer, H. Hvid-Hansen, F. Tågehøj Jensen, P. Charles, J. Marqversen and J.C. Riis Jørgensen

In order to evaluate the possibilities for using liposomes for scintigraphy, the in vitro stability of small unilamellar ^{99m}Tc-labelled liposomes of eight different compositions has been studied in plasma. Liposomes were prepared as described previously (Battelle Memorial Institute, 1979; Frøkjaer et al., 1982), and the technetium label was associated to preformed liposomes using a stannous chloride method (Richardson et al., 1979), and the preparations controlled by a gel chromatography column scanning method (Darte and Persson, 1979).

The in vitro stability after incubation in porcine plasma for 1 hour at 37°C (10 nmol P/ml plasma) was studied by chromatography on Sepharose CL-6B. The results are shown in Table 1. When incubated in a saline solution, pH 7.4, more than 91% ^{99m}Tc-radioactivity is liposome-associated.

Measured as the ability to maintain ^{99m}Tc-associated in presence of plasma, liposomes containing phosphatidic acid show a greater stability than the other liposome compositions.

TABLE 1

In vitro stability of ^{99}Tc-labelled liposomes in plasma

Composition (molar ratio)	^{99m}Tc-radioactivity (%)		
	Liposome-associated	Plasma protein-associated	Low mol
PC: cholesterol (2:1)	13	67	20
PC:PS (4:1)	23	57	20
PC:PG (4:1)	39	53	8
PC:PA (4:1)	51	47	2
PC:PA:cholesterol (3:1:1)	61	36	3
PC:PA:cholesterol (3:1:4)[a]	81	17	2
PG	27	64	9
PA[a]	75	23	2

[a] Aggregation after ^{99m}Tc-labelling.

The in vivo distribution of ^{99m}Tc-labelled liposomes and a ^{99m}Tc-labelled commer
cial sulfur colloid kit was followed after interstitial administration to rabbits. The
γ-camera images show the potential of using liposomes containing phosphatidic acid
for imaging the draining primary and secondary lymph nodes.

References

Battelle Memorial Institute (1979) British Patent Appl. No. 200 1929 A.

Darte, L. and Persson, B.R. (1979) J. Liq. Chromatogr. 2, 499–509.

Frøkjaer, S., Hjorth, E.L. and Wørts, O. (1982) in Optimization of Drug Delivery (Bundgaard, H.,
Hansen, A.B. and Koford, H., Eds.), pp. 384–401, Munksgaard, Copenhagen.

Richardson, V.J., Ryman, B.E., Jewkes, R.F., Jeyasingh, K., Tattersall, M.N.H., Newlands, E.S. and
Kaye, S.B. (1979) Br. J. Cancer 40, 35–43.

Microspheres and Drug Therapy. Pharmaceutical, Immunological and Medical Aspects
edited by S.S. Davis, L. Illum, J.G. McVie and E. Tomlinson
© *1984, Elsevier Science Publishers B.V.*

Macromolecular Rifamycin conjugates for the local treatment of rheumatoid arthritis

L. Molteni, G. Bruno, M. Garufi, I. Caruso and M. Fumagalli

The antibiotic Rifamycin SV has been used recently for the treatment of rheumatoid arthritis by intraarticular administration. The possible mechanism of action of the drug is related to its site of injection, and it enters the blood stream following its metabolic and excretion pathways. The injection is painful, and consequently the drug cannot be administered more frequently than once a week. In order to obtain soluble, long-lasting Rifamycin SV derivatives, which might be taken up by cells (macrophages, synoviocites, etc.) of the inflammatory infiltration, three macromolecular conjugates were synthesized, linking the antibiotic to a γ-globulin, to a dextran and contemporaneously to a dextran and a γ-globulin. The conjugates are endowed with an antibiotic potency and, in consequence, a possible therapeutic activity, related to the content of Rifamycin SV in the macromolecule. It is possible to determine the quantity of the linked Rifamycin SV microbiologically by evaluating the antibiotic potency of the macrocompounds (*Staphylococcus aureus*, 6528 P) or by spectrophotometric analysis.

The molecule of Rifamycin does not contain any radical which is able to perform the homopolar bond with the macromolecules: for this reason the formyl derivative of Rifamycin SV was used, because it reacts very easily and retains the complete antibiotic. The reaction between 3-formyl-Ryfamycin SV (4 g) and γ-globulin (2 g) occurs directly.

To link 3-formyl-Rifamycin SV to dextran, a new activated dextran was prepared: hydrazine-hydroxy-propyl-dextran: the hydrazone-hydroxy-propyl-dextran of formyl-Rifamycin SV is afterwards reduced to a (methyl-Rifamycin SV) (hydrazine-hydroxy-propyl-dextran).
It is possible to link the same dextran chain to the γ-globulin and to formyl-Rifamycin SV by a two-step conjugation reaction.

The macromolecular conjugates of Rifamycin SV are endowed with pharmacokinetics and bioavailability which differ from the free antibiotic. The intramuscular injection of Rifamycin dextran in the dog shows initial lower, but longer-lasting serum levels. The (γ-globulin-)(Rifamycin SV-methyl-hydrazine)-hydroxy-propyl-dextran 70,000 is practically non-bioavailable.

In the guinea pig, the sinovial concentration, after in situ injection of Rifamycin dextran conjugate, is much higher and longer lasting than the free Rifamycin SV, while the serum levels are lower.

A clinical trial with the dextran 5000 conjugate of Rifamycin SV, by intraarticular injection in the small joints of arthritic patients' fingers, to compare its therapeutic activity to free Rifamycin SV, is in progress. However, because of the poor water solubility of the Rifamycin SV γ-globulin conjugate, the initial trial with this compound was interrupted.

Section 4

Active targeting in vivo and in vitro — Homing with antibodies and magnetic particles

Microspheres and Drug Therapy. Pharmaceutical, Immunological and Medical Aspects
edited by S.S. Davis, L. Illum, J.G. McVie and E. Tomlinson
© 1984, Elsevier Science Publishers B.V.

CHAPTER 1

Drug targeting using monoclonal antibody-coated nanoparticles

Lisbeth Illum, P.D.E. Jones and S.S. Davis

1. Intravenous administration of colloidal particles

Colloidal particles administered via the intravenous route will find their way to different organs, depending on the size and surface characteristics of the particle (Illum et al., 1982). Particles larger than about 7 μm in diameter will normally be trapped in the capillary networks of the lungs. This effect has been exploited in radiodiagnostic imaging (Davis and Taube, 1978) as well as in drug targeting (Yoshioka et al., 1981; Illum and Davis, 1982). Particles in the size range 100 nm–5 μm tend to be removed efficiently by the cells of the reticuloendothelial system in the liver and to a lesser extent in the spleen. In general, the process of uptake is very rapid, with a half time of clearance from the blood of less than 1 minute. The rate and degree of uptake of particles can be reduced either by changing the surface characteristics of the particles by a coating process (Illum and Davis, 1983) or by preblocking the reticuloendothelial system with excess of placebo colloid (Murray, 1963). In such instances greater lung and bone marrow uptakes are observed.

Particles less than 100 nm can possibly leave the systemic circulation through gaps or fenestrations in the endothelial cells lining the blood vessels. The fenestrations are of different sizes, depending on the capillary bed considered. The capillary endothelium of pancreas, intestines and kidney has fenestrations of 50–60 nm while that of the liver, spleen and bone marrow has fenestrations of about 100 nm, for example, allowing particles such as chylomicrons to escape from the blood to the liver hepatocytes (Knook and Wisse, 1982) and particles to be taken up into the bone marrow (Frier, 1981). The blood vessels that supply some tumours are also believed to be leaky, thereby allowing the escape of small particles into the tumour tissue (Grislain et al., 1983). Indeed, one animal tumour, the Lewis lung carcinoma, has capillary beds where the endothelial cells are absent, thereby allowing good access of blood (and possibly particles contained therein) to the tumour cells (James and Salsbury, 1974).

The uptake of colloidal liposomal particles into tumours has been reported by Ryman and colleagues (Richardson et al., 1977; Ryman et al., 1978). Their investigations using the Walker 256 tumour showed that well sonicated (small) charged (preferably negatively) fluid liposomes could be localised in the tumour. However, Kimelberg et al. (1975) and Anghileri et al. (1976) have reported little evidence of uptak of liposomes into the tumour tissue of tumour-bearing mice. More recently, Grislai et al. (1983) have described the tissue distribution and blood clearance of biodegrad able polycyanoacrylate nanoparticles. After intravenous administration to mice bear ing a subcutaneously grafted Lewis lung carcinoma, progressive accumulation of th carrier in tumour tissue was observed using whole body autoradiography. Further more, a high level of activity was found in the metastatic lungs of cancerous animals No lung accumulation was found in healthy mice.

In a similar study Kreuter (Section 3, Chapter 12) has also claimed the uptake o nanoparticles into tumour tissues. Such results suggest that colloidal particles con taining cytotoxic agents could be beneficial in cancer chemotherapy. However, th reported uptakes of particles are not large when the data are considered as a percent age of the total dose administered. Thus, ways need to be found to increase the selec tivity of targeting of microspheres and nanoparticles if they are to be used clinicall to deliver cytostatic agents to tumour sites. In our work we have brought togethe two potential approaches for drug targeting: nanoparticles and monoclonal antibo dies.

2. Monoclonal antibodies and drug targeting

The antigen-antibody reaction is one of the most specific interactions that occurs i biological tissue. Monoclonal antibodies have been produced which specify antigen associated with human tumours, including carcinoma of the lung (Sikora an Wright, 1981) and osteogenic sarcoma (Embleton et al., 1981). Thus, in theory i should be possible to deliver a drug bound to an antibody specifically to tumour cells Until recently, this approach has had only limited success in practice since it has bee difficult to produce antisera with sufficient specificity (Rowland, 1983). The adven of hybridoma technology makes it possible to overcome these problems (Kohler an Milstein, 1975).

Monoclonal antibodies to human tumours can now be prepared in many labora tories and these have been used with success in radiodiagnostic imaging (Farrand et al., 1982) and drug targeting (Rowland, 1983; Arnon and Hurwitz, 1983). The re sults of recent studies indicate that antibodies or their immunologically active frag ments (F(ab)) may serve as carriers for drugs to tumour cells either by a direct conju gation of drug to antibody or through the use of a linking molecule, such as dextran

3. Monoclonal antibodies attached to colloidal particles

Various workers have linked monoclonal antibodies to liposomes in order to improv tissue selectivity in drug targeting. Various methods of linking have been described ranging from simple adsorption to covalent bonds (Leserman et al., 1979; Huang an

Kennell, 1979; Endoh et al., 1981; Heath et al., 1981). These antibody-liposome systems have shown specific binding in in vitro experiments (Leserman et al., 1979; Cohen et al., 1976; Weissmann et al., 1975), but the few results from in vivo studies have been disappointing (Weissmann et al., 1978; Torchilin, 1983).

Antibodies can also be coupled to microspheres by direct adsorption (Bagchi and Birnbaum, 1981; Illum et al., 1983) or via protein A adsorption (Widder et al., 1981; Couvreur, 1983) as well as by covalent linkage (e.g., carbodiimide, cyanogen bromide and glutaraldehyde reactions) (Molday et al., 1975; Yen et al., 1979; Rembaum et al., 1976; Rembaum and Margel, 1978). Such systems have been used mainly for immunological studies and cell separation (Illum and Jones, 1984).

4. Monoclonal antibody-nanoparticle systems

Although drug-antibody conjugates have the ability to target to tumour sites, the linking of the drug can be a difficult procedure that may result in inactivation of the drug and/or the antibody (Pimm et al., 1982b). In addition, there must be sufficient antibody to deliver the required concentration of the attached therapeutic agent to the target site. A colloidal system in the form of nanoparticles with a large carrier capacity coated with monoclonal antibodies has been proposed as an alternative (Illum et al., 1983). Polyhexylcyanoacrylate nanoparticles have been prepared using Dextran 70 as a stabiliser. The particles were coated with monoclonal antibodies and their interaction with target cells in vitro and in vivo has been investigated.

The physical adsorption of an antibody onto a solid particle can occur in two different ways. The adsorption can occur via the antigen binding sites (F(ab)) with the Fc portion protruding into the medium. In this configuration the antibody will not be able to bind with an antigenic target cell. Alternatively, the antibody can bind the other way round, with the Fc site adsorbed to the particle surface, thereby leaving the F(ab) binding sites free to interact with antigenic cells. Clearly, the second configuration is required for targeting purposes. This type of binding can be achieved if the surface of the nanoparticle is relatively hydrophobic (Bagchi and Birnbaum, 1981).

4.1. In vitro studies

Nanoparticles coated with monoclonal antibody were prepared according to Scheme 1 (Illum et al., 1983). Hexyl-2-cyanoacrylate was dispersed in acidified normal saline containing Dextran 70 as a stabiliser. After the polymerisation was complete, the resultant suspension of average particle size 170 nm was neutralised.

The anti-osteogenic sarcoma monoclonal antibodies (791T/36 and 791T/48) which recognise different epitopes on 788T osteogenic sarcoma cells were prepared as supernatants from in vitro cultured cells as described by Pimm et al. (1982a). In order to detect antibody-antigen binding the nanoparticles were also labelled with fluorescent bovine serum albumin.

356

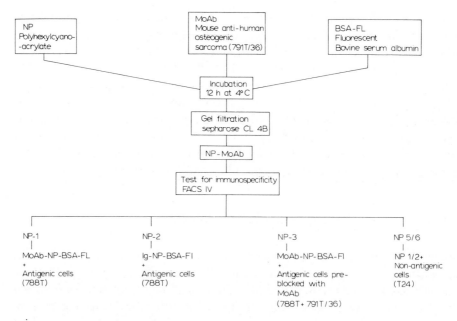

Scheme 1. In vitro studies on nanoparticles (NP) and monoclonal antibodies (MoAb).

Proteins (monoclonal antibody or normal immunoglobulins) and fluorescent conjugates were adsorbed together onto the surface of the nanoparticles by overnight incubation (equilibrium conditions). The coated nanoparticles were separated from the adsorption mixture by gel filtration on Sepharose CL-4B columns. This gave elution profiles with two distinct peaks. The first of these corresponded to the nanoparticles and the second to the adsorption mixture. The stability of the binding of the antibody to the nanoparticles in phosphate-buffered saline was good.

An adsorption isotherm study showed that, as expected (Bagchi and Birnbaum, 1981), the binding isotherm was Langmuirian in nature. Calculations made using surface area values based on a monodisperse distribution of nanoparticles of size 170 nm in diameter and the estimated area of 38 nm^2 per adsorbed immunoglobulin molecule (monoclonal antibody) at a pH value of 7 (Bagchi and Birnbaum, 1981) allowed an estimation of 2000 as the theoretical maximum number of monoclonal antibodies on each individual nanoparticle.

The target cells used in the in vitro cell binding assay were the human osteogenic sarcoma cell lines 788T and T24 as negative controls. These were grown in vitro as monolayers and then prepared as monodisperse cell suspensions.

The binding of coated nanoparticles to tumour cells was measured by flow cytofluorimetry using a Fluorescence Activated Cell Sorter, FACS IV. The specificity of the binding was assessed by inclusion in the assay of antigenically inappropriate target cells and the capacity of pretreatment of the target cells with antibody to block subsequent binding of the nanoparticles.

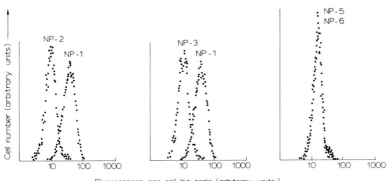

Figure 1. Flow cytofluorimetric graphs of the log normal fluorescence distribution of 788T and T24 tumour cells derived from cell cultures pretreated with media or antibody and incubated with either antibody- or immunoglobulin-coated fluorescent bovine serum albumin nanoparticle (NP) conjugates.

Figure 1 shows the shift in fluorescence intensity that occurs when nanoparticles coated with monoclonal antibody (but not when coated with normal immunoglobulin) interact specifically with the appropriate target cells (788T). The binding of antibody-coated nanoparticles to 788T cells could be inhibited by pretreatment of the cells with non-conjugated antibody. No shift in fluorescent intensity was observed for nanoparticles incubated with T24 cells.

The capacity of the coated nanoparticles to bind specifically to the target 788T cells was retained for up to 4 days after coating of the nanoparticles, but by 7 days specific binding of the nanoparticles to the cells was no longer demonstrable. It was also shown that pretreatment of the cells with antibody recognising a different epitope on the 788T cells to that recognised by the antibody coating the nanoparticles did not affect the specific binding of the coated nanoparticles to the cells.

The results of the in vitro study showed that monoclonal antibody was well adsorbed onto the surface of the polyhexylcyanoacrylate nanoparticles and that nanoparticles thus coated interacted in a specific way with antigenic tumour cells in vitro. Therefore, some (or all) of the antibody was adsorbed to the surface of the particle via the Fc portions leaving the F(ab) sites free to interact with antigenic cells.

4.2. In vivo studies

On the basis of the in vitro results, the applicability of the system to tumour targeting in vivo was investigated. Pimm et al. (1982b) have already shown that the same monoclonal antibodies are preferentially taken up in vivo by osteosarcoma tumour tissue xenografts in mice, as compared with muscle, bone or visceral organs.

The experimental procedure is shown in Scheme 2. The nanoparticles were prepared using a ^{14}C-labelled monomer in order to be able to follow the distribution of the nanoparticles in the body. The ^{14}C was incorporated into the backbone of the polymer. A mixture of Pluronic F68 (a non-ionic surface active agent) and Dextran

358

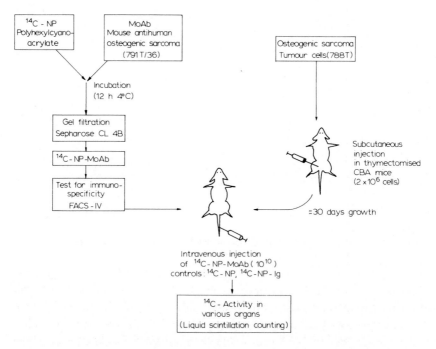

Scheme 2. In vivo studies on nanoparticles (NP) and monoclonal antibodies (MoAb).

70 was used as the stabiliser. The nanoparticles (of average size 130 nm) were dialysed against distilled water in order to obtain a sufficiently hydrophobic surface for adsorption of the antibodies. The monoclonal antibodies were adsorbed onto the nanoparticles by overnight incubation and the coated nanoparticles separated from the free protein by gel filtration as before.

The human tumour cell line osteogenic sarcoma 788T was used for producing tumour xenografts in mice. CBA mice were immunodeprived (thymectomized and irradiated) and xenograft growths were initiated by subcutaneous (flank) injection of 2×10^6 tumour cells. After 1 month the mice were examined and placed in nine groups of four so that all groups were as similar as possible with regard to tumour sizes. Then, naked nanoparticles, normal immunoglobulin-coated nanoparticles or monoclonal antibody-coated nanoparticles were injected intravenously into the tail vein. 4 hours, 24 hours and 4 days later, the groups of mice were killed and dissected. Tumour, spleen, kidney, liver, heart, lungs, bone and blood samples were weighed and assayed for radioactivity.

Figure 2 shows the distribution of naked, normal immunoglobulin G- and monoclonal antibody-coated nanoparticles in various tissues 4 hours, 24 hours and 4 days after intravenous injection. All three systems were mainly distributed in the liver and spleen and no significant uptake was found in the tumours for either naked or coated nanoparticle systems. Thus, the particles were apparently removed very effectively by the reticuloendothelial system (Kupffer cells).

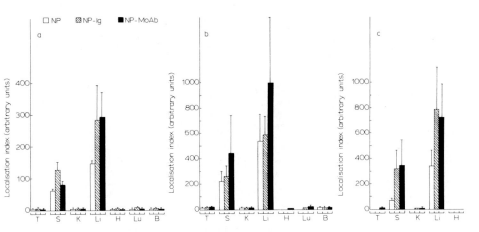

Figure 2. Distribution of naked and normal immunoglobulin G (Ig) or monoclonal antibody (MoAb) coated ^{14}C-labelled poly(hexyl-2-cyanoacrylate) nanoparticles (NP) in bone, tumour and visceral organs of mice (*n* = 4, mean ± S.E.) a 4 hours; b, 24 hours; c, 4 days, after injection. T, tumour; S, spleen; K, kidney; Li, liver; H, heart; Lu, lungs; B, bone.

The results for the naked nanoparticles do not agree with the findings of Grislain et al. (1983), who reported significant uptake of nanoparticles into tumours (Lewis lung carcinoma). They suggested that some of their small particles were able to escape the reticuloendothelial system (RES) and to reach the tumour by passing through the blood vessel endothelium. However, the Lewis lung carcinoma has been described as having poorly formed sinusoidal vascular channels in which an endothelial lining is absent and blood cells are in direct contact with tumour cells (James and Salsbury, 1974). A number of reasons for a lack of targeting of monoclonal antibody-coated particles to the tumours have been proposed (Illum et al., 1984).

1. Any monoclonal antibodies adsorbed with their Fc portion protruding outwards would be expected to enhance the clearance of the particles by the RES (Van Oss et al., 1975), thereby reducing any tumour targeting propensity.

2. Competitive displacement of the adsorbed monoclonal antibody by blood component could take place after the monoclonal antibody-coated nanoparticles are injected into the bloodstream.

3. A secondary coating process might occur where the monoclonal antibody-coated particles receive an opsonic layer that allows them to be taken up by the RES.

4. The size of the particles may be too large to allow their escape to extravascular sites.

5. The capillary endothelium in the region of the tumour is not sufficiently leaky to admit the escape of particles or that the blood supply to the tumour is not sufficient to allow effective targeting.

6. The liver and spleen may contain antigens originating from the xenograft and the particles are bound preferentially at these sites.

Aspects 1 and 2 can be resolved by the attachment of the antibody onto the particle

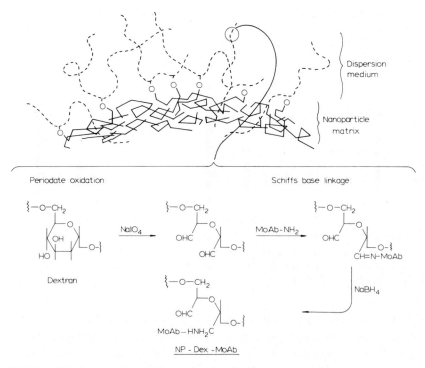

Scheme 3. Covalent attachment of monoclonal antibodies to nanoparticles.

using a covalent bond. Aspect 3 can be considered in terms of surface coatings that will extend the lifetime of particles in the blood as well as divert a proportion of them away from the liver and spleen to other sites.

4.3. Covalent attachment of monoclonal antibodies to nanoparticles

The formation of polyalkylcyanoacrylate nanoparticles occurs through an anionic polymerisation mechanism involving initiation by nucleophilic attack (Coover and McIntire, 1977). Normally, under aqueous conditions OH⁻ is the attacking species, resulting in a hydroxyl terminated polymer. However, when dextran is used as the stabilising agent it is possible for dextran itself to be incorporated into the nanoparticle through a covalent linkage (Scheme 3) (Douglas et al., 1984). Analysis has shown that about 10% of dextran can be incorporated in this way. The surface-bound dextran can be oxidized to provide free aldehyde groups that can then be linked to the monoclonal antibody through a Schiff's base linkage.

4.4. Surface coatings and the reticuloendothelial system

Following intravenous administration the uptake of particles by the cells of the reticuloendothelial system in the liver and spleen will be determined mainly by the physicochemical characteristics of the particles; in particular, their size, surface charge and surface hydrophobicity (Van Oss et al., 1975). Coating of particles with polymers and macromolecules can alter organ uptake considerably (Wilkins, 1967). Studies on emulsion systems by Jeppsson and Rossner (1975) and Geyer (1967) have demonstrated that non-ionic surfactants of the Pluronic (poloxamer) series can modify the kinetics of blood clearance and Illum and Davis (1983), using gamma scintigraphy and organ analysis, showed that blood clearance and organ deposition of polystyrene microspheres (1.27 μm) could be altered using Pluronic F108 (poloxamer 338). Coated particles had a reduced uptake in the liver with a corresponding increase in the lungs. These studies have now been extended using much smaller particles of polystyrene (i.e., 60 nm) and a wide range of coating agents (e.g., phospholipids, IgA, surfactants) (Illum and Davis, 1984). The uncoated particles were taken out of circulation rapidly by the liver and spleen. Approximately 90% of the particles were deposited in these organs and the half-time for clearance was of the order of 50 seconds. The amounts deposited in the lung and heart, as well as the carcass and remaining in the blood were small (Fig. 3). Coating the particles with poloxamer 338 had a dramatic effect. Although some particles were still taken up rapidly by the liver and spleen, the total uptake in these organs was greatly reduced and much larger quantities of activity were found in the lung and heart regions and the carcass and blood (Fig. 3). The blood clearance profiles for the uncoated and coated systems were also very different. In the absence of the surfactant the particles were cleared rapidly

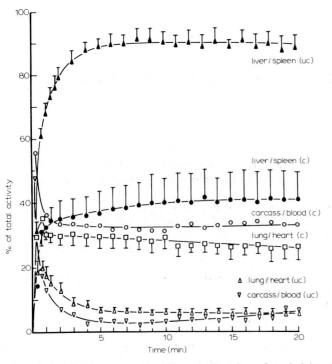

Figure 3. Activity-time profiles for different body regions after administration of uncoated (uc) and poloxamer 338-coated (c) polystyrene latex particles (50 nm) ($n = 3$, mean ± S.E.).

362

from the blood, while for coated particles significant sustained levels of activity were observed. The change in distribution of the particles and the deposition of particles in the bone marrow of the animal could be clearly demonstrated in scintiscans of rabbits. The effect of the non-ionic surfactant has been related to the hydrophilic nature of the coating material and the decreased adhesion of poloxamer-coated particles to cell surfaces (Illum and Davis, 1984).

These results demonstrate clearly that it is possible to divert small particles away from the reticuloendothelial systems of the liver and spleen by the use of appropriate surface coatings.

5. Conclusions

Small particles (nanoparticles) can be coated noncovalently with monoclonal antibodies which are well adsorbed to the particle surface. Although coated nanoparticles bind specifically to target cells in vitro, in vivo the particles are localised, in a similar manner to the naked particles, to the liver and spleen with no significant uptake in the tumour. This is probably due to loss of immunospecificity or failure to avoid clearance by the RES, as discussed. Particles coated with a non-ionic surface active agent and monoclonal antibodies covalently attached to their surface may have a greater chance of reaching tumour sites following intravenous administration, due to diversion of the surfactant-coated particles away from the RES.

Acknowledgements

This work was supported in part by the NATO Science Foundation and the Cancer Research Campaign.

References

Anghileri, L.J., Firusian, N. and Brucksch (1976) J. Nucl. Biol. Med. 20, 165–167.

Arnon, R. and Hurwitz, E. (1983) in Targeted Drugs (Goldberg, E.P, Ed.), pp. 23–55, Wiley-Interscience, New York.

Bagchi, P. and Birnbaum, S.M. (1981) J. Colloid Interface Sci. 83, 460–478.

Cohen, C.M., Weissmann, G., Hoffstein, S., Awasthi, Y.C. and Srivistava, S.K. (1976) Biochemistry 15, 452–460.

Coover, H.W. and McIntire, J.M. (1977) in Handbook of Adhesives (Skeist, I., Ed.), pp. 569–580, Van Nostrand, Rheinhold, New York.

Couvreur, P. (1983) in Topics in Pharmaceutical Sciences (Breimer, D.D. and Speiser, P., Eds.), Elsevier Biomedical Press, Amsterdam, pp. 305–316.

Davis, M.A. and Taube, R.A. (1978) J. Nucl. Med. 19, 1209–1213.

Douglas, S.J., Illum, J. and Davis, S.S. (1984) J. Colloid Interface Sci., in press.

Embleton, M.J., Gunn, B., Byers, V.S. and Baldwin, R.W. (1981) Br. J. Cancer 43, 582–587.

Endoh, H., Suzuki, Y. and Hashimoto, Y. (1981) J. Immunol. Meth. 44, 79–85.

Farrands, P.A., Perkins, A., Sully, L., Hopkins, J.S., Pimm, M.V., Baldwin, R.W. and Hardcastle, J.D. (1982) Lancet ii, 397–400.

Frier, M. (1981), in Progress in Radiopharmacology, (Cox, P.H., Ed.), Vol. 2, pp. 249–260, Elsevier/North Holland Biomedical Press, Amsterdam.

Geyer, R.P. (1967) Fette Med. 6, 59–61.

Grislain, L., Couvreur, P., Lenaerts, V., Roland, M., Deprez-Decampeneere, D. and Speiser, P. (1983) Int. J. Pharmaceut. 15, 335–345.

Heath, T.D., Macher, B.A. and Papahadjopoulos, D. (1981) Biochim. Biophys. Acta 640, 66–81.

Huang, L. and Kennell, S.J. (1979) Biochemistry 18, 1702–1707.

Illum, L. and Davis, S.S. (1982) J. Parent. Sci. Tech. 36, 242–248.

Illum, L. and Davis, S.S. (1983) J. Pharm. Sci. 72, 1086–1089.

Illum, L. and Davis, S.S. (1984) FEBS Lett. 167, 79–82.

Illum, L. and Jones, P.D.E. (1984) in Methods in Enzymology; Drug and Enzyme Targeting (Widder, K.J. and Green, R., Eds.), Academic Press, New York, in press.

Illum, L., Davis, S.S., Wilson, C.G., Thomas, N.W., Frier, M. and Hardy, J.G. (1982) Int. J. Pharmaceut. 12, 135–146.

Illum, L., Jones, P.D.E., Kreuter, J., Baldwin, R.W. and Davis, S.S. (1983) Int. J. Pharmaceut. 17, 65–76.

Illum, L., Jones, P.D.E. and Davis, S.S. (1984) J. Pharmacol. Exp. Therap., in press.

James, S.E. and Salsbury, A.J. (1974) Cancer Res. 34, 839–842.

Jeppsson, R. and Rossner, S. (1975) Acta Pharm. Toxicol. 37, 134–144.

Kimmelberg, H.K., Mayhew, E. and Papahadjopoulos, D. (1975) Life Sci. 17, 715–724.

Knook, D.L. and Wisse, E. (Eds.) (1982) Sinusoidal Liver Cells, Elsevier Biomedical Press, Amsterdam.

Kohler, G. and Milstein, C. (1975) Nature 256, 495–497.

Leserman, L.D., Weinstein, J.N., Blumenthal, R., Sharrow, S.O. and Terry, W.D. (1979) J. Immunol. 122, 585–591.

Molday, R.S., Dreyer, W.J., Rembaum, A. and Yen, S.P.S. (1975) J. Cell Biol. 64, 75–88.

Murray, I.M. (1963) J. Exp. Med. 117, 139–147.

Pimm, M.V., Embleton, M.J., Perkins, A.C., Price, M.R., Robins, R., Robinson, G.R. and Baldwin, R.W. (1982a) Int. J. Cancer 30, 75–85.

Pimm, M.V., Jones, J.A., Price, M.R., Middle, J.G., Embleton, M.J. and Baldwin, R.W. (1982b) Cancer Immunol. Immunother. 12, 125–134.

Rembaum, A. and Margel, S. (1978) Br. Polymer J. 10, 275–280.

Rembaum, A., Yen, S.P.S., Cheong, E., Wallace, S., Molday, R.S., Gordon, I.L. and Dreyer, W.J. (1976) Macromolecules 9, 328–336.

Richardson, V.J., Jeyasingh, K., Jewkes, R.F., Ryman, B.E. and Tattersall, M.H.N. (1977) Biochem. Soc. Trans. 5, 290–291.

Rowland, G. (1983) in Targeted Drugs (Goldberg, E.P., Ed.), pp. 57–72, Wiley-Interscience, New York.

Ryman, B.E., Jewkes, R.F., Jeyasingh, K., Osborne, M.P., Patel, H.M., Richardson, V.J., Tattersall, M.H.N. and Tyrrell, D.A. (1978) Ann. New York Acad. Sci. 308, 281–306.

Sikora, K. and Wright, R. (1981) Br. J. Cancer 43, 696–700.

Torchilin, V.P. (1983) in Targeted Drugs (Goldberg, E.P., Ed.), pp. 127–152, Wiley-Interscience, New York.

Van Oss, C.F., Gillam, C.F. and Neuman, A.W. (1975) Phagocytic Engulfment and Cell Adhesiveness, Dekker, New York.

Weissmann, G., Bloomgarden, R., Kaplan, C., Cohen, C., Hoffstein, S., Collins, T., Gottlieb, A. and Nagle, D. (1975) Proc. Natl. Acad. Sci. U.S.A. 72, 88–92.

Weissmann, G., Korchak, H., Finkelstein, M., Smolen, J. and Hoffstein, S. (1978) Ann. N.Y. Acad. Sci. 308, 235–249.

Widder, K.J., Senyei, A.E., Ovadia, H. and Paterson, P.Y. (1981) J. Pharm. Sci. 70, 387–389.

Wilkins, D.J. (1967) J. Colloid Interface Sci. 25, 84–89.

Yen, S.P.S., Rembaum, A., Molday, R.W. and Dreyer, W. (1979) in Emulsion Polymerisation, A.C.S. Symposium Series, Vol. 24 (Piirman, J. and Gordon, J.L., Eds.), pp. 236–257, Washington.

Yoshioka, T., Hashida, M., Muranishi, S. and Sezaki, H. (1981) Int. J. Pharmaceut. 8, 131–141.

Microspheres and Drug Therapy. Pharmaceutical, Immunological and Medical Aspects
edited by S.S. Davis, L. Illum, J.G. McVie and E. Tomlinson
© 1984, Elsevier Science Publishers B.V.

CHAPTER 2

Preparation and biomedical applications of monodisperse polymer particles

J. Ugelstad, A. Rembaum, J.T. Kemshead, K. Nustad, S. Funderud
and R. Schmid

1. Introduction

Magnetizable polymer particles may be used in cancer therapy for biophysical targeting of antitumour agents (Widder et al., 1979b, Mosbach and Schröder, 1979) and for in vitro separation of tumour cells from normal cells.

In most biochemical and biomedical applications of magnetic polymer particles a major problem lies in the preparation of polymer particles which are well characterized regarding size as well as content of magnetizable material. For use in cell separation procedures, the particles should, in addition, allow the establishment of an effective binding of the magnetic particles to the cancer cells, with little non-specific binding to other cells.

Most procedures for preparation of magnetic particles have included the use of finely divided iron, Fe_3O_4 or other ferrites, which in various ways has been covered with or introduced into synthetic or natural polymers.

Polymerization of a mixture of acrylate monomers by emulsion polymerization in the presence of finely divided Fe_3O_4 with ordinary initiators or cobalt irradiation has been described (Molday et al., 1977; Rembaum et al., 1979). The particles formed are of different sizes and contain different amounts of Fe_3O_4. Quite recently, it was reported that particles of polyacrolein containing magnetite may be prepared by controlled anionic polymerization of acrolein in the presence of colloidally dispersed Fe_3O_4 (ferro fluid) (Margel et al., 1982). Another recent method for preparation of polymer particles containing Fe_3O_4 involves a microsuspension process where Fe_3O_4 or other ferrites are made hydrophobic and added to the monomer mixture containing oil-soluble peroxide initiators. Then this mixture is suspended in water and polymerized. Small particles of hydrophobic polymer in the size range $0.1–1$ μm containing 1% by weight of Fe_3O_4 (Daniel et al., 1982) as well as larger particles, $10–100$ μm, with up to 30% Fe_3O_4 (Buske and Götze, 1983) have been prepared by variations of this method.

Preparation of natural polymers containing magnetizable materials has involved mixing of an aqueous solution of natural polymers such as starch (Mosbach and Schröder, 1979), dextran, agarose (Schröder and Mosbach, 1983) and albumin

(Widder et al., 1979a; Morimoto et al., 1981) with Fe_3O_4. Formation of particles is then achieved by pouring these mixtures while stirring into a water-insoluble, organic liquid followed by a possible insolubilization of the polymer by crystallization (Schröder and Mosbach, 1983), heat denaturation or cross-linking. Cellulose-based particles have been prepared starting with water-soluble cellulose and Fe_3O_4 (Forrest and Landon, 1978). Furthermore, it has been claimed that the Fe_3O_4 in the form of ferro fluid can be absorbed directly into already formed porous particles of Sepharose (Mosbach, 1982). An interesting method for covering Fe_3O_4 particles suspended in water with polymer involves the polymerization of the vinyl monomer with $K_2S_2O_8$, in which case the radicals are initiated at the surface of the Fe_3O_4 particles by a redox reaction (Kronick et al., 1978). Quite recently, very small magnetic iron-dextran particles have been prepared by addition of Fe^{2+} and Fe^{3+} salt mixtures to an aqueous solution of dextran, followed by heating at pH 11–15 (Molday and Mackenzie, 1982). After a relatively extensive separation and cleaning procedure, dextran particles of about 40 nm with up to 50% magnetite by weight were obtained.

Some of the particles described above have been tested in magnetic cell separation processes, including separation of cancer cells from normal cells, although they have not actually been used in cancer therapy yet. In cancer therapy removal of cancer cells by magnetic means has already been tried using very fine colloidal dispersions of cobalt. In this case the secondary antibody was bound directly to the metal surface by physical adsorption (Poyn et al., 1983).

The methods described above for formation of polymer particles containing magnetizable materials usually lead to a relatively broad particle size distribution, which results in different amounts of magnetizable material per particle. In addition, the concentration of magnetizable material in the particles will often vary too.

Ugelstad et al. (1980, 1983a–c) have described new methods for polymerization which allow the preparation of polymer particles which are completely uniform in size. The particles have been prepared in sizes from 0.5 to 100 μm. Also, the method allows the use of practically any kind of vinyl monomer and vinyl monomer mixtures for the preparation of monodisperse particles.

Core and shell particles are easily prepared, which in turn allows the preparation of particles of controlled low density combined with a surface containing suitable functional groups for covalent coupling to proteins. The method has also been used to prepare microporous and macroporous particles and combinations of these structures. Core and shell particles and porous particles have already found wide applications in immunoassays and in liquid chromatography (Nustad et al., 1982a,b; Johansen et al., 1983; Ugelstad et al., 1983a).

Quite recently Ugelstad et al. (1983d) developed various methods for rendering the monosized polymer particles magnetic by formation of magnetizable materials as Fe_3O_4 and other ferrites in already preformed monosized polymer particles. This chapter discusses the binding of different immunoglobulins to these particles, the biological activity of the bound immunoglobulins, the coupling of the particles to different cancer cells and the use of magnetic particles in cell separation. In addition, the preparation of highly monodisperse radioactive particles is described.

2. Materials and methods

2.1. Preparation of particles

Several types of magnetic particles have been prepared. The methods have in common that one starts with monosized polymer particles which in a second step are made 'magnetic' by formation of Fe_3O_4 or other ferrites in the particles. Macroporous magnetic particles have been prepared by formation of Fe_3O_4 inside the pores of the modified macroreticular styrene-divinylbenzene particles. Particles with up to 50% by weight of Fe_3O_4 may easily be formed. These particles have a pore volume of about 50% and a surface area of 100–200 m^2 per gram, dependent upon the amount and type of inert solvent used in the preparation of the particles and the content of Fe_3O_4. The pore size distribution has been shown to be very broad and includes pores from a few nm up to about 100 nm in diameter. The macroporous magnetic particles described in this chapter have a diameter of 3 μm and contain either 27 (SDM 27) or 40% (SDM 40) of magnetite by weight. These particles have also formed the bases for other types of particles. After the introduction of Fe_3O_4, the pores were filled with different types of polymers, including hydrophobic and hydrophilic polymers. In the latter case, the particles contain functional groups suitable for covalent binding of antibodies. In this chapter we describe compact particles made on the basis of the macroporous particles (SDM 40). These compact particles, denoted SDMC 40, were prepared by polymerizing a mixture of acrylates, including hydroxyethyl acrylate and ethylene dimethacrylate, in the presence of the SDM 40 particles. The resulting particles still had the same diameter as the starting particles. The surface area, however, was reduced to 4.8 m^2/g.

In addition, we here describe the use of compact, uniformly hydrophilic 'magnetic' particles with 30% by weight of Fe_3O_4. These particles, denoted AHMC 30, were prepared by formation of Fe_3O_4 inside hydrophilic monosized particles based upon mixtures of acrylates. In this case too, antibodies may be covalently bound to the monomer-derived OH groups on the surface of the particles. Introduction of aldehyde groups on the surface of these particles is described below.

Figure 1 shows a scanning electron micrograph of the magnetic macroporous 3-μm particles, SDM 40. Figure 2 shows an optical micrograph of the 3-μm hydrophilic compact magnetic particles, AHMC 30. The 'hole' in the AHMC 30 particles stems from the fact that the particles, which were prepared by swelling a seed of monodisperse polystyrene particles about 1 μm in diameter with hydrophilic monomers, expel the polystyrene seed during polymerization of the hydrophilic monomers (Ugelstad et al., 1983c).

2.2. Immunoglobulins

2.2.1. Sheep anti-rabbit IgG
This antiserum was prepared and immunopurified on a rabbit IgG-Sepharose 4B as described by Nustad et al. (1982b).

368

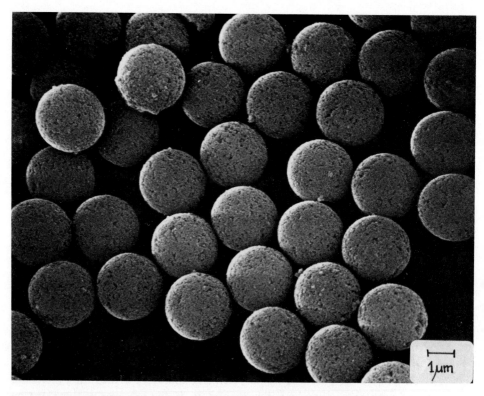

Figure 1. Scanning electron micrograph of magnetic macroporous 3-μm particles, SDM 40.

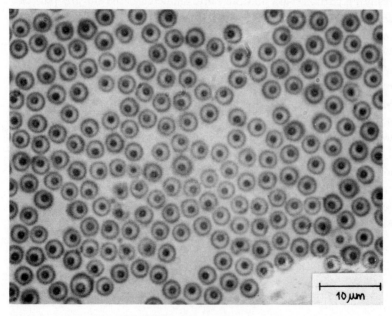

Figure 2. Optical micrograph of hydrophilic compact magnetic 3-μm particles, AHMC 30.

2.2.2. Sheep anti-mouse IgG

A mixture of protein A-Sepharose-purified monoclonal mouse IgG (20%) and poly-clonal mouse IgG (80%) was used to immunize a sheep. The sheep antiserum was immunopurified as described for the sheep anti-rabbit IgG.

2.2.3. Monoclonal antibodies and cell lines in the study of binding of particles to Burkitt lymphoma cells

Monoclonal antibodies AB-1 and AB-3 were developed at the Department of Immunology, The Norwegian Radium Hospital, Oslo. AB-1 (IgM) is a B-lymphocyte-specific antibody and AB-3 (IgG 2a) is an anti-DR framework antibody. The cell lines applied were Raji, a human Burkitt lymphoma-derived cell line, and X-63 Ag 8.653, a mouse myeloma cell line. The latter one was used in control experiments only.

2.2.4. Monoclonal antibodies for separation of neuroblastoma cells

The preparation of the monoclonal antibodies used in the separation of neuroblastoma cells was carried out by J. Kemshead at The Institute of Child Health, London.

2.2.5. Iodination of proteins

Purified IgG was iodinated as described by Fraker and Speck (1978). Normally, one molecule of iodine per molecule of IgG was obtained (Paus et al., 1982).

2.3. Binding of antibody to the particles

In all the experiments the amount of antibody bound was calculated from the distribution of the iodinated antibody.

2.3.1. Physical adsorption of antibody

Different amounts of sheep anti-rabbit IgG or sheep anti-mouse IgG (containing trace amounts of iodinated antibody) were added to 2 mg of particles suspended in 1 ml of phosphate buffer (0.1 M, pH 7.7). The reaction mixture was sonicated for 30 seconds in an ultrasonic bath and then rotated end-over-end overnight at room temperature. The particles were then washed repeatedly with 1 ml of Tris buffer (0.05 M Tris/0.1 M NaCl/0.01% bovine serum albumin/0.01% merthiolate/0.1% Tween 20, pH 7.7) until a constant value of bound protein was obtained. In each washing cycle the particles were suspended in 1 ml of buffer solution, rotated end-over-end for 24–72 hours, centrifuged, and decanted. (See note added in proof.)

2.3.2. Antibody bound to polyacrolein-coated particles

Grafting of polyacrolein to the particles was carried out by cobalt γ-irradiation of a mixture of an aqueous solution of acrolein and particles, as described previously (Rembaum et al., 1982). The grafting procedure was effective both for particles with hydrophobic and with hydrophilic surfaces.

Binding of antibody to the polyacrolein-coated particles was carried out in phosphate buffer. To 2 mg of particles suspended in 1 ml buffer (0.1 M, pH 5.2) were added different amounts of sheep anti-rabbit IgG (containing trace amounts of iodinated antibody).

The reaction mixture was sonicated for 30 seconds in an ultrasonic bath and then rotated end-over-end overnight at room temperature. After coupling, the reaction mixture was centrifuged. The particles were resuspended in 1 ml of a 1 M ethanol amine/0.1% Tween 20 solution (pH 9.5) and rotated for 3–4 hours to block the remaining reactive groups. Then the particles were washed twice with 1 ml of the Tris buffer described above by end-over-end rotation for 20–24 hours at room temperature.

2.3.3. Antibody bound to particles with hydroxy groups

2.3.3.1. Activation with p-toluene sulphonyl chloride. A modified version of the procedure described by Nilsson and coworkers (Nilsson et al., 1981; Nilsson and Mosbach, 1981) was used. The particles (100 mg) were transferred to acetone by sequential washings with 5-ml portions of acetone/water (3:7, 4:6 and 8:2, v/v) and finally three times with 5 ml of acetone followed by resuspension in 5 ml of acetone and sonification for 3 minutes in an ultrasonic bath. The washing procedure implied centrifugation and removal of the supernatant liquid before resuspending in the next 5 ml of liquid. To the final suspension were added, with shaking, 0.4 ml of pyridine and 0.4 g of p-toluene sulphonyl chloride, dissolved in about 1 ml of acetone. The reaction mixture was then rotated end-over-end overnight at room temperature. Then excess reagents were removed and the particles transferred back to a water suspension by reversing the washing scheme described above followed by washing three times with water. The suspension was stored at 4°C.

2.3.3.2. Coupling of antibody to tosylated particles. Immunopurified antibody (normally, 15 mg/g particles, containing trace amounts of iodinated antibody) dissolved in 3 ml of phosphate-buffered saline (0.01 M sodium phosphate/0.15 M NaCl, pH 7.5) was added to 2 ml of borate buffer (0.5 M, pH 9.5). Then 5 ml of the particle suspension were added with shaking. The reaction mixture was rotated end-over-end overnight at room temperature. After coupling, the reaction mixture was centrifuged and the particle pellet washed once with 2.5 ml of phosphate-buffered saline. Then the particles were resuspended in 5 ml of a 1 M ethanol amine/0.1% Tween 20 solution (pH 9.5) and rotated 2–4 hours to block the remaining reactive groups. Then the particles were washed twice by end-over-end rotation for 10–20 hours at room temperature with 5 ml of the Tris buffer described above. (See note added in proof.)

2.4. Determination of the binding capacity of the immobilized antibodies

The ability of sheep anti-rabbit IgG to bind rabbit IgG was tested and expressed in units as described by Nustad et al. (1982b). 1 unit, U, is defined as the rabbit IgG-binding capacity of 1 mg immunopurified sheep antibody using poly(ethylene glycol) as precipitating agent according to the procedure. The mouse IgG-binding capacity of sheep anti-mouse antibody was tested in a similar assay and expressed in corresponding units.

3. Results and discussion

3.1. Binding of protein to macroporous magnetic particles (SDM 40)

The results of binding of sheep anti-rabbit antibody to 3-μm monosized macroporous magnetic particles (SDM 40) are shown in Figure 3. The amount of antibody adsorbed is given as a function of the amount of antibody added. The points represent the values obtained after the fourth washing cycle. The decay of radioactivity during the experiment is not taken into account. The amount of antibody adsorbed increases towards an upper limit with increasing amount of antibody added. This is in agreement with previously reported measurements of adsorption isotherms of proteins on polystyrene particles (Norde and Lyklema, 1978; Bagchi and Birnbaum, 1981). It has been reported that this maximum quantity of IgG and other proteins is irreversibly bound, in that further dilution does not lead to any noticeable desorption of adsorbed protein. A slow desorption of already adsorbed protein has been observed in the presence of a relatively high concentration of albumin in the water phase, indicating a protein-mediated desorption (Brash et al., 1974; Morrissey, 1977). Therefore, it was verified by separate experiments that the content of albumin used in our washing buffer did not influence the results of adsorption.

The amount of antibody 'irreversibly' bound to this type of particle (SDM 40) was at maximum about 90 mg per g of particles. In comparison, a compact particle of polystyrene of the same size, which would have a surface area of 2 m^2/g, would, according to Bagchi and Birnbaum (1981), be expected to bind about 12 mg per g of particles in a monolayer. Experiments of binding IgG to the surface of polystyrene tubes indicate that a monolayer of IgG corresponds to 3.1 mg/m^2 (Cantarero et al., 1980). The high value of binding observed for the porous particles is obviously due

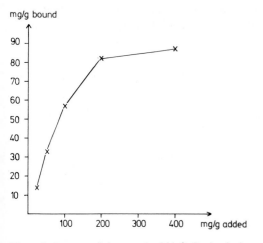

Figure 3. Amount of sheep anti-rabbit IgG adsorbed on magnetic macroporous 3-μm particles (SDM 40) as a function of the amount of antibody added.

TABLE 1

Percentage of the adsorbed antibody desorbed during 24 hours by a 6 M guanidine hydrochloride/0.5 M NaCl/0.05 M Tris solution, pH 7.0.

Particle type	% desorbed
Compact polystyrene particle with a smooth surface	84.6
Macroporous polystyrene particle	34.8
Macroporous magnetic particle	20.2

to the high surface area. However, expressed in mg per m², the macroporous particles adsorb only 0.6 mg/m², which is about one tenth to one fifth of what would be expected with a smooth surface. Apparently, only about one tenth to one fifth of the total surface is available for adsorption of the antibody, while the rest of the surface originates from pores too small to be accessible to the antibody.

Similar results as the ones given above were obtained with goat anti-rabbit, goat anti-mouse and sheep anti-mouse antibody.

To test the strength of the binding of protein by physical adsorption, particles coated with antibody were rotated end-over-end for about 24 hours with a guanidine solution (6 M guanidine hydrochloride/0.5 M NaCl/0.05 M Tris, pH 7.0). The guanidine solution was the only medium that caused noticeable desorption from macroporous particles. It appears from Table 1 that the adsorption of the antibody is much stronger on the macroporous particles than on the compact polystyrene particles. The high strength is mainly due to the porosity of the particles and not to the presence of magnetite.

Figure 4 shows the activity of the adsorbed sheep anti-rabbit antibody to bind rabbit IgG for the macroporous magnetic particles described above. The activity per g of particles as a function of the amount of antibody added is shown in Figure 4a, and the mean activity of each mg of the adsorbed antibody as a function of the

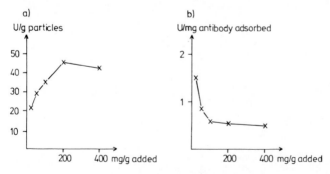

Figure 4. Activity of the adsorbed sheep anti-rabbit IgG to bind rabbit IgG as a function of the amount of antibody added. a, Activity per g of particles (SDM 40); b, mean activity of 1 mg of adsorbed antibody.

amount of antibody added is shown in Figure 4b. In spite of a quite low mean activity of adsorbed antibody, the activity per g particles increases towards an upper limit as high as 45 U/g with increasing amount of antibody added. The activity per g particles is much higher than the maximum activity observed on compact particles of the same size and is obviously caused by the high amount of antibody adsorbed. The low mean activity may be caused by the fact that a considerable part of the adsorbed antibody is hidden in pores no longer accessible to rabbit IgG. This phenomenon may be expected to be even more pronounced in the interaction of the immobilized antibody with objects as big as cells. It may be expected that only antibody adsorbed on the outer hemisphere of the particles can interact with the antigen determinants on the cell surface. Therefore, an even smaller fraction of the adsorbed antibody is involved in such interactions. When the porous particles have less than the maximum amount of antibody bound to them, it may in fact be anticipated that the antibody adsorbed may preferentially be adsorbed in the pores. In this case, the porous particles may be inferior to compact particles, even when the total amount of antibody bound is higher on them.

As has been demonstrated by Rembaum et al. (1982), reactive groups may be introduced to the particle surface by grafting polyacrolein onto it. The reactive groups permit a covalent binding of the antibody and may possibly also have a spacer arm effect. The results of binding of sheep anti-rabbit IgG to polyacrolein-coated 3-μm monosized macroporous magnetic particles are shown in Figure 5. The amount of antibody bound is given as a function of the amount of antibody added. The decay of radioactivity during the experiment is not taken into account. Also, in the case of polyacrolein-coated particles the amount of antibody bound increases towards an upper limit of about 90 mg per g of particles with increasing amount of antibody added. This limiting value is practically equal to the one observed with physical adsorption on uncoated macroporous magnetic particles. The polyacrolein-coated

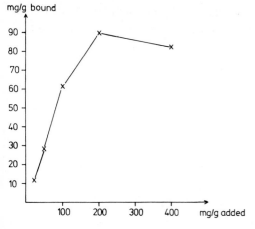

Figure 5. Amount of sheep anti-rabbit IgG bound to polyacrolein-coated magnetic macroporous 3-μm particles as a function of the amount of antibody added.

particles were treated with a 1 M ethanol amine/0.1% Tween 20 solution, pH 9.5, after the coupling procedure, to block remaining reactive groups. This difference in treatment did not have any effect on the amount of antibody adsorbed on macroporous magnetic particles.

Figure 6 shows the activity of the bound sheep anti-rabbit antibody to bind rabbit IgG for the polyacrolein-coated magnetic particles. Figure 6a gives the activity per g of particles as a function of the amount of antibody added. Figure 6b gives the mean activity of the bound antibody as a function of the amount of antibody added. The activity per g of particles is higher for polyacrolein-coated particles than for uncoated particles, in spite of the fact that the two types of particles have bound the same amount of antibody. This may possibly be explained both by a spacer arm effect of the polyacrolein chains, rendering the antibody more accessible to the rabbit IgG, and by a more favourable orientation of the covalently bound antibody. The activity per g of particles does not approach an upper limit with increasing amount of antibody added, but reaches a maximum value at 100 mg/g added. It seems that at higher amounts of antibody bound steric hindrance becomes of importance. The effect of steric hindrance is also evident from the marked decrease in the mean activity of the bound antibody with increasing amount of antibody added. This mean activity is higher for polyacrolein-coated particles than for uncoated particles up to 100 mg/g added, but is equally low for coated and uncoated particles when more than 100 mg antibody per g of particles are added. Therefore, up to 100 mg/g added the polyacrolein-coated particles seem to be superior to uncoated particles, in that higher activity of the bound antibody is attained with the same amount of antibody added.

The effect of various amounts of detergent in the coupling buffer on the amount of antibody adsorbed or covalently bound was examined for polyacrolein-coated and uncoated 3-μm macroporous magnetic particles with Tween 20 as detergent. The amount of antibody bound and the activity per g of particles as a function of the amount of detergent in the coupling buffer are shown in Figure 7. Only small amounts of detergent caused a noticeable decrease in the amount of antibody bound. Also, the activity per g of particles decreases in the presence of detergent. Both effects

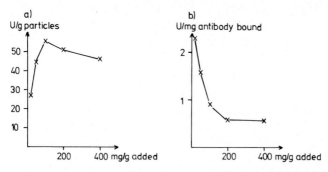

Figure 6. Activity of the bound sheep anti-rabbit IgG to bind rabbit IgG as a function of the amount of antibody added. a, Activity per g of polyacrolein-coated particles; b, mean activity of 1 mg of bound antibody.

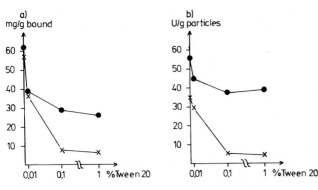

Figure 7. a, Amount of sheep anti-rabbit IgG bound to magnetic macroporous 3-μm particles as a function of the amount of detergent in the coupling buffer. b, Activity of the bound sheep anti-rabbit IgG to bind rabbit IgG as a function of the amount of detergent in the coupling buffer. x, Uncoated particles; ●, polyacrolein-coated particles.

are much less marked for the polyacrolein-coated particles. In the case of physical adsorption on uncoated particles, the protein is competing with the non-ionic detergent, resulting in a combined equilibrium adsorption layer determined by the relative strength of the adsorptive bonds of the two materials. In the case of covalent coupling to the polyacrolein, the decrease in observed binding of antibody may perhaps be due to a decrease in the rate of the coupling reaction caused by steric hindrance. The possibility of binding antibody in the presence of a small amount of detergent without too much decrease in activity per g of particles is advantageous, because the presence of emulsifier prevents agglutination of the particles. Therefore, in this respect also the polyacrolein-coated particles seem to have an advantage compared to the uncoated particles. The difference between physical adsorption of antibody and covalently bound antibody with respect to the effect of emulsifier is even more pronounced in the case of compact particles.

3.2. Binding of proteins to compact particles

3.2.1. SDMC 40
The compact magnetic particles with hydroxy groups at the surface, SDMC 40, were prepared, as described above, from the macroporous particles SDM 40. The antibody was covalently bound to SDMC 40 particles by the tosyl chloride method. Several experiments with variation of the amount of protein added revealed that maximum efficiency of the particles could be achieved with as little as 15 mg of antibody added per g of particles. This gave an amount of antibody bound equal to 4.5 mg per g of particles, with a mean activity per mg of antibody bound of 2.4 U.

3.2.2. AHMC 30
The compact hydrophilic magnetic particles, AHMC 30, were covered with a polyacrolein layer as described above. With 15 and 60 mg of antibody added per g of particles the amount of antibody bound was 4.1 and 11.2 mg/g, respectively. The mean

activity per mg of antibody bound was 2.6 and 2.3 U, respectively. These results confirm previous results with compact polystyrene particles, namely, that coverage of the particles with polyacrolein increases the capacity for binding of protein as compared with physical adsorption and also gives a relatively high activity of bound antibody.

3.3. Binding of particles to cancer cells

3.3.1. Removal of neuroblastoma cells from bone marrow

Kemshead and coworkers (Treleaven et al., 1984a,b) have applied the magnetic particles for in vitro removal of neuroblastoma cells from bone marrow. Until now, the work has been centered around the 3-μm macroporous particles, SDM 27, to which the antibody has been bound by physical adsorption.

The bone marrow was incubated with a cocktail of mouse monoclonal antibodies. Then a large excess in number (200:1) of magnetic particles with physically adsorbed sheep anti-mouse antibody was added. During mixing the cancer cells became coated with a layer of magnetic particles. Then the mixture was passed through a magnetic device where the cancer cells covered with magnetic particles as well as the excess of magnetic particles were retained while the normal cells passed through. By this method, Kemshead was able to remove at least 99.9% of the neuroblastoma cells from the bone marrow. It is interesting to note that the best results were achieved by use of 100 mg of sheep antibody per g of particles during the process of binding antibody to the particles. This is in accordance with the results of the measurements of binding capacity of antibody to the particles as described in this chapter. It was found that a direct binding of the monoclonal antibodies to the particles was far less effective.

To date, the method has been used clinically in treatment of a few patients with neuroblastoma. A portion of the bone marrow is taken out and treated in the way described above before the cleaned marrow is retransfused into the patient. The patient has, in the meantime, been treated with cytotoxic drugs and whole body irradiation to destroy cancer cells as completely as possible. Reinfusion of the treated bone marrow has resulted in the reappearance of normal production of blood cells. A few patients have had clinical remission for more than 6 months. None of the patients treated so far has had recurrence of disease.

The technique could in principle be used for removal of any tumour cells against which monoclonal antibodies are available.

3.3.2. Binding of magnetic particles to Burkitt lymphoma cells

3.3.2.1. Binding of particles with sheep anti-mouse IgG to Burkitt lymphoma cells coated with monoclonal antibody AB-3 (IgG 2a)

The Raji cells were treated with excess AB-3 for 45 minutes at 4°C in RPMI medium, followed by removal of unbound antibody by washing three times in the same medium. The porous particles (SDM 40) with adsorbed sheep anti-mouse IgG (60 mg antibody per g particles added) gave a maximum binding to the cells after 15 minutes when using about 100 particles per cell. However, the compact tosylated SDMC 40 particles and the compact acrolein-activated AHMC 30 particles showed a more rapid reaction. The final binding pattern was practically the same for all types of particles.

Figures 8 and 9 show pictures of Burkitt lymphoma cells covered with SDMC 40 and AHMC 30 particles, respectively. In both cases a ratio of particles to cancer cells of 100:1 was used.

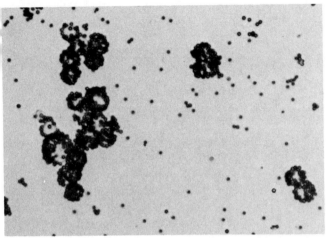

Figure 8. Binding of SDMC 40 particles with coupled sheep anti-mouse IgG to monoclonal anti-DR framework antibody (AB-3) on Raji cells. Magnification, × 280.

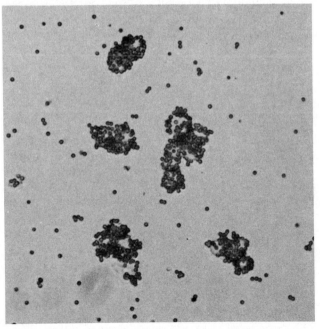

Figure 9. Binding of AHMC 30 particles with coupled sheep anti-mouse IgG to monoclonal anti-DR framework antibody (AB-3) on Raji cells. Magnification, × 280.

Non-specific binding of particles to the cells was investigated with Raji cells without specific monoclonal antibody. With the macroporous particles SDM 40 the degree of non-specific adsorption was very dependent upon the amount of antibody bound to the particle surface. To achieve an 'acceptable' low non-specific binding the amount of antibody added should be in excess of 50 mg/g. However, in the case of the compact SDMC 40 particles no non-specific binding was observed even with as little as 15 mg protein added per g of particles. The non-specific binding of cells to the particles AHMC 30 grafted with acrolein was also low at the same low level of antibody added.

3.3.2.2. Binding of magnetic particles with monoclonal antibodies directly to cells The AB-3 antibody, which is an IgG 2a, and the AB-1 antibody, which is an IgM, were both adsorbed on SDM 40 particles and coupled chemically to tosylated SDMC 40 particles. Non-specific adsorption was measured with the mouse myeloma cell line given in section 2.

The particles covered with AB-3 were compared with the indirect system described above, and were found to give identical results as regards binding to the Raji cells. Again the SDM 40 particles must be saturated with antibody to avoid non-specific binding of particles to the control cells. Figure 10 shows the binding of SDMC 40 particles with covalent bound AB-3 (15 mg antibody per g particles added) to Burkitt lymphoma cells using 100 particles per cell. It can be seen that the tumour cells are very effectively covered with the particles. Non-specific binding to the myeloma cells was negligible. Therefore, we conclude that direct coupling of monoclonal antibodies to cells is as efficient as an indirect method, using a second antibody on the particles, when working with cell lines with a single antigen. This is not in contrast to the results cited above using neuroblastoma cells, which are antigenic divergent and therefore

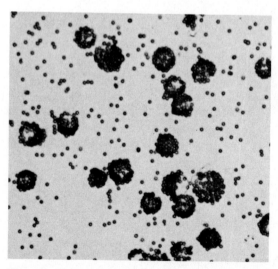

Figure 10. Binding of SDMC 40 particles with coupled monoclonal anti-DR framework antibody (AB-3) directly to Raji cells. Magnification, × 280.

necessitate the use of a monoclonal antibody cocktail. In these experiments an efficient binding of magnetic particles is only obtained using a second antibody on the particles.

It is interesting to note that one gets a more rapid binding to the cells with IgM bound directly to the particles than with IgG 2a. Preliminary data indicate that this cannot be explained by a difference in either the binding constants for the IgM and IgG 2a antibody or the number of antigens on the cell surface, which in fact is higher for the IgG 2a antibody. The more rapid binding with IgM may possibly be explained by a difference in the number of binding sites accessible on IgM and IgG 2a.

It is worth noting that a particle IgM complex is more sensitive than fluorescein-labelled IgM for cell-labelling of cells with low antigen concentration. These results will be presented in more detail in a forthcoming publication (Funderud, S. and Nustad, K., in preparation).

Full saturation of cells with magnetic particles was obtained using 100 particles per cell. However, preliminary experiments with hepatocytes which are 8 times larger than Raji cells showed that one there had to use 1000 particles per cell to obtain maximal binding (Danielsen, H., personal communication).

As a conclusion from the results with magnetic particles cited above, it may be stated that the ideal magnetic particles for use in cell separation have not yet been made. However, the experiments have given important hints as to the desired properties one should aim for.

1. The particles should be monodisperse and contain an identical amount of magnetic material. This has already been accomplished.

2. The antibody should be coupled to the particles in such a way that it has free access to antigenic sites on the cell surface. This has apparently been accomplished with the tosylated SDMC 40 particles, that is, by filling the pores of the SDM 40 particles with a hydrophilic polymer. The results hitherto obtained with the hydrophilic AHMC 30 particles with the antibody bound via a polyacrolein layer seem to indicate that this type of particle may be at least as good as SDMC 40.

It may be noted that AHMC 30 particles coated with polyacrolein also show low non-specific binding of low-molecular-weight haptens such as triiodothyronine (T_3), whereas all other magnetic particles prepared so far have high non-specific binding of T_3. Therefore, these particles may also be of value in immunoassays with magnetic separation.

4. Monosized radioactive particles

Monosized radioactive particles in the size range 10–15 μm are extensively used in circulation studies in animals. Such particles are usually prepared from styrene-divinylbenzene particles. After polymerization -SO_3H groups are introduced into the benzene rings. A fraction of the protons is exchanged with radioactive isotopes of metal ions and the particles are then treated in different ways to reduce leakage of radioactive ions during use. A high degree of monodispersity is essential for the application of these particles in circulation studies.

Previous methods for preparation of such particles have involved suspension polymerization of styrene-divinylbenzene monomers. This gives a broad particle size distribution and an extensive separation process is necessary to obtain a sufficient degree of monodispersity. This results in low yields of particles with the correct size, and even the most extensive separation gives standard deviations in size in the order of 10%.

The new processes for preparations of monodisperse particles developed by Ugelstad et al. (1980, 1983a–c) allow a direct and easy preparation of particles of any desired size with a standard deviation of about 1%. H. Moore at New England Nuclear (personal communication) has introduced various radioactive metal ions into these particles. Leakage of radioactive metal ions was hindered by coating the particles with a skin of polyfurfuryl alcohol. In Figure 11 is shown an optical micrograph of such radioactive particles of exactly 15 μm. Examination of the properties of these radioactive particles with regard to their use in circulation studies indicates a high degree of biotolerability.

A possible use of radioactive particles in cancer therapy involves irradiation of local metastases when injected into the abdominal cavity. It is essential for this application that the particles are not transported out of the abdominal cavity. Investigations with rats at the Norwegian Radium Hospital have shown that similar 15-μm particles

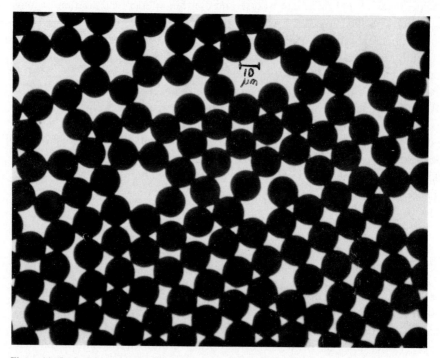

Figure 11. Optical micrograph of highly monodisperse radioactive particles of 15 μm.

without radioactivity were not transported out of the abdominal cavity and did not create any harmful effects over a period of 8 months.

Note added in proof

Recently we have found that it is favourable to disperse the particles in pure water or water with only a slight amount of buffer in a first step. This mixture is then added to a solution of the antibody in phosphate-buffered saline. Finally, a more concentrated buffer is added, to give a final buffer concentration of 0.1 M. This procedure involves the particles being covered with antibody before being brought in contact with the strongly buffered solution, and leads to a better dispersion of the particles (Nustad et al., 1984).

Acknowledgements

The authors wish to thank T. Ellingsen and L. Holm at SINTEF for the preparation of the different particles described in this paper.

References

Bagchi, P. and Birnbaum, S.M. (1981) J. Colloid Interface Sci. 83, 460–478.
Brash, J.L., Uniyal, S. and Samak, Q. (1974) Trans. Am. Soc. Artif. Intern. Organs 20A, 69–76.
Buske, N. and Götze, T. (1983) Acta Polymerica 34, 184–185.
Cantarero, L.A., Butler, J.E. and Osborne, J.W. (1980) Anal. Biochem. 105, 375–382.
Daniel, J.-C., Schuppiser, J.-L. and Tricot, M. (1982) U.S. Patent, 4,358,388.
Forrest, G.C. and Landon, J.R. (1978) Clin. Biochem. Anal. 7, 567–594.
Fraker, P.J. and Speck, J.C. (1978) Biochem. Biophys. Res. Commun. 80, 849–857.
Johansen, L., Nustad, K., Ørstavik, T.B., Ugelstad, J., Berge, A. and Ellingsen, T. (1983) J. Immunol. Methods 59, 255–264.
Kronick, P.L., Campbell, G.L. and Joseph, K. (1978) Science 200, 1074–1076.
Margel, S., Beitler, U. and Ofarim, M. (1982) J. Cell Sci. 56, 157–175.
Molday, R.S. and Mackenzie, D. (1982) J. Immunol. Methods 52, 353–367.
Molday, R.S., Yen, S.P.S. and Rembaum, A. (1977) Nature 268, 437–438.
Morimoto, Y., Okumura, M., Sugibayashi, K. and Kato, Y. (1981) J. Pharm. Dyn. 4, 624–631.
Morrissey, B.W. (1977) Ann. N.Y. Acad. Sci. 283, 50–64.
Mosbach, K. and Schröder, U. (1979) FEBS Lett. 102, 112–116.
Mosback, K.H. (1982) U.S. Patent, 4,335,094.
Nilsson, K. and Mosbach, K. (1981) Biochem. Biophys. Res. Commun. 102, 449–457.
Nilsson, K., Norrlöw, O. and Mosbach, K. (1981) Acta Chem. Scand. Ser. B35, 19–27.
Norde, W. and Lyklema, J. (1978) J. Colloid Interface Sci. 66, 257–265.
Nustad, K., Johansen, L., Schmid, R., Ugelstad, J., Ellingsen, T. and Berge A. (1982a) Agents Actions Suppl. 9, 207–212.

382

Nustad, K., Ugelstad, J., Berge, A., Ellingsen, T., Schmid, R., Johansen, L. and Børmer, O. (1982b) I.A.E.A. (SM) 259/19, 45–55.

Nustad, K., Johansen, L., Ugelstad, J., Ellingsen, T. and Berge A. (1984) Eur. Surg. Res. 16, Suppl. 2, 80–87.

Paus, E., Børmer, O. and Nustad, K. (1982) I.A.E.A. (SM) 259/18, 161–171.

Poyn, C.H., Dicke, K.A., Culbert, S., Frankel, L.S., Jagannath, S. and Read, C.L. (1983) Lancet, 524.

Rembaum, A., Yen, S.P.S. and Molday, R.S. (1979) J. Macromol. Sci., Chem. A13, 603–632.

Rembaum, A., Yen, R.C.K., Kempner, D.H. and Ugelstad, J. (1982) J. Immunol. Methods 52, 341–351.

Schröder, U. and Mosbach, K. (1983) PCT Int. Appl. WO83 01.738.

Treleaven, J.G., Gibson, F.M., Ugelstad, J., Rembaum, A. and Kemshead, J.T. (1984a) Magn. Sep. News 1, 103–109.

Treleaven, J.G., Gibson, F.M., Ugelstad, J., Rembaum, A., Phillip, T., Caine, G.D. and Kemshead, J.T. (1984b) Lancet 1, 70–73.

Ugelstad, J., Mørk, P.C., Kaggerud, K.H., Ellingsen, T. and Berge, A. (1980) Adv. Colloid Interface Sci. 13, 101–140.

Ugelstad, J., Söderberg, L., Berge, A. and Bergström, J. (1983a) Nature 303, 95–96.

Ugelstad, J., Mørk, P.C., Mfutakamba, H.R., Soleimany, E., Nordhuus, I., Schmid, R., Berge, A., Ellingsen, T., Aune, O. and Nustad, K. (1983b) in Science and Technology of Polymer Colloids (Poehlein, G.W., Ottewill, R.H. and Goodwin, J.W., Eds.), Vol. 1, pp. 51–99, Martinus Nijhoff, Boston.

Ugelstad, J., Mfutakamba, H.R., Mørk, P.C., Ellingsen, T., Berge, A., Schmid, R., Holm, L., Jørgedal, A., Hansen, F.K. and Nustad, K. (1983c) J. Polym. Sci., in press.

Ugelstad, J., Ellingsen, T., Berge, A. and Helgée, B. (1983d) PCT Int. Appl. WO83/03 920.

Widder, K., Flouret, G. and Senyei, A. (1979a) J. Pharm. Sci. 68, 79–82.

Widder, K.J., Senyei, A.E. and Ranney, D.F. (1979b) Adv. Pharmacol. Chemother. 16, 213–271.

Microspheres and Drug Therapy. Pharmaceutical, Immunological and Medical Aspects
edited by S.S. Davis, L. Illum, J.G. McVie and E. Tomlinson
© *1984, Elsevier Science Publishers B.V.*

Cell labeling and separation by means of monodisperse magnetic and nonmagnetic microspheres

A. Rembaum, J. Ugelstad, J.T. Kemshead, M. Chang and G. Richards

1. Introduction

Attempts to separate cell subpopulations using magnetic microspheres were summarized in the preceding chapter by J. Ugelstad et al., whose monodisperse magnetic microspheres were successfully used by Rembaum, Kemshead and coworkers (Kemshead et al., 1982, 1983) to eliminate neuroblastoma cells from human bone marrow. The removal of tumour cells from bone marrow destined for autologous transplantation constitutes a new approach to this disease (Treleaven et al., 1984). In this approach a mixture of several monoclonal antibodies has been used to sensitise neuroblastoma cells. Polystyrene magnetic microspheres, 3 μm in diameter, carrying sheep anti-mouse antibodies on the surface were targeted to the tumour cells to render these magnetic. A flow system was then employed using permanent magnets to effect the rapid and efficient removal of magnetic tumour cells from bone marrow. In the 15 bone marrow samples treated to date (in which tumour cell infiltration ranged from 0.1 to 3.0%), no neuroblastoma cells could be detected after the magnetic treatment. This was assessed by indirect immunofluorescent assays as well as by histological and cytological procedures. Before reinfusion of 'cleansed bone marrow', the patients received lethal chemotherapy and total body radiation.

In view of the promising potential success of this method and the possibility of 'cleansing bone marrows' invaded by other kinds of tumour cells, a continuation of the study of the procedure, i.e., mainly the binding of anti-mouse antibodies to the magnetic microspheres, was considered essential since loss of immobilized antibody was observed in certain cases. In this chapter we describe a method which reduces the amount of antibody leaching from the magnetic and nonmagnetic polystyrene microspheres. Thus far, the successful binding of sheep anti-mouse to magnetic microspheres has been due to strong adsorption of the antibody to microspheres made highly porous and having a surface area of the order of 100–200 m^2/g (for 3-μm particles) compared to the surface area of compact, non-porous magnetic particles of the same size of about 1 m^2/g. Adsorption of antibodies to such compact spheres was not satisfactory for efficient cell separation. In order to increase the amount of binding to compact spheres, these were functionalized by radiation grafting of acrolein to the surface. It was expected that the antibodies would react with the aldehyde or acetal groups of polyacrolein by covalent bonding, thereby resulting in microspheres with minimum leaching and sufficient antibody concentration. This was indeed found to be the case.

2. Materials and methods

2.1. Radiation grafting of polyacrolein

Preformed polymeric microspheres used in this study were 11.1-μm compact polystyrene, 3-μm magnetic porous polystyrene and 1.5-μm magnetic compact polystyrene. Acrolein (Eastman Kodak) was distilled at atmospheric pressure at 53°C before use. Poly(ethylene oxide) (PEO) of molecular weight 100,000 (Polysciences) and sodium dodecyl sulphate (SDS) (Fisher Scientific) were both used as received.

Cobalt γ-radiation source of 0.12 Mrad/hour dosage rate was used for initiation of the grafting and polymerization reaction.

A typical composition for this study was: porous magnetic polystyrene, 0.1 g; 0.4% PEO/H_2O solution, 4.0 ml; 20 wt.% of acrolein/H_2O, 2.0 ml; SDS, 0.01 g.

All reactions were carried out in 20-ml screw-capped scintillation vials. At least 10 minutes of nitrogen bubbling into the reaction mixture was necessary to remove dissolved oxygen prior to the initiation of polymerization. Total irradiation time was about 7 hours. During the first 3 hours, samples were removed from the γ source every 20 minutes for 5 minutes shaking. For the remaining time, this was repeated every 40 minutes.

After the irradiation was completed, the crude product, in the case of non-magnetic microspheres, was centrifuged at a speed of 1000 × g for no more than 5 minutes so that homopolyacrolein particles (500–1000 Å) could be separated from the polyacrolein-grafted microspheres. The grafted product was washed with distilled water and resuspended in PEO solution. This process was repeated at least four times to ensure the complete removal of homopolymer particles. When the grafting reaction was implemented on magnetic microspheres, the product was isolated by means of a magnetic field.

2.2. Reaction of polyacrolein-grafted microspheres with m-aminophenol
m-Aminophenol (Aldrich Chemicals) was recrystallized from water twice, before use. All reactions were performed at 65°C in water (5 ml) for 30 minutes. After reaction, all samples were washed with distilled water three times before they were examined under the fluorescence microscope (Fig. 1).

2.3. Characterization of polyacrolein-grafted microspheres
Scanning and transmission electron microscopes were used to study the morphology of products. Quantitative determination of the amount of polyacrolein in the micro-

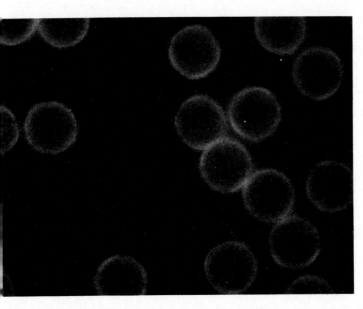

Figure 1. Magnetic polystyrene spheres (8 μm in diameter) with polyacrolein on the surface. Acrolein was grafted by means of ionizing radiation. The presence of polyacrolein was proven by reaction with *m*-aminophenol, which resulted in fluorescent surfaces. The magnetic polystyrene spheres immersed in acrolein and washed with distilled water, then reacted with *m*-aminophenol did not yield fluorescent surfaces (control).

spheres was carried out by infrared analysis using a Fourier Transform Infra Red spectrophotometer (MO91-0121 DIGILAB).

2.4. The binding of antibodies to microspheres

Lyophilyzed mouse IgG and rabbit IgG were obtained from Sigma Chemical Co., St. Louis, MO. Affinity purified goat anti-rabbit IgG (G ∝ R) was obtained from TAGO Inc., Burlingame, CA. The mouse IgG was resuspended and dialyzed (to remove chloride ion) against 0.05 M potassium phosphate buffer, pH 7.5. The rabbit IgG, being salt free, was resuspended in the same phosphate buffer and used without further treatment.

The G∝R was desalted in a Sephadex G25-150 (Sigma Chemical Co.) column equilibrated with 0.05 M potassium phosphate, pH 7.5, according to the method of Neal and Florini (1973).

The protein concentrations of the above reagents were determined by the method of Lowry et al. (1951), using bovine serum albumin as the standard (Sigma 905–10).

Na^{125}I was obtained from New England Nuclear, Boston, MA. All the immunoglobulin reagents were radioactively labeled with ^{125}I using Chloramine-T (Greenwood et al., 1963). Unreacted iodine was removed by desalting.

Buffers used for coupling protein to the microspheres were: 0.1 M sodium acetate, pH 5.3; 0.1 M potassium phosphate, pH 7.5; 0.1 M sodium bicarbonate, pH 9.4.

TABLE 1

Protein binding to microspheres: Effect of acrolein grafting

Type of microsphere	% Polyacrolein by weight	Buffer (% Tween-20)	μg mouse IgG bound per 1×10^6 beads	Mouse IgG bound (% by weight of beads)
11.1-μm compact polystyrene	≈ 3	0	15	1.8
		0.1	10	1.3
		1	9.8	1.2
	0	0	6.7	0.83
		0.1	0.34	0.03
		1	0.51	0.06
3-μm porous magnetic	15	0	1.9	9.5
		0.1	1.3	6.6
		1	1.2	5.9
	0	0	3.2	16.1
		0.1	1.4	7.0
		1	1.2	6.2

These buffers were used with or without Tween-20® (ICI American Inc., Wilmington, DE) as stated in the procedures below.

Buffers used for washing were either 0.05 M potassium phosphate, pH 7.5, with 0.05% Tween-20® (KHPO₄-Tween) or KHPO₄-Tween containing 0.15 M NaCl and 0.1% sodium azide (PBS-Tween).

2.5. Coupling of mouse IgG to microspheres

Grafted and nongrafted samples of 11.1-μm compact polystyrene or 3-μm magnetic porous polystyrene microspheres were reacted with excess radioactively labeled mouse IgG at pH 7.5 with 1.0%, 0.1% and 0% Tween-20 for 2 hours at room temperature with continuous shaking, then the samples were incubated overnight at 4°C (Table 1).

Ungrafted, once-grafted and thrice-grafted 1.5-μm magnetic compact polystyrene microspheres were reacted with excess mouse IgG at either pH 5.3, 7.5 or 9.4, with or without Tween-20, for either 2 hours with periodic vortexing at 37°C (ungrafted microspheres) or at room temperature (grafted microspheres), and then incubated overnight at 4°C.

Each sample was washed by centrifugation (Eppendorf 5412) at least three times with KHPO₄-Tween. During each wash, the samples were sonicated in a bath sonicator ('Ultrason', L&R Manufacturing Co., Kearny, NJ) for up to 5 minutes, as well as vortexed, to redisperse the pellet. The washed samples were counted in either a gamma counter or liquid scintillation counter (Table 2).

TABLE 2

Binding of mouse IgG to 1.5-μm compact magnetic beads

	Amount of mouse IgG bound per 10^6 beads			
	Buffer (% Tween-20)	pH 5.3	pH 7.5	pH 9.4
Control (no grafting)	0.2	2.0		0.58
	0	13.0		7.2
Grafted once	0.2	4.9	2.5	0.71
	0	22.2	17.0 ·	14.2
Grafted thrice	0.2	9.7		2.0
	0	16.2		8.5

2.6. Specific activity of an antibody after covalent coupling to acrolein-grafted polystyrene (PS) beads

10 μg of G $\propto$ R or radioactively labeled G $\propto$ R was reacted with 2.6 × 10^5 11.1-μm grafted compact PS microspheres for 50 minutes at room temperature at pH 5.3, 7.5 or 9.4 in the presence of 0.2% Tween-20. Then, an excess of bovine serum albumin (BSA) was added to quench any further binding of G $\propto$ R to the microspheres, by competitively binding the remaining available aldehyde groups. The samples were then washed three times (as above) with PBS-Tween, and the amount of G $\propto$ R bound was determined by radioactive counting. 20 μg of radioactively labeled rabbit IgG in PBS-Tween containing 5% normal goat serum were then added to the microspheres which had been reacted with the unlabeled G $\propto$ R. These were then incubated at room temperature for 5 hours with periodic vortexing. The samples were then washed and counted as described above (Table 3).

3. Results and discussion

3.1. Grafting of polyacrolein by means of ionizing radiation

Radiation grafting of acrolein onto polymer microspheres was evidenced by the infrared spectra of products which showed absorption peaks at 1725 cm^{-1}, which can be ascribed to the aldehyde carbonyl group. Furthermore, fluorimetric determination of polyacrolein with *m*-aminophenol also showed positive results for all three systems (Fig. 1). The presence of polyacrolein resulted in fluorescent microspheres. A method of quantitative determination of the amount of polyacrolein in the grafted copolymer was developed, using the 'peak height ratio' of Fourier Transform Infrared selected wavelengths. For example, to analyse the polyacrolein/porous magnetic polystyrene system, we selected peaks at 1725 and 1540 cm^{-1}. A calibration curve was constructed

TABLE 3

Specific activity of antibody (G ∝ R IgG) after covalent coupling to acrolein-grafted polystyrene beads (11.1 μm)

First step			Second step			
pH	G ∝ R IgG bound (μg)	Number of G ∝ R molecules per cm^2	Rabbit IgG bound			Molar ratio (μg rabbit IgG: μg G ∝ R IgG)
			cpm		μg	
			Test	Control		
5.3	0.40	1.6×10^{12}	2242	2114	0.16	0.4
7.5	0.18	0.7×10^{12}	1584	1435	0.11	0.6
9.4	0.06	0.24×10^{12}	932	746	0.06	1.0
Beads reacted with BSA only (control)						
5.3			178			
7.5			149			
9.4			186			

by plotting the peak height ratio (1725 cm^{-1}/1545 cm^{-1}) of various polymer blends of known compositions. These polymer blends were made simply by mixing homopolyacrolein with untreated magnetic polystyrene. A linear relation between peak height ratio and concentration of polyacrolein was obtained. Using this technique, we found that aldehyde contents can be effectively increased by increasing (a) surfactant concentration, (b) frequency of mixing during radiation, (e) monomer concentration and (d) surface area of the preformed polymeric microspheres.

We have also examined the morphology of these products under an electron microscope. Theoretically, acrolein-treated polymeric microspheres may be in either of the following two forms: A. A core-shell form where polymerization occurs at particle/water interface. Polyacrolein forms a thin film and wraps the preformed microsphere. Eventually, the substrate particles 'core' will be coated with a 'shell' of polyacrolein. In this case, the grafted spheres appear smooth in the scanning electronmicrographs. B. Hybrid beads morphology. This involves a two-step reaction. Polyacrolein was generated from aqueous phase polymerization and formed small microspheres, which collided with substrate particle due to Brownian motion and subsequently grafted onto substrate particle by γ radiation.

The morphology of these products may be governed by a number of factors: A. Solubility of substrate polymer in acrolein — higher solubility favours interfacial polymerization. B. The size of polyacrolein microspheres. C. The susceptibility of substrate polymer under radiation. D. The porosity of substrate polymer.

Our electron microscope results showed that the actual morphology is in between these two forms. Electron micrographs can only display the hybrid beads structure. Since the grafted polyacrolein beads do not account for all the polyacrolein covalently bound to substrate polymer, we have concluded that the remaining amount of polyacrolein not revealed by the electron microscope is probably introduced into the core-shell form.

3.2. Fluorometric determination of polyacrolein with m-aminophenol

A fluorometric method has been reported in the literature to measure acrolein and related compounds through their reaction with *m*-aminophenol. The fluorescent compound was identified to be 7-hydroxyl quinoline. Polymeric microspheres grafted with polyacrolein were found to react like acrolein with *m*-aminophenol to yield fluorescent microspheres (Fig. 1). The original non-grafted microspheres after reaction with *m*-aminophenol remained non-fluorescent.

3.3. Binding of antibodies to non-modified and acrolein-modified microspheres

Acrolein grafting completely changed the binding characteristics of the 11.1-μm compact PS microspheres (Table 1). This is readily seen by comparing the amount of mouse IgG bound in the presence and absence of Tween-20. Non-activated PS binds protein hydrophobically. In RIA and ELISA systems, the mild detergent Tween-20 is used extensively to minimise hydrophobic binding of proteins to polystyrene (as well as to other plastics). In the present case Tween-20 reduced the binding of mouse IgG to the ungrafted compact PS microspheres to 5–8% of its 'non-Tween' value. A look at the binding data for acrolein-grafted compact PS (Table 1) shows that these microspheres no longer 'behave' like pure PS. Not only do they bind twice as much mouse IgG in the absence of Tween, but there is also no sharp drop in binding in the presence of Tween-20: Tween only reduced the binding to 66% of its 'non-Tween' value, suggesting that most of the binding of mouse IgG to the grafted compact PS microspheres is covalent (via aldehyde) rather than hydrophobic in nature.

The best indicator of the effect of polyacrolein grafting on these compact PS microspheres is a comparison of the amount of mouse IgG bound in the presence and absence of Tween-20. For the compact PS microspheres this difference in grafted to non-grafted binding is a factor of 20 (0.51 vs. 9.8 μg, see Table 1).

The inability of the Tween-20 to cause a major reduction in the binding of the non-grafted magnetic porous PS microspheres is indicative that these microspheres are binding protein in a different manner (qualitatively or quantitatively) than pure PS. The grafting of even 15% (by weight) of acrolein on these microspheres had no effect on the mouse IgG-binding capacity in the presence of Tween, and actually reduced the mouse IgG-binding capacity in the absence of Tween. Although the quantity of mouse IgG protein bound to the magnetic porous PS microspheres was not improved with polyacrolein grafting, it remains to be determined if there is a qualitative change in the protein bound to the microsphere, i.e., a change in the amount of denatured protein. It should be noted that all the acrolein-grafted microspheres tested, compact PS, magnetic porous PS and the magnetic compact PS, showed superior dispersability after centrifugation in buffer without detergent.

Table 2 summarizes the results for the binding of mouse IgG to the 1.5-μm magnetic compact polystyrene microspheres. The data show that the amount of protein bound to the microspheres increased with the repeated radiation grafting. There is also a definite pH effect for both the ungrafted and grafted magnetic compact PS spheres: more mouse IgG bound at the lower pH values.

Since the results of the previous experiments showed that the 11.1-μm compact polystyrene microspheres exhibited the most dramatic positive change in protein binding, and the presence of polyacrolein on the spheres could be confirmed by FTIR, these microspheres were chosen for testing in a 'second step' experiment. The ability of a microsphere to bind large amounts of protein is superfluous if the bound protein is denatured. This experiment was designed to give some indication as to the ability of an active affinity purified antibody to retain its affinity for antigen when bound to a grafted microsphere.

According to the manufacturer (TAGO Inc.), this antibody reagent (goat anti-rabbit IgG) contained 74% active antibody. Table 3 shows that the goat anti-rabbit IgG remained very active upon being bound to the grafted compact microspheres. The maximum molar ratio of antigen bound in the second step per antibody covalently bound in the first step is 1:1. This indicates the bound goat anti-rabbit IgG is at least 50% active (a fully active antibody molecule could be expected to bind two molecules of antigen).

3.4. Binding of sheep anti-rabbit IgG (S$\propto$R) to acrolein-coated and uncoated 3-μm polymeric microspheres

The finding that a high concentration of antibodies could be bound to modified microspheres, i.e., to microspheres coated with polyacrolein by radiation grafting, was confirmed independently using different antibodies; in particular the binding of S$\propto$R to polyacrolein-coated and uncoated microspheres reproduced the results obtained by the use of G$\propto$R. However, the experimental procedure was somewhat altered and is described below. To 2 mg of nonmagnetic compact cross-linked polymethylstyrene microspheres cross-linked with divinylbenzene and coated with polyacrolein, 40 μg of S$\propto$R were added in 1 ml of a buffer (0.1 M phosphate, pH 5.2). The low pH of the medium was used to maximize the amount of bound antibody (see Table 3). The same procedure was repeated with a 5-fold increase of S$\propto$R (200 μg). For uncoated microspheres a pH 7.7 phosphate buffer was used in this control experiment. After coupling the beads were rotated end-over-end in a 1 M ethanolamine solution (pH 9.5) containing 0.1% Tween 20 for 3 hours and twice in a Tris buffer (0.05 M Tris/0.1 M NaCl/0.01% bovine serum albumin/0.01% merthiolate/0.1% Tween 20; pH 7.7) for 20–24 hours. The results are shown in Table 4.

It should be emphasized that the results shown in Table 4 obtained in a different laboratory confirmed our own data (Tables 1 and 2). About a 2-fold amount of S$\propto$R could be bound to polyacrolein-coated microspheres (35% compared with 17.2%). This does not necessarily imply an increased surface area of the microspheres; in fact, scanning electron microscopy showed a smooth instead of an irregular surface, indicating that the binding is covalent rather than hydrophobic in nature. Furthermore,

TABLE 4

Binding of sheep anti-rabbit IgG (S $\propto$ R) to acrolein-coated and uncoated compact 3-μm beads (methylstyrene-divinylbenzene)

Amount of S $\propto$ R added (mg/g)	Percent of S $\propto$ R bound to:	
	Acrolein-coated beads	Uncoated beads
20	49.6	21.5
100	35.0	17.2

in a separate study, the same radiation grafted spheres showed low nonspecific adsorption in a radioimmunoassay of triiodotyronine (unpublished observations). The reaction of polyacrolein-covered microspheres with proteins is simple and direct. Furthermore, acrolein can be grafted on a variety of hydrophilic or hydrophobic commercially prepared microspheres. Therefore, it offers a possibility of numerous biological applications.

Acknowledgements

This report represents one phase of research carried on at the Jet Propulsion Laboratory, California Institute of Technology, under Contract NAS7-918, sponsored by the National Aeronautics and Space Administration, and by Grant No. 1R01-CA20668-04 awarded by the National Cancer Institute, DHEW, and Grant No. 70-1859 awarded by the Defense Advanced Research Project Agency.

References

Greenwood, F.C., Hunter, W.M. and Glover, J.S. (1963) Biochem. J. 89, 114–123.

Kemshead, J.T., Rembaum, A. and Ugelstad, J. (1982) ASCO Meeting Abstracts, St Louis, MO.

Kemshead, J.T., Gibson, F.J., Ugelstad, J. and Rembaum, A. (1983) AACR Meeting Abstracts, San Diego, CA.

Lowry, O.H., Rosebrough, N.T., Farr, A.L. and Randall, R.J. (1951) J. Biol. Chem. 193, 265–275.

Neal, M.W. and Florini, J.R. (1973) Anal. Biochem. 55, 328–330.

Treleaven, J.G., Gibson, F.M., Ugelstad, J., Rembaum, A., Philip, T., Caine, G.D. and Kemshead, J.T. (1983) Lancet 1, 70–73.

Microspheres and Drug Therapy. Pharmaceutical, Immunological and Medical Aspects
edited by S.S. Davis, L. Illum, J.G. McVie and E. Tomlinson
© 1984, Elsevier Science Publishers B.V.

CHAPTER 4

Magnetic albumin microspheres in drug delivery

Kenneth J. Widder and Andrew E. Senyei

1. Introduction

Selective targeting of anti-tumour agents with concomitant elimination of toxic side effects has been a major goal in cancer chemotherapy. The clinical outcome of systemic therapy rests on an exquisite balance between the ability of the administered antineoplastic agents to destroy aberrant tumour cells and doing relatively less damage to normal host cells. Currently, the therapeutic index of most of the antineoplastic agents used in systemic therapy remains marginal, despite efforts to modify the drugs to achieve tumour specificity. The lack of success of systemic therapy to achieve tumour specificity is based on the fact that biochemical differences between tumour and host cells are minimal and are almost always quantitative rather than qualitative (Rowland et al., 1975). In addition, various surface properties of malignant cells interfere with recognition by the host immune system (Byers and Levin, 1976). Despite various chemical modifications made on chemotherapeutic agents, such as altering their partition coefficient (thus affecting tissue distribution), attaching an immunologic ligand or altering charge density, only variable success has been achieved in increasing specificity. A detailed comparison of the various methods of drug delivery has been reviewed elsewhere (Widder et al., 1979a, 1982).

A number of problems exist for successful targeting of biodegradable carriers. The first and perhaps the most significant obstacle is the rapid sequestration of intravascularly administered drug carriers by mononuclear phagocytes of the reticuloendothelial system (Segal et al., 1974; McDougall et al., 1974). Because of their rapid clearance, only a small fraction of injected carrier is available to localize at the tumour site, thus producing a weak local drug gradient. Two approaches have been pursued to alleviate this problem. The first consists of blocking the reticuloendothelial system prior to administering the drug carrier. Gregoriadis and Neerunjun (1974) administered carbon particles intravenously. Paradoxically, these increased rather than decreased the hepatic localization of liposomes. More recent attempts have employed concomitant treatment with either a large number of non-drug-bearing liposomes (McDougall et al., 1974; Gregoriadis and Neerunjun, 1974) or a high dose of methyl palmitate (Tanaka et al., 1975). Both modes of blockage delayed the clearance of a smaller number of concomitantly administered drug-containing liposomes.

However, blockage of the reticuloendothelial system in cancer patients is undesirable. These patients have an increased susceptibility to infections and the reticuloendothelial system acts as the first-line clearance mechanism against infectious agents.

Another approach to impart specificity to drug carriers such as liposomes involves the incorporation of specific ligands onto the external surface of the carrier. Such components include desialylated fetuin (Gregoriadis and Neerunjun, 1975), erythrocyte membrane glycoprotein (Marchesi et al., 1972; Juliano and Stamp, 1976), heat-aggregated immunoglobulins (Weissman et al., 1975) and native immunoglobulins (Gregoriadis et al., 1981).

The first of these, desialylated fetuin, has been shown to alter the organ distribution of liposomes by associating with receptors on hepatocytes. Though this does not modify the usual organ distribution of liposomes after intravascular administration, it accentuates rather than solves the problem of hepatic sequestration.

Efforts have been made to impart specificity by incorporating either purified receptor molecules or anti-receptor molecules into the external surface of liposomes (Juliano and Stamp, 1976; Weissman et al., 1975). Incorporation of the major sialoglycoprotein receptor of the red cell membrane into liposomes results in selective binding to erythrocytes in the presence of multivalent plant lectins that cross-link the common sialoglycoprotein. This system is not practical for in vivo use due to intravascular agglutination. However, the possibility of drug carrier localization based on complimentary interactions between carrier-bound glyoproteins and tissue glycoprotein receptors has significant future potential (Prieels et al., 1978).

Another approach taken to impart an element of specificity involves the observation that a high proportion of mononuclear phagocytes have surface receptors for denatured immunoglobulins. The incorporation of heat-aggregated IgG into liposomes results in their preferential uptake by these cells (Weissman et al., 1975). Although attaching this ligand provides another mechanism for cell-specific targeting, it also increases rather than decreases reticuloendothelial clearance.

Finally, antibodies directed against cell surface determinants have been bound to microspheres as well as liposomes (Gregoriadis and Neerunjun, 1975; Gregoriadis and Meehan, 1981; Illum et al., 1984). The antibody associated with the carrier can interact with specific antigens on the target cell surface. The molecular orientation of the antibody embedded in the carrier theoretically minimizes its own antigenicity by burying the most antigenic Fc portion in the lipid bilayer. The question of antigenicity is important in that most of the immune sera that are generated are done so in unrelated animals. The administration of this foreign protein to a sensitized recipient can, in theory, result in severe immune-complex disease. In vivo tests using liposomes bearing anti-HeLa cell IgG have demonstrated a 25-fold increase in the uptake of encapsulated bleomycin by HeLa cells compared to non-cross-reactive fibroblasts (Gregoriadis and Neerunjun, 1975). Although in vitro results appear encouraging, the usefulness of this approach for in vivo targeting is limited again by the rapid clearance of the carrier by the reticuloendothelial system. In another system, human lymphocytes precoated with kappa light chain were reacted in vitro with liposomes bearing anti-human IgG (kappa chain). It demonstrated that liposomal interaction with antigen-bearing lymphocytes was dependent on both antibody and antigen concentrations. The usefulness of this approach in vivo remains to be seen. If this problem of clearance could be overcome, antibody-mediated targeting could well provide a valuable approach to cell-specific focusing of chemotherapeutic agents.

Another obstacle in targeting particulate drug carriers is the vascular system itself. The endothelial cells lining the capillary-level vasculature have severely frustrated attempts at in vivo targeting which are based on cell surface differences between normal and malignant cells. In order for a drug carrier to be able to recognize a tumour cell, it must first transverse the vascular system into the extra-vascular space. However, with the possible exception of the endothelial cells of an angiosarcoma, there is not necessarily a similarity between the surface antigens of endothelial cells lining the vasculature of a tumour and those of the tumour cell. Thus, not only do endothelial cells create a mechanical barrier for the particulate carriers, but, in addition, they 'shield' the carrier from target cell recognition. This markedly impairs the efficiency of drug targeting using carriers directed against tumour-associated antigens. Consequently, targeted carriers must either take advantage of naturally occurring differences in permeability of the tumour neovasculature or selectively induce changes in that permeability.

In order to circumvent the reticuloendothelial system and provide for a method of site-specific drug delivery, we developed a magnetically responsive drug carrier composed of albumin (Widder et al., 1978). Because of their magnetic characteristics, these microspheres are capable of area-specific localization when subjected to an external magnetic field over a specific target site. In restricting the carrier by biophysical means, one can effectively eliminate the problems associated with clearance by reticuloendothelial cells.

Microspheres composed of albumin and Fe_3O_4 (magnetite) were designed with the following rationale. Small albumin spheres (approximately 1.0 μm), slowly degradable in vivo by endogenous proteases and hydrolases, can be injected intravascularly without occlusion of the microvasculature. Moreover, the microspheres are minimally reactive with blood components, and clinically nontoxic from the standpoints of chemical and immunological reactivity. The carrier is capable of accommodating a wide variety of water-soluble agents. In contrast to liposomes, the albumin matrix can be stabilized by heating or chemical cross-linking to afford a braod spectrum of release kinetics (Widder et al., 1979b). Magnetite was found to have the desired degree of magnetic responsivity and is readily available from commercial sources. Furthermore, the individual Fe_3O_4 particles are much smaller (10–20 nm) than the microsphere and, consequently, occupy a fraction of the potential drug space.

Adriamycin (doxorubicin HCl) was chosen as a prototype drug for several reasons. It has demonstrated activity against a broad range of tumours (Blum, 1975) and also has direct activity at a tumour site, thus not requiring hepatic microsomal activation. The high degree of water solubility of the drug results in its extensive entrapment within the spheres (Widder et al., 1980).

Magnetic targeting of the microspheres was developed to overcome the two major problems previously discussed: reticuloendothelial clearance and target site specificity. Microspheres are infused into an artery supplying a given in vivo target site. A magnet of sufficient field strength to retard the microspheres solely at the capillary level vasculature is placed externally over the target area. Restriction of the microspheres at the microvascular level can be achieved by taking advantage of the physiological difference between the linear flow velocity of blood in large arteries (approximately 30 cm/second) versus that in capillaries (0.05 cm/second). A greater field is necessary to retard the microspheres in the faster moving arterial system as opposed to intracapillary retention.

Restriction of the microspheres within the capillary circulation is essential for two reasons. First, drug diffusion occurs maximally in capillaries and venules; secondly, one ideally would like to facilitate transit of the microspheres from the microvasculature into the extravascular compartment. Accomplishing this would create a depot for sustained drug release in the target area. Moreover, as the carrier is removed from the vasculature, drug slowly released from the microspheres would not immediately be washed away by the circulation, but rather bathe the local tumour environment with a highly focused local concentration of the released drug. By restricting the activity of the targeted drug to the tumour site, one may use a much lower concentration of drug than is needed if systemic therapy is given. Moreover, a significantly lower dosage should minimize or eliminate the adverse toxic side effects associated with high-dose systemic chemotherapy.

2. Magnetic microspheres

2.1. Method of preparation

The microspheres are prepared by heat denaturation via a phase separation emulsion polymerization method (Widder et al., 1978, 1979b). Alternatively, microspheres may be prepared at room temperature by stabilizing the albumin matrix with aldehyde cross-linking agents that have been stabilized in the organic phase (Widder et al., 1979b). In general, an aqueous solution of human serum albumin, bulk purified adriamycin (in the case of adriamycin-containing microspheres; Adria Laboratories) and 10–20 nm particles of magnetite (Ferrofluidics Corporation) is emulsified with 30 ml of cottonseed oil. Trace amounts of ^{125}I-labelled bovine serum albumin are added if a radioactive label is desired. The emulsion is homogenized by sonication for 1 minute at 100 W at 27°C with a Heat Systems (model W 185D) sonifier with a 0.635 cm titanium probe inside a recirculating attachment chamber. This procedure generates small non-cross-linked microspheres containing both Fe_3O_4 and the entrapped drug. Matrix stabilization is subsequently achieved by one of two methods: heat denaturation at temperatures between 100 and 165°C or treatment with oil-soluble carbonyl reagents such as 0.2 M 2,3-butanedione or glutaraldehyde. The degree of matrix stabilization is varied by altering the temperature and time in the case of heat denaturation, or duration of exposure time to chemical cross-linkers. Oil and cross-linking agents are removed by multiple diethyl ether washings and the resulting microspheres are stored in powder form at 4°C. The resulting microspheres range in size from 0.2 to 1.35 μm in diameter, with an average diameter of 1 μm (see Fig. 1). The average adriamycin content of standard microsphere preparation is approximately 10% (w/w). Of this, approximately 40–50 mg of adriamycin are capable of slow release per mg of albumin carrier.

The kinetics of release of biologically active drug was assayed by analyzing the supernatants of prewashed microspheres (1 mg/ml) stabilized by heating either at 115 or 135°C. Both preparations demonstrated a biphasic release pattern; however, the rate of release was subsequently slower for the 135°C preparation (see Fig. 2).

The effect of carrier stabilization on the biological activity of released adriamycin was quantitated by a dose-response analysis using an in vitro rat fibrosarcoma system (Widder et al., 1980). A standard dose-response curve was generated using known concentrations of free adriamycin and the ID_{40} was found to be 1 mg/ml. The 115 and 135°C preparations released 20.0 and 9.5 mg/ml equivalents of biologically active drug, respectively, after 240 minutes of incubation (see Fig. 3). The resulting ratios of biological activity to chemically determined activity were 1.00 (20 mg/ml:20

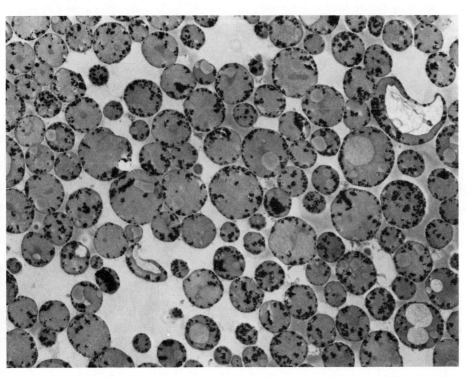

Figure 1. Transmission electron micrograph of magnetically responsive albumin microspheres. Magnification, × 7140 (Widder et al., 1979a).

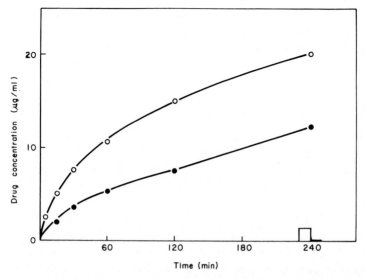

Figure 2. Kinetic release of chemically determined adriamycin from albumin microspheres stabilized at 115 (○) and 135°C (●). Both preparations contained 40 μg of slowly diffusable adriamycin per mg of carrier prior to onset of release. Drug concentrations represent μg of adriamycin per ml of RPMI 1640 release medium. Actual values at 240 minutes were 20.0 and 12.2 μg/ml, respectively, for the 115 and 135°C preparations. The proportions of slowly releasable drug that travelled with and subsequently diffused from magnetically responsive microspheres (circles at 240 minutes) versus unresponsive microspheres (bars at 240 minutes) were 15:1 and 147:1, respectively, for the 115 and 135°C preparations (Widder et al., 1979a).

mg/ml) for the 115°C preparation and 0.78 (9.5 mg/ml : 12.1 mg/ml) for the 135°C preparation. Hence, heat stabilization at 115°C produced no degradation of the released drug, and stabilization at 135°C produced a 22% decrease. This value corresponds well to the known increase in aglycone formation with heat stabilization at 135°C (26% degradation of adriamycin to aglycones).

Further analysis of the 135°C preparation indicated that 20% of the active drug was released during the first hour, leaving 80% for subsequent release. Although relatively slow, this rate was considerably faster than the rate of in vitro matrix degradation (less than 3% in 48 hours) (Widder et al., 1979b). Hence, drug release corresponds more closely with the rate of hydration of the microspheres rather than matrix degradation. This may well vary, depending on the molecular weight of the agent entrapped within the microspheres.

2.2. In vivo distribution and tumour studies

The microspheres were next tested in vivo to assess the validity of this drug targeting concept. The subcutaneous tissue in the tail of Sprague-Dawley rats was chosen as the initial target site for microsphere localization (Widder et al., 1978). The ventral caudal artery was selected for microsphere infusion as it supplies the majority of the blood to the tail.

For purposes of the experiment, the tail was demarcated into four sections, each

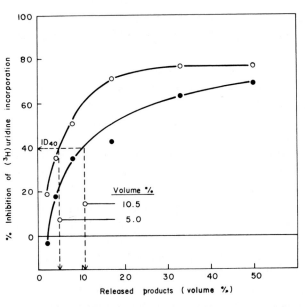

Figure 3. Dose-response quantitation of biologically active drug products released from 0 to 240 minutes of incubation by microspheres stabilized at 115 (○) and 135°C (●). Concentrations of biologically active drug are calculated at $(100/ID_{40}$ volume % of unknown supernatant) × $(ID_{40}$ equivalent of 1.00 μg/ml for free drug). The actual values are 20.0 and 9.5 μg/ml for the 115 and 135°C preparations, respectively. Both preparations were identical to those used in Figure 2, and contained 40 μg of slowly diffusible adriamycin per mg of carrier (Widder et al., 1979a).

measuring 3.5–4.0 cm in length. Microspheres were infused through a polyethylene catheter inserted into the ventral caudal artery, at tail segment 1. The target area for microsphere localization was in tail segment 3, 6.5 cm distal to the point of catheter insertion. A variable gap bipolar permanent magnet was used to magnetically localize the spheres at the target site.

Microspheres, labelled with ^{125}I, were infused at a rate of 0.6 ml/minute, a rate corresponding to the normal flow rate of blood within the ventral caudal artery. Following infusion, the catheter was removed and resumption of blood flow was verified using a transcutaneous Doppler device. The magnet remained in position for 30 minutes following microsphere infusion, after which time the animal was killed. The tail segments and major organs were then counted for gamma radiation to assess carrier distribution.

The localization of microspheres at the target site (tail segment 3) increased with the intensity of the magnetic field. At a magnetic field strength of 8000 Oe, more than 50% of the carrier was present in the target tail segment. The other segments, not influenced by the magnetic field, demonstrated negligible carrier retention. Failure to achieve greater retention of carrier in segment 3 is most probably due to physiological shunting of blood via perforating arterial branches connecting the superficial and deep branches of the caudal artery (Greene, 1968). Shunting can be minimized by advancing the catheter distally toward tail segment 3. As predicted by in vitro experiments, retention of microspheres decreased significantly at lower field strengths.

Magnetic targeting produced a significant effect on microsphere distribution. If one views carrier distribution in terms of μg of microspheres per g wet weight of tissue analyzed, the ratios of carrier localized to the target site compared to liver and heart were 8.6:1 and 215:1, respectively.

Further experiments following carrier distribution 24 hours after removal of the magnetic field have shown the same percentage retention of the microspheres at the target site as observed after 30 minutes. Hence, a 30 minute exposure to the field appears sufficient to restrict the carrier for a prolonged period at a designated site. Transmission electron microscopy of tail segment 3, performed after 30 minutes of exposure to the magnetic field, revealed microspheres entrapped between endothelial cells of small arterioles and capillaries as well as endocytosed by endothelial cells (Widder et al., 1978). No evidence of intravascular thrombosis or conglutination of the microspheres was observed. Hence, long-term retention of the microspheres at the target site appeared to be a result of the movement of the microspheres from the vascular space to the interstitial environment. Again, this would be desirable since the microspheres would then serve as extravascular depots for sustained drug release.

After it had been established that the drug carrier could be selectively targeted with a high degree of efficiency, we next investigated the extent of adriamycin targeting. As the drug is highly water-soluble, it was important to determine whether delivery of adriamycin could be quantitatively related to microsphere delivery. For this purpose, targeting experiments were repeated using the same rat tail system as described in the carrier distribution studies (Senyei et al., 1981). The drug carrier preparation in this study consisted of microspheres that were stabilized at 135°C and contained approximately 36 μg of slowly releasable adriamycin per mg of microspheres. Microspheres were infused through the ventral caudal artery. Experimental animals were killed 30 minutes after exposure of the target site to an 8000-Oe magnetic field. Tissue concentrations of adriamycin were determined using a modification of the method described by Bachur and Cradock (1970). Adriamycin was solubilized from the tail skin and other organs by an overnight extraction with 0.5 N acetic acid at 4°C. Quantitative adriamycin concentrations were determined by spectrophotofluorometry.

In the presence of an 8000-Oe magnetic field (field gradient, $\pm$ 4000 Oe/cm), 3.9 μg of carrier-delivered adriamycin was localized per g of target tail skin (Table 1) when the animals were killed 5 minutes after carrier infusion. No drug was detectable in the non-target tail segments or in the liver. By contrast, a 100-fold higher dose of systemically injected free adriamycin was required to obtain a comparable local tissue concentration (Table 1). Unlike the carrier-delivered drug, this resulted in a liver concentration of 15 μg of adriamycin per g of liver and a target to liver adriamycin ratio of 1:4.5. Carrier localization of one-hundredth of the systemic dose of adriamycin resulted in a dramatic reversal of the target:liver ratio, demonstrating a greater than 3.9:1 differential.

In experiments where the animals were killed 60 minutes after the microsphere

TABLE 1

In vivo distribution of carrier-delivered and free adriamycin

Form of drug	Dose (mg/kg)	Magnetic field[a]	Tissue concentrations (μg/g)[b]	
			Target tail skin	Pooled organs[c]
Carrier-delivered	0.05	0	1	1
	0.05	+	3.9	1
Free	0.05	0	1	1
	5.00	0	5.5	15.0

[a] A magnetic field of 8000 Oe was placed over tail segment 3 (target area) for 5 minutes.
[b] Limits of detection, $\leqslant 1$ μg of drug per g of tissue (wet weight).
[c] Organs consisted of liver, spleen, kidneys, lungs and heart. Adriamycin was found predominantly in the liver.

infusion (30 minutes after the magnetic field was removed from tail segment 3), an adriamycin concentration of 3.7 μg/g was found at the target site with no detectable levels of the drug to be found in adjacent tail segments or in any of the visceral organs examined. In contrast, the adriamycin tissue concentration at the target site decreased to 1.8 μg/g in animals receiving 5.0 mg/kg of free adriamycin intravenously, with a significant amount of drug still detectable in the pooled visceral organs. Thus, after 60 minutes, using 0.1% of the free intravenous dose, adriamycin targeted via magnetic microspheres yielded approximately twice the local adriamycin concentration at a preselected site, with no detectable systemic distribution.

Once we had established the feasibility of selectively localizing a significant amount of injected microspheres containing a biologically active drug, and that the drug could be concentrated to a significant degree at the desired site, the microsphere delivery system was used to treat established rat tumours (Widder et al., 1981a). Microspheres used for these experiments were prepared at 120–125°C. The encapsulation procedure resulted in the entrapment of 97% of the biologically active adriamycin, as determined by the methods previously described.

The ascitic form of the Yoshida rat sarcoma (generously supplied by Dr. Arthur Bogden, Mason Research Institute) was serially passed intraperitoneally in syngeneic Holtzman rats (200–270 g). This tumour was chosen for its known sensitivity to adriamycin and because of its aggressive biological behaviour. The solid form of the tumour can be obtained by inoculating tumour cells subcutaneously. Tumour nodules appeared approximately 3 days after implantation. The average time of death of the untreated animals was found to be 16 days post-tumour inoculation.

Prior to the microsphere experiments, animals (five per group) were inoculated with 2.9×10^7 tumour cells into the axillary region and treated with adriamycin intravenously to assess tumour sensitivity to the drug. Animals received either intravenous normal saline, 0.5 mg adriamycin per kg, or 5.0 mg of adriamycin per kg on days

1, 5 and 9 post-inoculation of the tumour. Animals were assessed for tumour size, weight change, and life span. Tumours were evaluated by measuring the tumour in two dimensions with a micrometer and values were stated as mm², the product of tumour width and length.

Only animals receiving the multiple high dose regimen, 5 mg adriamycin/kg, showed any evidence of tumour sensitivity to the drug. 6 days after tumour implantation, the animals receiving a high dose of adriamycin had an average tumour size 82% smaller than the saline control group and the low-dose adriamycin group (0.5 mg/kg) at day 12. The animals receiving saline or a low dose of adriamycin demonstrated a weight gain of 23.3 and 17.8 g, respectively. In contrast, animals receiving the 5 mg/kg dosage regimen had an average weight loss of 12 g, demonstrating evidence of systemic toxicity. No difference in life span was noted between any treatment group, with an average life span of 9.2, 9.6 and 10.2 days noted for the saline control, low-dose adriamycin group and high-dose adriamycin group, respectively. In summary, animals receiving multiple doses of adriamycin at a dose of 5 mg/kg demonstrated evidence of systemic toxicity, with weight loss and a scruffy coat. Moreover, no enhancement of life span was noted in this group.

Once tumour sensitivity had been established, experiments were designed to treat the Yoshida sarcoma with adriamycin targeted via magnetic microspheres. As previously, animals were inoculated with 3.5×10^8 tumour cells into the lateral aspect of the tail, but, unlike sensitivity experiments, animals were used for experiments 6–8 days after tumour implantation. By the time of experimental use, tumours were not only measurable, but on occasion showed evidence of necrosis. The average tumour size at the time of experimental use was 200 mm². At the time of treatment, animal weights ranged from 185 to 250 g. Regardless of the type of therapy given, animals received only single-dose treatment 6–8 days after tumour inoculation.

The experimental group consisted of 22 animals which received either drug-bearing microspheres at a dose of 0.5 mg of adriamycin per kg or 2.5 mg/kg with the tumour exposed to the magnetic field for 30 minutes. The method of microsphere infusion into the ventral caudal artery was identical to the methods described previously. The following groups of animals constituted the control groups. Ten animals received 'placebo' microspheres (without drug) infused in an identical manner with exposure of the tumour to the magnetic field application. Finally, free adriamycin was administered intraarterially (via the ventral caudal artery) at 0.5 and 5 mg/kg and intravenously at 5 mg/kg. The animals were observed for weight change, size of tumour, and deaths. All animals were killed 30 days after treatment. Complete autopsies were performed and organs were examined both grossly and microscopically for evidence of tumour.

The results of single-dose therapy with magnetically responsive microspheres are presented in Table 2. The tumour size increased markedly in all the animals treated with free adriamycin, regardless of the route of administration or dose. Control animals receiving either no treatment, placebo microspheres or drug-bearing microspheres without localization also demonstrated a significant increase in tumour size.

TABLE 2

Effect of magnetic microspheres containing adriamycin on Yoshida sarcoma-bearing rats

	Untreated control	Adriamycin		Placebo microspheres with magnet	Microspheres bearing 0.5 mg/kg adriamycin		Microspheres bearing 2.5 mg/kg adriamycin
		5 mg/kg intraarterially	0.5 mg/kg intraarterially		No magnet	With magnet	With magnet
Initial tumour size (mm^2)	423	496	459	254	502	413	226
Final tumour size (mm^2)	932	859	701	594	1,076	38	22
Deaths (%)	90	100	100	100	100	0	0
Regressions (%)	0	0	0	0	0	100	100
Total remissions (%)	0	0	0	0	0	75	80
Metastases (%)	100	100	100	100	100	0	0

In contrast, there was a significant (83%) decrease in tumour size in animals receiving adriamycin-containing microspheres (0.5 or 2.5 mg/kg) with the magnet placed adjacent to the tumour. The weights of all control animals increased during the course of the experiments, indicating no evidence of systemic toxicity. Animals receiving targeted therapy also showed an increase in weight.

In all groups of animals, except those receiving magnetically localized adriamycin microspheres, there was an 80–100% mortality rate and an 80–100% incidence of distant metastases during the 30 days that the animals were observed. In contrast, no deaths or metastases occurred in the animals given a single dose of magnetically targeted microspheres containing adriamycin. Moreover, 77% of the animals in this group had complete tumour remission as confirmed by microscopic examination of the tissues. An additional 13% had significant tumour regression. In comparison, there were no remissions or regressions in any control group.

In prior experiments performed to assess tumour susceptibility to adriamycin, it was found that the tumour would respond only when the therapeutic regimen consisted of multiple-dose intravenous adriamycin (5 mg/kg) given on days 1, 5 and 9 after tumour inoculation. Animals thus treated showed some evidence of tumour regression. However, these animals also experienced a weight loss, suggestive of toxicity due to the drug. Moreover, survival was not enhanced in animals treated in this fashion compared to untreated controls.

In contrast, when a single dose of adriamycin is administered in magnetically responsive microspheres and targeted to the tumour site, one can achieve 77% total remission of the tumour with no deaths or histological evidence of metastases in experimental animals. These animals were treated after the tumour load was evident (6–8 days after tumour inoculation) and with only a single dose of either 0.5 or 2.5 mg of adriamycin per kg as compared to multiple-dose therapy. Evidence of tumour necrosis was histologically evident as early as 3 days post-treatment.

Currently, we do not know the lower level of sensitivity of the delivery system as it relates to the adriamycin experiments. As 90–100% regressions were achieved with a single magnetically localized adriamycin dose of 0.5 mg/kg, with no significant improvement noted upon administration of a 5-fold higher dose, the lowest effective dose is unknown. By using magnetic localization, we are concentrating the drug significantly in a confined region, thereby creating high localized drug levels (Senyei et al., 1981).

In additional experiments, vindesine sulfate was encapsulated in the magnetically responsive microspheres and used for targeting to the Yoshida sarcoma (Morris et al., 1982). The same general experimental design was used as in the previously described adriamycin studies. Again, tumours were implanted subcutaneously in the tail of female Holtzman rats and allowed to grow to at least 450 mm^2 before initiation of the experimental treatment. Drug-bearing magnetic microspheres at a dose of 0.5 or 2.5 mg/kg were infused proximal to the tumour via the ventral caudal artery. A bipolar permanent magnet was placed adjacent to the tumour for a period of 30 minutes during the infusion to effect localization. Other groups of animals received either

0.5 or 2.5 mg/kg of free vindesine or drug-bearing microspheres without utilization of the external magnet to achieve localization. An untreated control group was monitored also.

Of the 20 animals receiving magnetically targeted vindesine, 75% had a total remission of the tumour. The remaining animals demonstrated marked tumour regression, representing an overall 95% regression rate. None of the 20 animals receiving localized treatment had metastatic disease and one of the animals died. In contrast, untreated animals as well as those receiving either free vindesine or non-localized vindesine spheres exhibited significant tumour growth with metastases, with subsequent death in 90–100% of the animals. The results from this experiment correlated closely with those from the adriamycin experiments in demonstrating rather dramatic regressions and remissions in animals treated in localized therapy.

In order to understand the interaction of targeted microspheres with tumour cells within a tumour bed, we performed electron microscopy on tumours from experimental animals (Widder et al., 1983). It is of importance from a mechanistic viewpoint to understand the ultrastructural relationships between the drug carrier and the tumour cell in order to optimize drug delivery by this system. Placebo spheres were used as opposed to adriamycin-containing microspheres due to the previously demonstrated rapid tumouricidal effect of the latter. The animals were killed at 5 minutes, 30 minutes or 24 hours after microsphere administration. Tumours were fixed in 4% glutaraldehyde in 0.15 M sodium cacodylate buffer (pH 7.4) processed routinely (Marino and Adams, 1980) and examined by transmission electron microscopy (JEOL 100B).

When the animals were killed 5 minutes after the microspheres had been targeted to the tumour, the microspheres were found in endothelial-type cells lining the vascular spaces. This early process of endocytosis by the endothelial cells was observed previously (Widder et al., 1978) when the microspheres were targeted to normal cutaneous tissue. Moreover, in those experiments, microspheres were also found lodged between adjacent endothelial cells in gap junctions. Thus, it is apparent that the initial step in carrier disposition, after the process of localization, is a migration of the microspheres out of the vasculature and their sequestration in the endothelial cells or the tumour cells lining vascular spaces. The mechanism by which this occurs is probably a result of an endocytic response secondary to mechanical pushing against the endothelial cells. As endothelial cells normally transport high-molecular-weight substances by endocytosis and subsequent vacuolization, microspheres pushed against endothelial cells by the magnetic field most probably are internalized by a similar process.

Electron micrographs obtained 30 minutes after the microspheres were targeted demonstrated a further migration of the microsphere from the endothelial cells into the interstitial compartment. As early as 30 minutes after the infusion of the carrier, microspheres were found adjacent to tumour cells or within tumour cells. As previously suggested, the drug is released from microspheres by radial diffusion (Senyei et al., 1981). As the microspheres were found in the interstitium surrounded by tumour cells, one microsphere can, in theory, release enough drug in a radial fashion to be tumouricidal to surrounding tumour cells. Hence, a one to one microsphere to tumour cell relationship is not a prerequisite for effective tumour destruction. Moreover, this mechanism essentially provides for an oncolytic amplification system where multiple tumour cells may be killed by the presence of only one drug carrier.

Microspheres were also endocytosed by tumour cells. The spheres within the cell were membrane-bound, indicating their intracellular processing as phagosomes. These microspheres can release their drug intracellularly and, in so doing, kill the target cell. As the tumour becomes damaged by the drug, drug released subsequently by the microspheres could diffuse out of the disabled cell through its 'leaky' plasma membrane and effect neighbouring tumour cells. Thus, two potential mechanisms exist to explain the rapid necrosis of the tumour observed when adriamycin was selectively targeted to the tumour via magnetic microspheres (Widder et al., 1981a).

24 hours after microsphere targeting, one can still observe intact microspheres within tumour cells. Thus, the carrier is still available to release drug to the tumour. The ability of microspheres to release encapsulated antineoplastic agents into the tumour environment over an extended period of time allows for the killing of tumour cells re-entering the cell cycle which are now more sensitive to many anti-tumour agents. Studies using ^{125}I-labelled microspheres have substantiated the presence of microspheres within the target site up to 21 days after localization. Hence, this method of drug delivery allows for sustained drug release over an extensive period of time.

A similar approach to drug delivery has been proposed where magnetically responsive mitomycin C microspheres were prepared (Kato et al., 1980). These studies demonstrated the entrapment and subsequent release of the entrapped drug. In addition, placebo magnetic microspheres were tested in vivo and selectively localized both to the lungs and the kidneys (Morimoto et al., 1980, 1981). These studies, as well as data generated from laboratories, demonstrate the feasibility of the magnetic drug delivery system.

Finally, we investigated the use of the biological response modifiers, poly(inosine cytosine) (PolyIC) and protein A, when localized selectively to the rat mammary adenocarcinoma 13762. PolyIC is known to induce interferon (Levy et al., 1969) and protein A has been shown to be a T and B cell mitogen (Sakane and Green, 1978) and induce gamma interferon (McCool et al., 1981). The mammary adenocarcinoma (2×10^6 cells) was transplanted subcutaneously in the tail and animals were treated when the tumour became palpable. Two groups of animals (ten animals per group) were treated with polyIC microspheres (polyIC = 7.2% of microsphere weight). Each animal received a single dose of 1 mg of microspheres. Animals received either polyIC microspheres intraarterially, or intraarterially with magnetic localization to the tumour.

Four groups of animals were treated with the protein A microspheres. Again, animals received only single dose treatment which consisted of 1 mg of protein A microspheres (protein A = 9% of microsphere weight). The groups consisted of animals receiving the microspheres intraarterially, intraperitoneally, intralesionally, or targeted directly to the tumour. Animals were followed for 30 days, or until death, and monitored for tumour size and the presence of metastases.

Results from these experiments are shown in Table 3. Both groups receiving polyIC microspheres, intraarterially or magnetically localized to the tumour, demonstrate a delay in appearance of flank metastases as well as some retardation of tumour growth rate. However, a prolongation of animal survival was not significantly enhanced compared to control animals. Nevertheless, protein A microspheres demonstrated a significant prolongation of animal survival specifically in the experimental group receiving magnetically targeted therapy. An increase in the lifespan was noted in the other groups receiving protein A microspheres intraperitoneally, intraarterially and intralesionally; but not to the extent of the magnetically localized group. Moreover, nine of the ten animals receiving localized protein A therapy showed a complete remission of the tumour (defined as complete clinical disappearance) 4 days post-treatment, with subsequent reappearance of the tumour. This decrease in survival time compares favourably with that seen in the group of animals receiving targeted adriamycin.

Linear regression analysis of tumour growth demonstrates a significantly decreased rate of tumour growth in animals receiving magnetically localized protein A compared to untreated and placebo control animals. This decrease in tumour growth

TABLE 3

Effect of magnetic microspheres, containing various biological response modifiers, on rat mammary adenocarcinoma 13762

Treatment	Death (days) from time of implant	Appearance of flank metastases from time of treatment (days)	Day tumour reaches 50 mm from date of treatment (LxW/2)
Untreated	32.9	–	–
Placebos			
Intraarterially	42.4	11.2	13.0
Localized[a]	42.0	13.7	7.9
PolyIC			
Intraarterially	43.2	22.4	11.4
Localized	40.1	26.0	16.4
Protein A			
Intraperitoneally	41.6	21.0	11.5
Intraarterially	37.1	19.8	10.0
Intralesionally	40.1	17.3	8.0
Localized	51.3	26.8	15.6
Adriamycin, localized	52.8	33.8	31.0

All animals received 1 mg of microspheres. The implant was a rat mammary adenocarcinoma 13762 passaged in Fisher 344 rats. Animals were inoculated with 1×10^6 tumour cells subcutaneously in the tail. PolyIC = 7.2% and protein A = 9% weight of microspheres.
[a] Magnetic exposure time = 20 minutes.

is not as pronounced as is seen in the animals receiving targeted adriamycin (the curve for which actually demonstrates a negative slope). However, it must be remembered that animals received a single dose of either protein A or adriamycin microspheres consisting of only 1 mg of microspheres. It is encouraging to note tumouricidal activity of a biological response modifier if specifically localized to a given tumour site. Perhaps with a higher dose or multiple doses, permanent tumour remission may be accomplished. We believe this is the first demonstration of the efficacy of localized immunomodulators in the treatment of primary tumours when the agent is anatomically restricted to the tumour site.

3. Conclusions

It is hoped that the magnetic carrier system may find utility in the treatment of patients with tumours limited to and localized in anatomical regions with well-defined blood supplies. Two major advantages of this carrier over other delivery systems are its high efficiency of in vivo targeting and its controllable release of drug at the microvascular level. Its protracted residence within a tumour affords long-term sustained therapy. In addition, the carrier exhibits minimal toxicity at doses required for the therapy of large tumours (unpublished results, using BDF_1 mice). The carrier represents a universal vehicle that is potentially compatible with a wide spectrum of chemotherapeutic agents as well as low- and high-molecular-weight synthetic and natural products. It affords a mechanism to achieve uniform target distribution of water-soluble immuno-potentiating agents such as protein A and polyIC. In the case of weakly antigenic tumours or tumour-induced immuno-suppression, the microspheres also may permit the localized delivery of inflammatory agents, such as histamine, or macrophage-activating substances, such as BCG, muramyl dipeptide and lymphokines (Fidler, 1980). This could initiate the directed chemotaxis and inflammatory activities of blood monocytes, neutrophils and T lymphocytes. Directed immunotherapy may well offer a solution for the general treatment of metastases without directly targeting microspheres to each foci of metastatic tumour.

The versatile nature of the microspheres allows for the simultaneous delivery of multiple agents. Moreover, the ease and rapidity of drug-carrier preparation potentially allows for the delivery of combination chemotherapy, or chemo-immunotherapy to tumours whose drug sensitivities are determined by prior biological analysis of resected tumour. Many short-term tissue culture systems are currently used to assess tumour sensitivity to chemotherapeutic agents as well as in vivo systems involving the inoculation of human tumours into nude mice.

Targeting of highly toxic chemotherapeutic agents to tumour sites, with the subsequent reduction of the systemically available drug, should minimize any compromise of the host immunity. In fact, immune potentiation by various antineoplastic agents has been recently reported where properly timed administration of low doses of the respective drugs resulted in the selective destruction of T lymphocyte suppressor cells

(Tomazic et al., 1980; Hengst et al., 1980). Low levels of adriamycin released from the tumour site in animals treated with targeted therapy may well have resulted in T suppressor cell cytotoxicity. This perhaps may be one explanation for the observed lack of metastatic disease in this experimental group.

Finally, the albumin matrix is capable of incorporating a variety of radionuclides for use in antitumour therapy. This can potentially afford an optimal homogeneous distribution of radioactivity confined within a given tumour with the elimination of radiation damage to adjacent critical organs and tissues.

The ability to entrap a variety of drugs suggests potential uses in a number of other localized disease states. It may be of particular value for the delivery of antibiotics in patients with bacterial or fungal abscesses and other sequestered infections, such as prostatitis and osteomyelitis. Prior studies in which microspheres were targeted to non-tumour tail tissue resulted in 40% of the targeted microspheres being present in bone and associated connective tissue (Widder et al., 1978). Hence, the carrier should achieve and maintain high therapeutic concentrations of drug within bone tissue.

Another potential use of the microspheres involves the delivery of fibrinolytic agents in the treatment of deep venous thrombosis and pulmonary embolism. To date, we have entrapped urokinase, a potent fibrinolytic enzyme, with no reduction of the enzymatic capability of the protein. As urokinase is a potent activator of plasmin, bleeding can result from its systemic administration. Currently, its use is restricted to treating pulmonary embolism. Clearly, a mechanism to target a smaller quantity of the enzyme would be advantageous in achieving a high localized enzyme concentration with a subsequent reduction of possible systemic bleeding.

Magnetic microspheres have already proven to be valuable in the laboratory as a research tool (Widder et al., 1979c, 1981b). By incorporating protein A (SpA), a staphylococcal surface coat protein, into the matrix of microsphere, one can rapidly and efficiently bind most subclasses of immunoglobulin G to the surface of the protein A microsphere by incubation alone. This is accomplished by virtue of two receptor sites per molecule of SpA for the Fc portion of IgG. Thus, all the resultant IgG bound to the microsphere is properly oriented with the F(ab) arms available to interact with antigen. No chemical coupling agents or spacer groups are necessary using this system. We have already demonstrated the utility of these microspheres for cell sorting utilizing the magnetic property of the microspheres. This is accomplished by binding the microsphere surface with antibodies of appropriate specificity for a particular cell type. Cells that bear complimentary surface determinants bind with the microspheres and are magnetically separated from the cell suspension. This is accomplished with a high degree of sensitivity and specificity. The system is applicable to the isolation of any organism (i.e., bacterium, virus) or molecular structure as long as an antibody exists to the desired product.

In conclusion, magnetically responsive microspheres offer a new approach in accomplishing the goal of drug targeting. Scale-up of the system is required before this system will find clinical utility. With the advent of computerized axial tomography and other sophisticated diagnostic techniques, the rapid and exact localization of small lesions is possible. Hence, it would appear that the diagnostic capability exists to proceed with targeted chemotherapy on an experimental clinical basis. Based on the targeting capabilities and release characteristics of the available drug carriers, it appears that magnetically responsive small albumin microspheres currently represent an optimal prototype system for the area-specific delivery of antitumour agents.

References

Bachur, N.R. and Cradock, F.C. (1970) J. Pharmacol. Exp. Therap. 175, 331–337.

Blum, R.H. (1975) Cancer Chemother. Rep. 6, 247–257.

Byers, V.S. and Levin, A.S. (1976) in Basic and Clinical Immunology (Fudenberg and Stites, D.P., Eds.), p. 242, Lange Medical Publications, Los Altos.

Fidler, I.J. (1980) Science 208, 1469–1470.

Greene, E.C. (1968) The Anatomy of the Rat, Hafner, New York.

Gregoriadis, G. and Neerunjun, E.D. (1974) Eur. J. Biochem. 47, 179–185.

Gregoriadis, G. and Neerunjun, E.D. (1975) Biochem. Biophys. Res. Commun. 64, 537–544.

Gregoriadis, G. and Meehan, A. (1981) Biochem. J. 200, 211–216.

Gregoriadis, G., Meehan, A. and Mah, M.M. (1981) Biochem. J. 200, 203–210.

Hengst, J.C.S., Mokyr, M.D. and Dray, S. (1980) Cancer Res. 40, 2135–2141.

Illum, L., Jones, P.D.E., Kreuter, J., Baldwin, R.W., and Davis, S.S. (1984) Int. J. Pharmaceut., in press.

Juliano, R.L. and Stamp, D. (1976) Nature 261, 235–237.

Kato, T., Nemoto, R., Mori, H., Unno, K., Goto, A. and Homma, M. (1980) Nippon Ganchirogaku Kaishi. 15, 58–62.

Levy, H.D., Law, L.W. and Rabson, A.S. (1969) Proc. Natl. Acad. Sci. U.S.A. 62, 357–361.

Marchesi, V.T., Tillack, T.W., Jackson, R.L., Segrest, J.P. and Scott, R.E. (1972) Proc. Natl. Acad. U.S.A. 69, 1445–1449.

Marino, P.A. and Adams, D.O. (1980) Cell Immunol. 54, 11–25.

McCool, R.E., Catalona, W.J., Langford, M.P. and Ratliff, T.L. (1981) J. Interferon Res. 1, 473.

McDougall, L.R., Dunnick, J.K., McNamee, M.S. and Kriss, J.P. (1974) Proc. Natl. Acad. Sci. U.S.A. 71, 3487–3491.

Morimoto, Y., Sugibayashi, K., Okumura, M. and Kato, Y. (1980) J. Pharm. Dyn. 3, 264–267.

Morimoto, Y., Okumura, M., Sugibayashi, K. and Kato, Y. (1981) J. Pharm. Dyn. 4, 624–631.

Morris, R.D., Poore, G.A., Howard, D.P. and Sefranka, J.A. (1982) Proceedings 13th International Cancer Congress.

Prieels, J.P., Pizzo, S.F., Glasgow, L.R., Paulson, J.C. and Hill, R.L. (1978) Proc. Natl. Acad. Sci. U.S.A. 75, 2215–2219.

Rowland, G.F., O'Neill, G.J. and Davies, D.A.L. (1975) Nature 255, 487–488.

Sakane, T. and Green, I. (1978) J. Immunol. 120, 302–311.

Segal, A.W., Willis, E.J., Richmond, J.E., Salvin, G., Black, C.D.V. and Gregoriadis, G. (1974) Br. J. Exp. Pathol. 55, 320–327.

Senyei, A.E., Reich, S.D., Gonczy, C. and Widder, K.J. (1981) J. Pharm. Sci. 70, 389–391.

Tanaka, T., Taneda, K., Kobayashi, H., Okumura, K., Muranishi, S. and Sezaki, H. (1975) Chem. Pharm. Bull. 23, 3069–3074.

Tomazic, V.T., Ehrke, M.J. and Mihich, E. (1980) Cancer Res. 40, 2748–2755.

Weissman, C., Bloomgarden, D., Kaplan, A., Cohen, C., Hoffstein, S., Collins, T., Gotlieb, A. and Nagle, D. (1975) Proc. Natl. Acad. Sci. U.S.A. 72, 88–92.

Widder, K.J., Senyei, A.E. and Scarpelli, D.G. (1978) Proc. Soc. Exp. Biol. Med. 158, 141–146.

Widder, K.J., Senyei, A.E. and Ranney, D.F. (1979a) in Advances in Pharmacology and Chemotherapy (Garattini, S., Goldin, A., Hawking, F., Kopin, I.J. and Schnitzer, R.J., Eds.) pp. 213–217, Academic Press, New York.

Widder, K.J., Flouret, G. and Senyei, A.E. (1979b) J. Pharm. Sci. 68, 79–81.

Widder, K.J., Senyei, A.E., Ovadia, H. and Paterson, P.Y. (1979c) Clin. Immunol. Immunopath. 14, 395–400.

Widder, K.J., Senyei, A.E. and Ranney, D.F. (1980) Cancer Res. 40, 3512–3517.

Widder, K.J., Morris, R.M., Poore, G., Howard, D.P., Jr. and Senyei, A.E. (1981a) Proc. Natl. Acad. Sci. U.S.A. 78, 579–581.

Widder, K.J., Senyei, A.E., Ovadia, H. and Paterson, P.Y. (1981b) J. Pharm. Sci. 70, 387–389.

Widder, K.J., Senyei, A.E. and Sears, B. (1982) J. Pharm. Sci. 71, 379–387.

Widder, K.J., Marino, P.A., Morris, R.M., Howard, D.P., Poore, G.A. and Senyei, A.E. (1983) Eur. J. Cancer Clin. Oncol. 19, 141–147.

Microspheres and Drug Therapy. Pharmaceutical, Immunological and Medical Aspects
edited by S.S. Davis, L. Illum, J.G. McVie and E. Tomlinson
© *1984, Elsevier Science Publishers B.V.*
413

CHAPTER 5

Localization of magnetic microspheres in 36 canine osteogenic sarcomas

J.M. Bartlett, R.C. Richardson, G.S. Elliott, W.E. Blevins, W. Janas,
J.R. Hale and R.L. Silver

1. Introduction

The selective delivery and retention of drugs at specific target sites within the body pose a substantial problem in drug design and formulation. The availability of directed drug delivery systems may facilitate the use of therapeutic agents which have significant systemic toxicity at blood levels required for therapeutic efficacy. By limiting drug delivery to a specific region or structure in the body, therapeutic drug levels may be achieved at the local site while toxic systemic concentrations may be avoided. This concept is of considerable utility in the administration of cancer chemotherapeutic agents, which frequently exhibit serious systemic side effects at therapeutic levels.

A number of approaches to the problem of selective drug delivery have been suggested, and an extensive literature review has been published (Widder et al., 1979b). Among these proposals was the concept of using magnetically guided albumin microspheres (Senyei et al., 1978) as a directed drug delivery system. Typically, these microspheres are prepared by an emulsion polymerization technique (Widder et al., 1979a). In this procedure a mixture containing human serum albumin, a water-soluble drug, such as doxorubicin, and nanoparticles of magnetite (an insoluble iron oxide, Fe_3O_4) is homogenized in cottonseed oil, which serves as the external phase of the emulsion. Uniform, spherical particles 1–3 μm in diameter and containing both the drug and the magnetite are formed by irreversible heat denaturation of the albumin in the cottonseed oil. The presence of magnetite in the spheres causes them to be magnetically responsive.

Reports of in vivo studies using this drug delivery system have been promising. Using the Yoshida sarcoma tumour model implanted in rat tails, Widder et al. (1981) reported that 12 animals dosed intraarterially with 0.5 mg/kg of doxorubicin entrapped in magnetically localized microspheres all demonstrated either total or partial tumour remission. Control groups were treated with free doxorubicin administered intraarterially at 0.5 and 5.0 mg/kg, free doxorubicin administered intravenously at 5.0 mg/kg, and placebo microspheres administered intraarterially. These control groups all experienced significant tumour growth, widespread metastases and, in most cases, death of the animal.

In a similar study Sugibayashi et al. (1982) compared the antitumour effects of intravenously administered doxorubicin-entrapped magnetically localized bovine serum albumin microspheres and free doxorubicin on AH7974 lung metastases in rats. The doxorubicin concentration in the lung tissue of the microsphere-treated group was eight times the concentration in the group treated with the free drug. Histopathologic examination of lung tissue showed that the microsphere-treated lungs exhibited greater antitumour drug effects than did lungs treated with the free drug. Increases in the lung weight resulting primarily from tumour growth did not occur as rapidly in the microsphere-treated group as they did in either the free drug group or the untreated controls. Finally, the mean survival times of the group treated with magnetically localized drug-bearing microspheres were significantly longer than either the control group or the group treated with free doxorubicin.

Using a nontumour-bearing rat-tail model, Widder et al. (1978) determined the in vivo distribution of intraarterially administered ^{125}I-labeled magnetic microspheres. 24 hours after magnetic localization of the microspheres within the tail, approximately 50% of the radioactivity remained at the target side. Microspheres that passed through the tail target site were found primarily in the liver, spleen and lungs, the organs which normally sequester foreign particulates from the blood. In a separate study (Senyei et al., 1981), it was observed that 0.05 mg/kg of intraarterially administered magnetic microspheres containing doxorubicin delivered a drug concentration in the target tissue equivalent to the tissue concentration achieved with 5.0 mg/kg of free intravenous doxorubicin. With the low dose of doxorubicin associated with the magnetic microspheres, the drug concentration in a pooled organ sample (liver, spleen, kidneys, lungs and heart) was less than the minimum detectable concentration (1 μg/g), while the 5.0 mg/kg dose of free doxorubicin demonstrated pooled organ concentrations three times that of the target site. This difference is especially important for drugs such as doxorubicin, which demonstrate severe systemic toxicity at normal doses of the free drug.

The objective of the work presented here is to determine the site-specific localization and retention of magnetically targeted human albumin microspheres (HAM). The model selected was a spontaneous canine osteosarcoma of the limb. Osteosarcomas in man and dog show marked similarities with respect to location, behaviour, and radiographic and histopathologic appearance (Owen, 1969). The advantage of using the canine osteosarcoma is that it frequently is located in a distal extremity, and therefore is easily accessible to an externally placed magnet.

2. Experimental procedures

2.1. Methods and materials

2.1.1. Radioactively labeled magnetic microspheres
The magnetic microspheres used for this study were provided by Dr. Robert Morris, Lilly Research Laboratories, Indianapolis, IN. The microspheres were composed of

20% (by weight) magnetite in a human albumin matrix.

Typically, the microspheres were prepared for radioactive labeling by mixing 300 mg of the HAM with 30 ml of ether containing 30 mg of stannous chloride dihydrate. The ether was removed using a rotary evaporator (Rotovapor, Buchi, Switzerland), leaving the stannous chloride in association with the microspheres. Immediately prior to infusion, a microsphere suspension was prepared in the following manner: (a) the dry, stannous chloride-treated microspheres were suspended in 3 ml of ethanol, USP; (b) this alcoholic suspension was diluted with 13.5 ml of 0.9% NaCl containing 0.1% (by volume) polysorbate 80 as a wetting and suspending agent; (c) the suspension was then further diluted with 12.5 ml of 0.9% NaCl; (d) the suspension was transferred to a 30 ml vial containing 200 μCi of sodium ^{99m}Tc-pertechnetate and incubated at room temperature for 5 minutes to allow the labeling reaction to go to completion. The reaction flask was sonicated briefly in an ultrasonic bath (Ultramet III, Buehler Ltd., Evanston, IL) after the first two steps. After the third step (immediately prior to radioactive labeling) the suspension was sonicated for 30 seconds at 100 W with a Heat Systems model W350 sonifier (Ultrasonics, Plainview, NY). The vial containing the radioactively labeled microspheres (^{99m}Tc-HAM) was again sonicated by immersion in the ultrasonic bath immediately prior to withdrawing the calculated volume for injection. These sonication steps were to ensure complete dispersion of the microspheres.

2.1.2. Animals
^{99m}Tc-HAM localization studies were conducted in 36 dogs of various breeds bearing spontaneous osteosarcomas of the limb. The dogs had been referred to the Purdue Comparative Oncology Program, a network of over 140 cooperating veterinarians from the Lafayette and Indianapolis (IN, U.S.A.) areas which is dedicated to the compassionate use of animals with spontaneous neoplasia as models for human as well as animal cancer. The diagnosis of osteosarcoma was confirmed by histopathology following clinical, radiographic, and laboratory evaluation of each subject. No animals were entered into the study unless preexperimental evaluation indicated that 6-week survivability was probable.

For the localization procedures, the dogs were premedicated with 0.04 mg/kg atropine sulfate given subcutaneously 20 minutes prior to the induction of anaesthesia, which was accomplished with 1.1 mg/kg xylazine (Rompun, Haver-Lockhart, Shawnee, KS) and 2.2 mg/kg ketamine hydrochloride (Ketaset, Bristol Laboratories, Syracuse, NY) given concomitantly as an intravenous bolus injection. Anaesthesia was maintained throughout the procedure using methoxyflurane (Metofane, Pitman-Moore, Washington Crossing, NJ).

2.2. Tumour localization experiments
^{99m}Tc-HAM localization was evaluated by three delivery routes: retrograde intravenous (eight dogs), intraarterial (11 dogs), and intramedullary (eight dogs). In addition, biodistribution studies were performed on nine dogs. The biodistribution studies included one control animal infused by the normograde intravenous route with-

out magnetic localization, eight animals infused by the intraarterial route with magnetic localization and three animals infused by the intramedullary route with magnetic localization. Biodistribution studies were not conducted for the retrograde intravenous delivery since radiographic contrast studies demonstrated that access by this route was primarily to large diameter superficial veins rather than to more diffuse tumour capillaries.

Retrograde intravenous delivery of ^{99m}Tc-HAM was accomplished by inserting a catheter proximal to the tumour in a direction counter to normal blood flow. The ^{99m}Tc-HAM suspension was infused under tourniquetted conditions so that the limb vascularity was back-filled with the injected material.

The intraarterial route was established by catheterizing either the carotid artery for delivery to rear limb tumours or the femoral artery for delivery to forelimb tumours. Under fluoroscopic control, the catheter tip was positioned in the arterial access to the tumour.

The intramedullary route of administration was accessed by installing a catheter normograde to blood flow in a superficial vein distal to the tumour. The limb was then wrapped as tightly as possible with an Esmarch bandage to eliminate venous return from the limb and force any injected material into the deep intramedullary vascular channels rather than into the normal superficial venous system.

For each dog studied, contrast angiography with diatrizoate meglumine (Hypaque Meglumine 60%, Winthrop Laboratories, NY) was used to demonstrate the vascularity of the tumour. Radiographs were made for both the cranial/caudal and the lateral projections. In general, it was observed that pre-examination of the access routes to the tumour using radiographic techniques served as a good predictor of the localization of ^{99m}Tc-HAM in the tumour.

^{99m}Tc-HAM was administered at a dose of 1 mg of microspheres per cubic centimeter of tumour volume. The tumour volume was calculated by assuming that the tumour was an ellipsoid with a volume equal to $4/3 \pi abc$, where a, b and c represent the semiaxes of the ellipsoid. These measurements were taken from radiographs of the tumour.

The magnet used to induce localization of the ^{99m}Tc-HAM in the tumour was a 5-kW electromagnet prepared at the Francis Bitter National Magnet Laboratory, Cambridge, MA. The single pole of this magnet had a 10-cm chisel-shaped tip that could be freely moved in all directions to facilitate external positioning over the tumour. Once the magnet was in position, the power was applied and infusion of ^{99m}Tc-HAM was begun. The tumour site was maintained under magnetic influence for 30 minutes post-infusion, and then the power to the magnet was turned off. Redistribution of radioactivity from the tumour site was monitored for 15 minutes after magnet shut-down by using a shielded 2 inch by 2 inch NaI(Tl) crystal scintillation detector and a Canberra Series 30 Multichannel Analyzer (Canberra Industries, Inc., Meriden, CT) set in the multichannel scaling mode. At the end of the redistribution study, the detector was reset to the pulse height analysis mode and 30-second counts were obtained over the tumour site, lungs, liver, paw distal to the tumour, and the contralateral paw.

2.3. Biodistribution studies

To determine the biodistribution of ^{99m}Tc-HAM, 12 dogs were killed immediately after the magnetic localization of the microspheres. One animal, serving as a control, was given radioactively labeled microspheres by the normograde intravenous route without the use of the magnet. At necropsy, samples of tissue from the lungs, liver, kidney, spleen, heart, brain, gut and blood were taken. The percentage of injected radioactivity per gram of tissue was determined by counting the samples with a NaI(Tl) well crystal and a single channel gamma-ray spectrometer (Mech-Tronics Nuclear, Addison, IL). In nine dogs the tumour-bearing limb was removed, cross-sectioned, and then imaged using either a Pho-Dot rectilinear scanner (Nuclear-Chicago, Des Plaines, IL) or a Pho-Gamma HP scintillation camera (Nuclear-Chicago, Des Plaines, IL). This was done to demonstrate the distribution of radioactivity within the tumour itself.

2.4. Evaluation procedures

Tumour localization of magnetically responsive ^{99m}Tc-HAM was evaluated using two separate criteria. The first criterion was a measure of the permanence of localization once the magnetic influence had been terminated, and was determined by monitoring the retention of radioactivity at the target site as a function of time after the treatment. Data collection was begun at the time the magnetic influence was removed and continued for 15 minutes. In general, the level of radioactivity was observed to stabilize within the 15-minute counting time, suggesting that redistribution of ^{99m}Tc-HAM out of the target site was essentially complete at this time. These data are reported as the retention value, which is the ratio of the count rate at the end of the monitoring period to the count rate at the start of the monitoring period.

The second criterion was a relative evaluation of the biodistribution of ^{99m}Tc-HAM between the target site and the lungs and the liver, the primary localization sites for ^{99}Tc-HAM that was not retained at the target site. Data were accumulated subsequent to the completion of the redistribution studies by resetting the multichannel analyzer to the pulse height analysis mode and accumulating 30-second counts over the target site, the lungs, and the liver. A tumour index value was generated by dividing the tumour count by the sum of the counts over the tumour, the lungs, and the liver, that is

$$\text{tumour index} = \frac{\text{tumour}}{\text{tumour} + \text{lung} + \text{liver}}$$

The value reported is a relative indicator of biodistribution and does not take into consideration either the total activity administered or any differences in counting geometries from dog to dog. However, when both the retention value and the tumour index are determined for a number of studies, they can serve as indicators of how the various routes of administration compare to one another with respect to the efficiency of drug carrier localization.

3. Results and discussion

3.1. Survival studies

3.1.1. Intravenous infusion of ^{99m}Tc-HAM

The results of the retrograde intravenous administration studies are shown in Table 1. Three dogs were given ^{99m}Tc-HAM while the tumour site was under the influence of the magnetic field. One dog (636-716) subsequently participated in a second study under this same protocol; the resultant data are treated as two independent studies since the elapsed time between the studies resulted in significant changes in the tumour and in tumour vascularity during that time. For these four studies, retention of the ^{99m}Tc-HAM at the target site after magnet shutdown ranged from 73 to 99%, and the tumour index (that is, the relative biodistribution) ranged from 0.40 to 0.86.

To determine the effect of the magnet on localization, ^{99m}Tc-HAM was administered to four dogs in the same manner as in the magnet studies, but without using magnetic localization. The tourniquet was released 30 minutes after ^{99m}Tc-HAM infusion, again as in the case of the magnet studies. The retention of ^{99m}Tc-HAM at the target site after the tourniquet was released ranged from 67 to 98% while the tumour index ranged from 0.49 to 0.96.

3.1.2. Intraarterial infusion of ^{99}Tc-HAM

Three separate modes of injection were examined in conjunction with the intraarterial studies, as shown in Table 2. In six dogs magnetic localization of microspheres infused over a 2-minute period was performed on nine separate occasions. The post-magnet retention of activity ranged from 84 to 97%, while the tumour index ranged from 0.05 to 0.91. In three cases the microspheres were administered over a period of 20 minutes to evaluate the hypothesis that slowing the rate of infusion would increase the relative amount of microspheres retained at the target site (tumour index).

TABLE 1

Retrograde intravenous administration of microspheres

Case No.	Percentage retention	Tumour index
A. Localization with magnet		
636-716	81	0.71
	99	0.86
637-827	73	0.51
638-075	92	0.40
B. Localization without magnet		
636-693	68	0.81
637-841	98	0.96
638-075	67	0.49
638-352	87	0.80

TABLE 2

Intraarterial administration of microspheres

Case No.	Percentage retention	Tumour index
A. Localization with magnet		
1. Injection time 2 minutes		
638-028	96	0.05
	89	0.64
638-219	94	0.16
637-430	87	0.57
	97	0.84
638-279	94	0.65
638-874	95	0.91
	84	0.86
639-083	93	0.56
2. Injection time 20 minutes		
637-790	97	0.68
637-839	93	0.88
637-942	94	–
3. Injection by infusion pump		
637-430	90	–
636-981	95	0.60
B. Localization without magnet		
636-864	32	–
	31	0.40
636-877	25	0.24
637-712	100	0.43
639-460	65	0.44

Post-magnet retention ranged from 93 to 97% while the tumour index, which was determined for two of the three dogs, was 0.68 for one dog and 0.88 for the other. In two separate studies, ^{99m}Tc-HAM was given with an infusion pump set to deliver 1 ml/minute. Retentions at the tumour site following magnet shutdown were 90 and 95%, respectively. The tumour index was obtained for only one study and was 0.60.

As a control for the intraarterial administration studies, four dogs were given ^{99}Tc-HAM without imposing a magnetic field over the tumour. One dog participated in this control study on two separate occasions. For this group of dogs, post-treatment retention of ^{99m}Tc-HAM ranged from 25 to 100%. The dog that exhibited the very high retention of ^{99m}Tc-HAM (637-712) was severely compromised in blood flow. This factor, compounded by an unusually large tumour volume and the resultant large dose of ^{99m}Tc-HAM, created an abnormal situation compared to other animals in the study. The tumour index for this group was lower than the tumour index seen with the magnet, ranging from 0.24 to 0.44.

3.1.3. Intramedullary infusion of ^{99}Tc-HAM

The third access route was the intramedullary route. By wrapping the tumour-bearing limb with an Esmarch bandage, a 3-inch wide strip of thin latex, it is possible practically to eliminate blood flow, either arterial or venous, in the limb. If a superficial vein is then accessed and the infusion is forced into the vessel, the infusion will traverse the vessel to the nearest joint space, where it will exit the vessel and, seeking the path of least resistance, enter the intramedullary space of the bone and exit the limb by traveling through the marrow space of the bone. This approach has been used in humans to treat osteomyelitis (Finsterbush and Weinberg, 1972), and the hypothesis was that it would be a better access route for tumours which arise from bone than the intraarterial or the retrograde venous routes, which tended to fill the more vascular soft tissue components of the tumour. Eight dogs were studied with this mode of access with magnetic localization in a total of ten separate experiments. The results are given in Table 3. Percentage retention of activity at the tumour site was somewhat less than seen by the intraarterial route, ranging from 48 to 96%. The tumour index was also somewhat lower, ranging from 0.07 to 0.70. Localization by the intramedullary route without magnetic guidance was quite similar to the data obtained with the magnet. Post-administration retention of the ^{99m}Tc-HAM ranged from 12 to 96%. The tumour index ranged from 0.27 to 0.49 and was very similar to that seen with magnetic localization.

3.2. Non-survival biodistribution studies

To determine the biodistribution of the ^{99m}Tc-HAM, non-survival studies were conducted in 12 dogs. One study was a normograde intravenous administration with no

TABLE 3

Intramedullary administration of microspheres

Case No.	Percentage retention	Tumour index
A. Localization with magnet		
638-790	96	0.19
639-000	84	0.50
638-945	48	0.07
	74	0.46
638-830	62	0.34
638-083	82	0.52
639-310	75	0.34
	92	0.59
639-506	–	0.70
639-730	79	0.53
B. Localization without magnet		
639-310	79	0.27
639-506	96	0.38
639-730	12	0.49

magnet and no tourniquet to confirm the normal distribution of the microspheres, eight were intraarterial studies with magnetic localization, and three were intramedullary administration studies with magnet. The results are given in Table 4. When ^{99m}Tc-HAM was administered intravenously without magnetic localization, the greatest concentrations of ^{99m}Tc-HAM were found in the lungs and in the liver. Lower concentrations were detected in the blood, the kidney and the spleen, while minimal levels were observed in the brain, the jejunum and the heart. Following either intraarterial or intramedullary administration with magnetic localization, the primary biodistribution of ^{99m}Tc-HAM outside the tumour was again to the lungs, liver, spleen, and kidneys. One dog (639-000) was killed while the tumour was still under magnetic influence. In this case, most of the ^{99m}Tc-HAM remained in the magnetic field and, as a result, minimal extra-tumoural biodistribution occurred.

In nine cases the tumours were examined for uniformity of ^{99m}Tc-HAM distribution Rectilinear or gamma camera images of radioactivity were made of tumour cross-sections. A typical example of ^{99m}Tc-HAM distribution in the tumour after intraarterial administration and magnetic localization is seen in Figure 1. The ^{99m}Tc-HAM localization, shown as darkened areas in the scan, was greatest near the pole tip of the magnet, in the soft tissue component of the tumour. Osseous regions of these cross-sections (those lighter regions in the center of the section) do not show the same concentration of ^{99m}Tc-HAM. A more striking illustration of this same effect is shown

TABLE 4

Biodistribution of magnetic microspheres

Case No.	% Injected dose per gram of tissue							
	Lung	Liver	Kidney	Spleen	Blood	Brain	Jejunum	Heart
1. Normograde intravenous administration, no magnetic localization								
639-474	0.25	0.04	0.03	0.02	0.03	0.002	0.006	0.008
2. Intraarterial administration, with magnetic localization								
636-864	0.08	0.01	0.002	0.004	0.002	0.0001	0.0004	0.001
637-823	0.02	0.02	0.02	0.01	0.01	0.0001	0.001	—
637-942	0.003	0.03	0.02	0.02	0.002	0.0004	0.002	0.001
638-075	0.04	0.02	0.003	0.02	0.004	0.0001	0.001	0.001
638-964	0.04	0.05	0.01	0.07	0.01	0.001	0.001	0.002
638-874	0.01	0.01	0.04	0.01	0.01	0.0002	0.002	0.002
639-083	0.01	0.01	0.02	0.01	0.005	0.0002	0.002	0.002
639-460	0.005	0.01	0.01	0,01	0.002	0.0001	0.008	0.001
3. Intramedullary administration, with magnetic localization								
638-876	0.05	0.06	0.02	0.02	0.01	0.001	0.004	0.003
639-000	0.0001	0.0001	0.0002	0.0001	0.00003	0.0002	0.00002	0.00002
626-964	0.03	0.01	0.02	0.01	0.003	0.0001	0.001	0.001

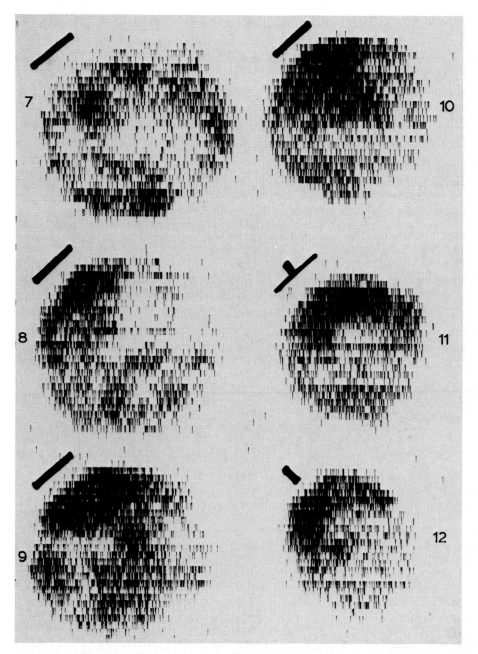

Figure 1. Rectilinear scan of a series of contiguous cross-sections through the tumour. Section 7 in this instance is the most distal cross-section and section 12 is the most proximal, with respect to the dog's leg. The external magnet placement over the tumour during magnetic localization is denoted by the black bar above the upper left quadrant of the cross-sectional scan. Section 11 was in contact with the proximal end of the magnet pole tip, while section 12 was proximal to the magnet position.

In Figure 2. This figure also shows tissue localization of ^{99m}Tc-HAM after intraarterial infusion and magnetic localization. In this study, only the periphery of the cross-sections demonstrate any ^{99m}Tc-HAM localization while the centre areas, which proved to be principally necrotic tissue, showed no uptake of ^{99m}Tc-HAM.

Intramedullary administration of ^{99m}Tc-HAM in conjunction with magnetic guid-

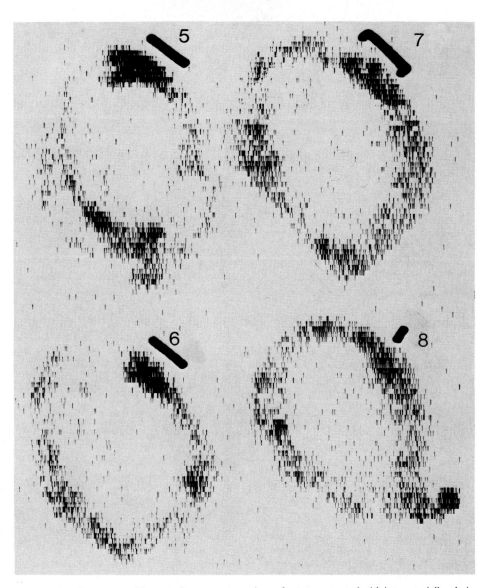

Figure 2. Rectilinear scan of four contiguous cross-sections of a tumour treated with intraarterially administered, magnetically localized ^{99m}Tc-HAM. The position of the externally positioned magnet is indicated by the black bar above the upper right hand quadrant of the scan. Section 7 shows the position of the proximal pole tip of the magnet, while section 8 was proximal to the magnet chisel tip.

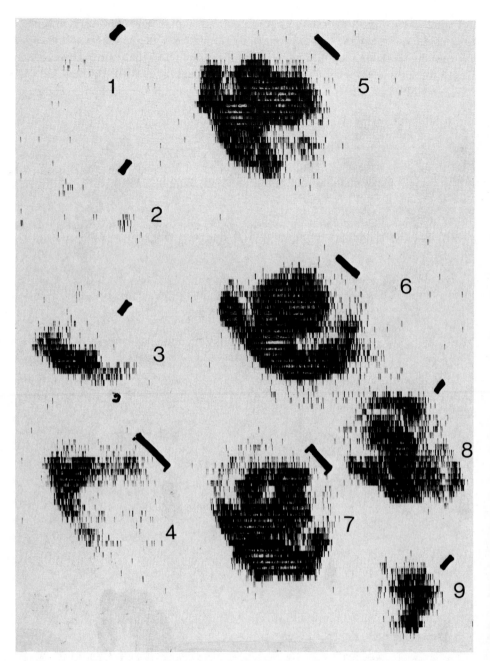

Figure 3. Rectilinear scan of the contiguous cross-sections of a tumour treated with ^{99m}Tc-HAM administered by the intramedullary access route and localized by magnetic guidance. Section 1 is the most proximal segment, and section 9 is the most distal segment. The external magnet placement is indicated by the black bar above the upper right quadrant. Sections 4–7 were in actual contact with the magnet pole tip.

ance greatly improved the localization of the ^{99m}Tc-HAM in the osseous portions of the tumour, as seen in Figure 3. This animal (639-000) was killed while the tumour was still under magnetic influence, and therefore represents the maximum magnetic effect on tumour localization. In animals that were killed subsequent to the removal of the magnetic influence, the localization was not as dramatic as seen in this particular case, but there was definite improved osseous localization of ^{99m}Tc-HAM compared to the intraarterial administration studies.

4. Conclusions

Biodistribution studies demonstrated that ^{99m}Tc-HAM accumulated in the tumour, lung, liver, spleen and kidneys; little activity was seen in the blood, brain, heart or jejunum. This indicates that the ^{99m}Tc remained in association with the human albumin microspheres rather than dissociating in vivo and distributing as the free pertechnetate. Unbound radioactivity would appear primarily in blood, gut and kidney. The biodistribution data obtained in this manner correlated well with the tumour index determinations in the survival studies, lending support to the tumour index as a relative indicator of tumour localization of microspheres.

For the eight antemortem studies in which ^{99m}Tc-HAM was administered by the retrograde intravenous route, no differences in tumour localization or retention of ^{99m}Tc-HAM could be discerned between the group that was infused with the tumour under magnetic influence and the group infused without the magnetic guidance of ^{99m}Tc-HAM.

The data from the dogs that were infused with ^{99m}Tc-HAM intraarterially demonstrated a definite improvement in tumour localization and retention of ^{99m}Tc-HAM when the tumour was under magnetic influence. From the rectilinear scans, it was evident that this localization was primarily in the well-perfused, soft tissue component of the tumour and not in either necrotic tissue or the osseous portions of the tumour. The mode of intraarterial infusion, that is, infusion pump as compared to bolus injection or 20-minute manual infusion, did not have any observable effect on tumour localization or retention of ^{99m}Tc-HAM.

The data from the intramedullary studies suggest that, as with the intravenous administration of ^{99m}Tc-HAM, the magnet is not particularly effective in increasing tumour retention of ^{99m}Tc-HAM. However, as seen in the rectilinear scans of the tumour cross-sections, this route of administration is effective in accessing the osseous portions of the tumour which are not accessible by the intraarterial route.

Acknowledgements

This work was supported by the Purdue Comparative Oncology Program, West Lafayette, IN, and by Eli Lilly and Company, Indianapolis, IN. The authors would like to express their appreciation to Mrs. Karen Klemme for typing the manuscript and to Dr. Wayne V. Kessler for his editorial comments.

References

Finsterbush, A. and Weinberg, H. (1972) J. Bone Joint Surg. 54, 1227–1234.

Owen, L.N. (1969) Bone Tumors in Man and Animals, Butterworths, London, pp. 29–52.

Senyei, A.E., Widder, K.J., and Czerlinski, G. (1978) J. Appl. Phys. 49, 3578–3583.

Senyei, A.E., Reich, S.D., Gonczy, C. and Widder, K.J. (1981) J. Pharm. Sci. 70, 389–391.

Sugibayashi, K., Okumura, M. and Morimoto, Y. (1982) Biomaterials 3, 181–186.

Widder, K.J., Senyei, A.E. and Scarpelli, D.G. (1978) Proc. Soc. Exp. Biol. Med. 58, 141–146.

Widder, K., Flouret, G. and Senyei, A. (1979a) J. Pharm. Sci. 68, 79–82.

Widder, K.J., Senyei, A.E. and Ranney, D.F. (1979b) in Advances in Pharmacology (Garattini, S., Goldin, A., Hawking, F., Kopin, J. and Schnitzer, R.J., Eds.), Vol. 16, pp. 213–271, Academic Press, New York.

Widder, K.J., Morris, R.M., Poore, G., Howard, D.P., Jr. and Senyei, A.E. (1981) Proc. Natl. Acad. Sci. U.S.A. 78, 579–581.

Microspheres and Drug Therapy. Pharmaceutical, Immunological and Medical Aspects
edited by S.S. Davis, L. Illum, J.G. McVie and E. Tomlinson
© 1984, Elsevier Science Publishers B.V.

CHAPTER 6

Crystallized carbohydrate spheres for slow release, drug targeting and cell separation

Ulf Schröder, Arne Ståhl and Leif G. Salford

1. Introduction

In order to avoid the problems of elimination, inactivation or low access to target areas, there is increasing interest in employing carrier systems for slow release and targeting of biologically active substances, such as drugs, thus avoiding frequent administrations, negative side effects and promoting higher concentrations in the target area.

Working with carrier systems for slow release and targeting, ideally the following criteria should be fulfilled before the possible use in humans (Langer and Peppas, 1981). The matrix should be: chemically inert in biological systems; biologically well-characterized; non-toxic and non-immunogenic; able to be eliminated from the body by normal routes; administered easily (i.e., by injection); capable of entrapment and release of biologically active substances of various molecular weights.

Traditionally, synthetic or semisynthetic polymers have been designed to be used as biodegradable matrix systems in agricultural as well as in veterinary and human medical areas. This kind of design involves covalent cross-linking of a polymer and often also a covalent attachment of the active substance to the matrix. However, covalently cross-linked biodegradable matrices are potentially harmful to organisms due to the possible production of toxic byproducts from the degrading matrix. Furthermore, the covalent attachment itself might introduce changes in the chemical structure of the substance, necessitating cumbersome and often expensive toxicological testing. In the area of slow-release preparations for low-molecular-weight substances there are a number of methods available (Langer, 1980). However, less progress has been made in finding a suitable system for proteins, peptides and other water-soluble substances, and it has been even more difficult to find a combination of targeting and slow release of biologically active substances.

In the work with proteins and their carrier systems, the proteins are normally coupled to the matrix by a covalent linkage, achieved after creation of reactive ligands on the matrix with subsequent attachment of the protein. Due to steric hindrance, all the reactive ligands will not react with the protein and are subsequently deactivated, normally by allowing ethanolamine or mercaptoethanol to be coupled to the reactive ligands. However, this substituted matrix may enhance the immunological system, creating antibodies against the coupled protein. On the other hand, carrying out the activation procedures on the protein surface creates hapten groups on the protein, with the possibility of antibody formation against the protein. Furthermore, it has been shown that low-molecular-weight dextran covalently attached to a protein is strongly immunogenic (Richter and Kågedal, 1972). All of these factors are equally unwanted if a slow-release system based on covalent coupling of autologous proteins is desired.

However, these factors are useful and desirable if a slow-release system for antigens is required, where the system is to be used for enhancement of the immunological response against a protein.

In this area, finding safer adjuvants with good effectiveness for the possible use in human vaccination, there have been extensive efforts during the last years due to the increasing number of specific antigens from various organisms (i.e., parasites) that have been produced with the help of the gene cloning technique. However, these antigens, despite having high specificity, often lack adequate immunogenicity. Consequently, there is presently a strong desire for adjuvants that could be used in humans. Adjuvants that have been tested include alumina and silica, mineral oils, vegetable oils, alginate, saponins and carotenoids, bacterial toxins and cell wall components. In some of the above systems the adjuvant effect is partly due to the sustained release of antigens from the matrix, i.e., mineral oil, alum and silica (Borek, 1979). The most popular adjuvants used in animals, i.e., Freund's, has not been considered safe in humans because of the long-term persistence of mineral oil in animals, the formation of disseminated focal granuloma, the induction of auto-immune reactions and the potentiation of plasma cell tumours in mice. Further, using aluminium hydroxide in vaccinations in humans, granulomas have been reported which might restrict their future use in humans to some extent (Slater et al., 1982).

With matrix systems giving slow release of active compound, it would also be desirable if the immunological response could be altered and/or enhanced with the help of different kinds of immunomodulators. Examples of such immunomodulators are DEAE- or sulphate-substituted dextrans where it has been shown that DEAE-dextran enhances the humoral antibody production, protecting animals against infection (Wittman et al., 1975). Dextran substituted with sulphate groups has, furthermore, an adjuvant effect on the T-cell-mediated immunological response (McCarthy et al., 1977).

In attempts to design 'magic bullets' for drug delivery, soluble and particulate carrier systems have been used. Examples of soluble carriers are the antibodies with attached drugs and the particulate system include all types of microspheres. The difficulties in avoiding uptake of the reticuloendothelial system is, however, a problem if the goal is to target microspheres, with their drug content, to other areas in the body. By co-entrapping magnetite in crystallized carbohydrate spheres this problem can be substantially reduced using arterial injection, with subsequent targeting of the magnetic spheres via external magnetic fields. The magnetic microspheres may also be used in magnetic cell separation, where affinity ligands are attached to the surface of the spheres, rendering a very efficient and simple separation method for use in immunology and cell biology.

This chapter describes a simple technique for the preparation of a slow-release bio-degradable matrix system, where drugs, proteins and magnetite particles are all entrapped in carbohydrate spheres stabilized by crystallization (Schröder, 1983a, 1983b; Schröder and Ståhl, 1983). The term crystallization is used in a broad sense, meaning that all chemical bonds apart from covalent bonds are used in the stabilization process (Fig. 1). However, the most important of these bonds are the hydrogen bonds, although the other weak bonds, such as Van der Waals forces and, in some circumstances, ionic bonds, are also involved.

2. Crystallized carbohydrate spheres (CCS) for slow release

Preparation of CCS with entrapped substances is as follows. An aqueous carbohydrate solution is thoroughly mixed with an aqueous solution of the substance to be entrapped. The substances are dissolved in their normal solvents, such as buffers, water, etc. An emulsifying medium (corn, rape seed or cottonseed oil) is added, and a coarse pre-emulsion formed by magnetic stirring. The pre-emulsion is further homogenized by probe sonication for 40 seconds while cooling on an icebath or by

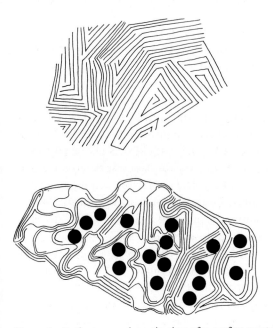

Figure 1. At the top a schematic view of a perfect crystalline polymer matrix, where the polymers are attached to each other via noncovalent bonds, such as hydrogen bonds, Van der Waals forces or, in some cases, ionic bonds. At the bottom a schematic view of a partially crystalline structure where drugs, proteins or magnetite are entrapped into the matrix.

high-pressure homogenization. The microdroplet emulsion is then slowly poured into acetone, containing 0.1% (w/v) Tween 80, while stirring at 1000 rpm. The carbohydrate spheres precipitate, and are then washed by centrifugation with 4×50 ml of 0.1% Tween 80-acetone and finally suspended in 2 ml 1% Tween-acetone, whereupon they are allowed to dry at room temperature. If sterile CCS are required, the last wash and the drying are performed under sterile conditions.

The highest concentration of the carbohydrate that can be used is determined by the increasing viscosity of the solutions, making them difficult to disperse in the emulsifying medium. This concentration corresponds to approximately 50% (w/v) for dextran T500, 100% for dextran T10 and the dextrin Awedex W90. Glucose, sucrose, maltose and other low-molecular-weight carbohydrates can be used up to concentrations of about 250% (w/v). At the lowest concentration, which is about one tenth of the above-mentioned, the CCS are rapidly redissolved when suspended in water.

The carbohydrates preferentially used are the dextrans (because of their well known and well documented use as plasma volume expanders) and the dextrins, i.e., acid-hydrolized starch (because of their biocompatability and biodegradability). Homogenization can be achieved by either probe sonication or high-pressure homogenization. Due to its simplicity and high reproducibility, high-pressure homogenization is the method of choice, especially when larger amounts of entrapped material are required. Another advantage of the method is the possibility of making CCS of various sizes and/or by a recycling procedure creating very narrow size-distributions.

2.1. Assay of the biological activity of the entrapped proteins

When making CCS from a 20% dextran T10, these CCS are rapidly dissolved when suspended in water, thus making determination of the biological activity of the proteins after entrapment and subsequent dissolution possible. Insulin was allowed to stimulate adipocytes to incorporate [^{3}H]glucose, and the production of ^{3}H-labelled fatty acids was determined by liquid scintillation (Moody et al., 1974). The anti-viral effect of interferon was assayed in a plaque-assay (Campbell et al., 1975). Plasmin was analysed using the substrate H-D-Val-Leu-Lys-pNA (S-2251, Kabi Diagnostika, Stockholm, Sweden) (Friberger et al., 1978). Beta-galactosidase was determined with the substrate ONPG (Sigma) (Craven et al., 1965). The monoclonal antibody against phytohaemagglutinin (PHA) was determined in an ELISA technique, using peroxidase-labelled anti-mouse IgG as second antibody and ABTS (Sigma A-1888) as chromogene and H_2O_2 as substrate to the enzyme (Engvall et al., 1971).

When the biological activity of the protein insulin, the enzymatic activity of the enzymes plasmin and beta-galactosidase or the binding capacity of the monoclonal antibody were assayed, they all retained approximately 70% of their activity as compared to the activity added for entrapment. Furthermore, when radioactively labelled insulin or human serum albumin (HSA) were entrapped, 70% of the added radioactivity was found to be entrapped within the spheres, implying that all of the proteins entrapped retained their biological activity.

Using dextran as the matrix and the vegetable oils as emulsifying systems, hydrophobic proteins were normally entrapped with a lower yield. This was seen with interferon, human growth hormone and myoglobin, where only about 20–40% of the protein was found to be entrapped. However, using the dextrin Awedex W90 as matrix and 0.1% of the emulgator Gafac PE-410 in the oil, the entrapment efficiency could be increased. Furthermore, no significant difficulties were seen in the preparation of the spheres whether the final protein content was 0.2 or 35% (dry weight) (as tested with a 30% solution of dextran T500 and ovalbumin).

2.2. Release studies

Crystallized dextran spheres, made from a 50% solution of dextran T40, suspended in water, withstand complete erosion over a period of more than 8 months at room temperature. When testing for in vitro release of radioactively labelled proteins in phosphate-buffered saline containing 1% HSA, 50% release was achieved in 15 days for human growth hormone, 8 days for HSA and myoglobin and for insulin a 50% release was obtained in about 4 days (Fig. 2). In the use of the dextrins as matrix material for the CCS, one would anticipate that the amount of α-amylase would influence the release rate. However, no such influence could be detected, even at enzyme concentrations that were 10,000 times higher than in human blood serum. The initial burst effect that is seen during the first 24 hours is probably due to the spheroid shape of the matrix, giving a high surface area.

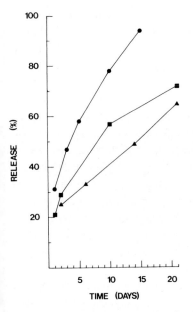

Figure 2. Release of entrapped insulin (●), HSA and myoglobin (■) and biosynthetic human growth hormone (▲) in phosphate-buffered saline containing 1% HSA at room temperature. 100 mg CCS contained 1 mg of insulin, 40 mg of HSA, 4 mg of myoglobin and 2 mg of biosynthetic human growth hormone, respectively. The insulin, HSA and myoglobin were entrapped in dextran T500 and the growth hormone was entrapped in the dextrin.

In these studies, no significant variations in the release rate were seen at the different levels of entrapment.

2.3. Assay of the immunological response to entrapped antigens

In the immunization studies (Schröder and Ståhl, 1983), groups of five mice were used, and each mouse was injected at a single site, subcutaneously above the left hind leg. Blood samples were taken from the tail and analysis of the antibody response was performed with serial duplicate dilutions of the samples with an ELISA technique using the same method as above when analysing PHA in the slow release experiments. Ovalbumin was chosen as a model antigen, and entrapped into dextran spheres. The mice receiving single subcutaneous injection of 80 μg of ovalbumin entrapped in dextran spheres had, after about 1 month, a peak in their antibody concentration, which then declined slowly to a level comparable to the highest level obtained in the mice that received 80 μg of the antigen dissolved in water. When injecting the ovalbumin dissolved in water together with a 5% solution of the dextran, no enhancement of the IgG-antibody level (as compared to water) could be detected.

As anticipated, co-entrapment of DEAE- or sulphate-dextran gave an even better enhancement of the IgG level as compared to using CCS made of non-substituted dextrans. When injecting the antigen and the substituted dextran in soluble form, the antibody response was again at a considerably lower level compared to the CCS formulations (Fig. 3).

Using bee venom entrapped in the CCS, compared with the mice that received the antigen dissolved in water, the CCS preparation of antigen was shown to enhance the IgG level to approximately that found with ovalbumin, suggesting about the same enhancement as with ovalbumin. When injecting 80 μg of the antigen dissolved in water, with subsequent administration of the same dose 2 weeks later, the IgG level reached the same level, a further 2 weeks later, as was achieved with a single injection of 8 μg entrapped in the CCS assayed 4 weeks after injection. Injecting 400 μg of bee venom entrapped in CCS (which is four times the LD_{50} in mice), the IgG response increased rapidly. For comparison, results from mice injected with 80 μg bee venom suspended in Freund's Complete Adjuvant (FCA) are shown in Figure 4. No mouse receiving the CCS-bee venom preparation, in this high dose group, showed any visible side reactions, i.e., inflammatory response or necrosis at the injection site, as compared to the mice receiving the bee venom in FCA, which had to be terminated after 8 weeks. This might imply the possibility of using CCS preparations when injecting high doses of toxic antigens without producing an escalation in toxic side reactions, and at the same time achieving a high antibody response.

When the antigens from schistosomiasis adult worm were entrapped in CCS and subsequently injected, the antibody response was of the same magnitude as for ovalbumin.

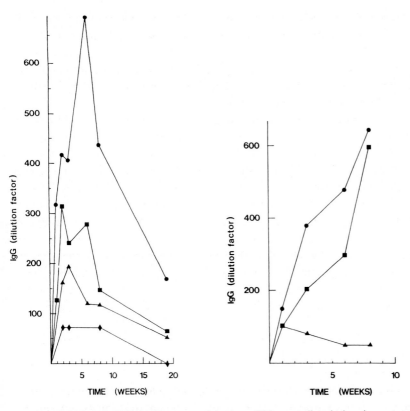

Figure 3. IgG response after subcutaneous injection of 80 μg ovalbumin in mice, entrapped in dextran spheres where 65% of the dextran was sulphate dextran (●), entrapped in dextran spheres where 35% of the dextran was DEAE-dextran (■), entrapped in dextran spheres of unsubstituted dextran (▲), and dissolved in water (◆).

Figure 4. IgG response after subcutaneous injection of 80 μg bee venom dissolved in water (▲), 80 μg suspended in Freund's complete adjuvant (■) and 400 μg entrapped in dextran spheres (●).

3. Magnetic microspheres for drug targeting

When preparing magnetic dextran spheres, the dextran is dissolved in Ferrofluid EMG 805 HGMS at 70°C for 1 hour. Instead of the dextran, it is also possible to use glucose, maltose or dextrins or any other carbohydrate that might be of special interest. To the Ferrofluid-carbohydrate suspension a solution of the drug is added and the mixture emulsified with the probe sonicator for 35 seconds in an emulsifying medium consisting of 25 ml of vegetable oil, 1.25 g Gafac PE-510 and 5 ml of chloroform. The carbohydrates are stabilized and washed as described above.

Radioactively labelled magnetically responsive microspheres have been used in a series of experiments on rats exposed to magnetic fields of 0.8–1.4 T produced by a bipolar magnet. A suspension of the microspheres was injected either intraarterially or intravenously while a selected part of the body was exposed to the magnetic field. With the goal of holding the magnetic spheres in the selected area, it is of utmost importance to utilize the gradient of the field. This can lead to arrest of the microspheres in the temporal muscle of the rats after intravenous injection and, after intraarterial injection, in the rat tail, with the highest concentration of microspheres in the segments closest to the edges of magnet.

In the brain tumour laboratory in Lund, major efforts have been directed towards the use of magnetically responsive microspheres for brain tumours. By intraarterial injection into the internal carotid artery, the microspheres can be arrested in a part of one hemisphere of the brain. Using radioactively labelled microspheres it has been proven that the spheres can be concentrated in the brain 100-fold compared to spheres studied without a magnetic field. The microspheres are held in the smallest vessels. Therefore, it is of importance that the microspheres are homogenous in size, having a diameter of 1 μm, allowing continuous blood circulation while the microspheres leak their content of appropriate therapeutic agents into the surrounding tissue. The fact that the magnetically responsive microspheres can be held in a highly vascularized tissue such as the brain gives promise for the future use of the method in both tumours and other tissues in any part of the body.

4. Magnetic microspheres for cell separation

The preparation of spheres for cell separation is the same as for the spheres used for drug targeting; however, in order to attach an affinity ligand to the magnetic spheres, an activation step is performed using tresylchloride (Nilsson, et al., 1981), creating reactive ligands on the surface of the spheres. These activated magnetic spheres are stable for at least 6 months when stored at room temperature.

The main benefits of the tresylchloride method are that the activation, which has to be carried out in water-free acetone, is largely a part of the normal washing procedure in the preparation of magnetic spheres. Secondly, the coupling of the affinity ligand (i.e., protein) is performed in 10–15 minutes at room temperature, a timing which is in contrast to most other coupling procedures.

To stabilize the magnetic spheres, 1,6-diaminohexane is added and internal cross-linking of the spheres carried out for a further 5 minutes. The spheres are washed and then used for cell magnetic separation. As a model, peripheral human lymphocytes and mouse monoclonal antibodies against T-suppressor (OKT8) and T-helper (OKT4) cells have been used. A rabbit anti-mouse antibody was covalently coupled to the surface of the magnetic spheres and the lymphocytes were incubated with the monoclonal antibodies. After washing away excess antibody, the magnetic spheres were incubated with the lymphocytes and then subjected to separation in a continuous flow system above a magnet. Cells were then analysed using a Fluorescein Activated Cell Sorter (FACS). Results indicate that the magnetic separation of cells could deplete the cell population of a specific cell type to a value below the detection limit of the FACS ($< 0.5\%$) and lead to a non-specific adsorption also below the detection limit of the FACS (Schröder and Borrebaeck, 1983).

5. Summary

Described in this chapter is a method for the preparation of a matrix for entrapment of substances, which when released retain their biological activities, and where the matrix materials are well known carbohydrates with documented low toxicity in human as well as in the veterinary medical fields. With co-entrapment of magnetic material it is also possible to use the spheres for magnetic drug targeting as well as cell magnetic separation. The method of manufacture using a high-pressure homogenization technique is easily scaled up to produce large amounts.

Release of the entrapped substances most probably occurs via erosion of the matrix, rendering unmodified products. A further advantage of this approach is that there is no enzymatic degradation of the matrix influencing the release, since the parameters capable of breaking the hydrogen bonds stabilizing the crystallized structure are mainly pH and ionic strength, both of which are stable in the human body.

Acknowledgements

This work was partially supported by the Swedish Board for Technical Development (83-4403) and the Swedish Cancer Society (83-211).

References

Borek F. (1979) in The Antigens, Vol. IV, (Sela, M., Ed.), pp. 369–428, Academic Press, New York.
Campbell J.B., Kochman M.A. and White S.L. (1975) Can. J. Microbiol. 21, 1247–1253.
Craven G.R., Steers, E.Jr. and Anfinsen C.B. (1965) J. Biol. Chem. 240, 2486.
Engvall E. and Perlman P. (1971) Immunochemistry 8, 871.
Friberger P., Knös M., Gustavsson S., Aurell L. and Claesson G. (1978) Haemostasis 7, 138–145.
Langer R.S. (1980) Chem. Eng. Comm. 6, 1–48.
Langer R.S. and Peppas, N.A. (1981) Biomaterials 2, 201–214.
McCarthy R.E., Arnold L.W. and Babcock G.F. (1977) Immunology 32, 963–974.
Moody, A.J., Stan M.A., Stan M. and Glieman (1974) J. Horm. Metab. Res. 6, 12–16.
Nilsson K. and Mosbach K. (1981) Biochem. Biophys. Res. Comm. 102, 449–457.
Richter W. and Kågedahl L. (1972) Int. Arch. Allergy 42, 887–904.
Schröder U. (1983a) PCT/SE83/00268.
Schröder U. (1983b) Biomaterials, in press.
Schröder U. and Ståhl A. (1983) J. Immunol. Methods, in press.
Schröder U. and Borrebaeck C.A.K. (1983) PCT/SE83/00106.
Slater D.N., Underwood J.C.E., Durrant T.E., Hopper T. and Hopper I.P. (1982) Br. J. Dermatol. 107, 103–108.
Wittman, G., Dietzschold B. and Bauer K. (1975) Arch. Virol. 47, 225–235.

Microspheres and Drug Therapy. Pharmaceutical, Immunological and Medical Aspects
edited by S.S. Davis, L. Illum, J.G. McVie and E. Tomlinson
© *1984, Elsevier Science Publishers B.V.*

CHAPTER 7

Methods of vascular access for delivery of microspheres to distal extremity tumors in dogs — A large animal model

G.S. Elliott, W.E. Blevins, R.C. Richardson, W. Janas, J.M. Bartlett, J.R. Hale and R.L. Silver

Angiography by three routes was used to evaluate spontaneous distal extremity tumors in dogs prior to infusion of 1–3-μm diameter human albumin microspheres containing magnetite (Fe_3O_4). The purpose of the study was to determine the usefulness of the dog as a large animal model of human disease for targeted drug delivery. To date, perfusion studies of (1) the normal limb, (2) hemangiopericytoma (a soft tissue sarcoma) and (3) osteogenic sarcoma have been conducted in 40 dogs.

Intravenous access under short-term tourniqueted conditions demonstrated venous-arterial shunting through both osseous and extra-osseous tumors; however, it demonstrated preferential filling of superficial large diameter non-tumor vasculature as compared to tumor vasculature and precluded visualization of the extent of tumor filling. This technique was the most simple to perform.

Intraarterial injection was accomplished by catheterization of the brachial artery or the femoral artery of the affected limb. It demonstrated the most uniform perfusion of extra-osseous tumor; however, osseous vasculature was inconsistently perfused. This technique was also simple to perform but required fluoroscopic control for proper catheter placement.

Intramedullary access to primary bone tumors was accomplished by venous catheterization distal to the tumor and pressure injection under whole-limb (Esmarch) tourniquet, thereby forcing the injected material into deep (intramedullary) vascular channels rather than the normal superficial venous system. When massive overlying extra-osseous tumor or normal soft tissue prevented complete occlusion of the superficial limb vasculature by the Esmarch tourniquet, distribution was superficial, as in the intravenous technique. This technique demonstrated the best delivery route for osseous tumors. It was usually not difficult to perform; however, vascular access was not possible in cases where the tumor had caused distal limb edema.

These studies precisely predicted microsphere delivery and localization. Extraosseous tumors of the distal extremity were best perfused by the intraarterial technique. Osseous tumors of the distal extremities were best perfused by the intramedullary technique. Primary bone tumors with a significant soft tissue component required a combined intraarterial and intramedullary technique to access the entire tumor.

As a large animal model, angiography of spontaneous distal extremity tumors in the dog demonstrated individual differences in tumor vascularity which may be present in humans. Tumor size and tumor/limb relationships approximated those of man. Dog size allowed angiography and sphere delivery techniques to approximate those of man. Correlation with microsphere deposition suggested that appropriate angiography should preceed attempts to deliver magnetic microspheres if they are to be used in targeted drug delivery.

Microspheres and Drug Therapy. Pharmaceutical, Immunological and Medical Aspects
edited by S.S. Davis, L. Illum, J.G. McVie and E. Tomlinson
© *1984, Elsevier Science Publishers B.V.*

CHAPTER 8

Selective targeting of magnetic albumin microspheres containing vindesine sulfate: Total remission in Yoshida sarcoma-bearing rats

R.M. Morris, G.A. Poore, D.P. Howard and J.A. Sefranka

Magnetically responsive microspheres containing 70% albumin, 20% magnetite and 10% vindesine sulfate were prepared by an emulsion polymerization process utilizing ultra-shear mixing to achieve a 1-μm sphere diameter. The spheres were selectively localized in Yoshida sarcoma tumors implanted subcutaneously in the tail of female Holtzman rats. The tumors were allowed to grow to at least 450 mm^2 before initiation of experimental treatment.

Drug-bearing magnetic microspheres at a dose level of 0.5 or 2.5 mg/kg were infused proximal to the tumor via the ventral caudal artery. A bipolar permanent magnet was placed such that both poles were adjacent to the tumor for 30 minutes during and post-infusion to effect localization. Other groups of animals (10 rats/group) received either 0.5 or 2.5 mg/kg of free vindesine sulfate or drug-bearing microspheres without utilization of the magnet. An untreated control group was also monitored.

Of the 20 animals receiving magnetically localized vindesine, 85% had total remission of the tumor. The remaining animals demonstrated marked tumor regression translating to an overall 95% regression rate with only one death and no evidence of distant metastases. No significant differences were noted in remission/regression results between the 0.5 and 2.5 mg/kg dose when both were magnetically localized.

In contrast, untreated animals as well as those receiving either free vindesine or non-localized vindesine spheres exhibited tumor growth, with widespread distant metastases and subsequent death in the majority of the animals. It was also noted that the group of animals receiving 2.5 mg/kg of free vindesine died within 72 hours of dosing, due to the overt toxicity of the drug; however, animals receiving the same dose as non-localized microspheres suffered no apparent acute toxicological problems. However, even with this high dose, non-targeted treatment of the tumor was ineffective.

The study illustrates, in a simple animal model, the potential to enhance the activity of oncolytic agents by magnetically concentrating the drug within the tumor. Additionally, the lower dose utilized for magnetic delivery should minimize side effects.

Microspheres and Drug Therapy. Pharmaceutical, Immunological and Medical Aspects
edited by S.S. Davis, L. Illum, J.G. McVie and E. Tomlinson

CHAPTER 9

Agarose-polyaldehyde microsphere beads and their use for specific removal of unwanted materials by haemoperfusion

S. Margel

The development and properties of a novel adsorbent system consisting of polyacrolein or polyglutaraldehyde microspheres encapsulated in agarose matrix will be described. The microspheres contain aldehyde groups through which various amino ligands, e.g., drugs, proteins, antibodies and enzymes, can be covalently bound in a single step under physiological pH. In a model system bovine serum albumin (BSA) was bound to the beads and the conjugates were used in vitro and in vivo for the removal of a specific antibody-anti-BSA. The immuno beads were found to be very efficient. Thus, relatively short periods of haemoperfusion are needed for quantitative removal of anti-BSA. The beads are biocompatible; there are negligible decreases in red blood cells, an up to 10% decrease in white blood cells and an up to 15% decline in platelets.

Microspheres and Drug Therapy. Pharmaceutical, Immunological and Medical Aspects
edited by S.S. Davis, L. Illum, J.G. McVie and E. Tomlinson
© *1984, Elsevier Science Publishers B.V.*

Immuno-isolation of organelles using magnetic beads — Binding properties with antibodies

K. Howell, W. Ansorge and J. Grünberg

Microspheres with specific antibodies bound offer promising new approaches and developments not only in drug therapy (targeting) but also in cell biology (specific isolation procedures). In both cases, it is critical to prepare an immunobead of high specificity.

We have established an immuno-isolation system for organelles using magnetic beads since recent advances in the understanding of membrane traffic in cells require procedures for the isolation of subcellular compartments on the basis of the distribution of exposed antigens rather than density (conventional fractionation). In order to determine and quantitate precisely the various parameters involved in the immunoadsorption step, a simple antibody/antigen model was used: isolation of the vesicular stomatitis virus (VSV) from a suspension of high concentrations (10 × excess or more) of various subcellular fractions. Optimization of the system resulted in three major advantages over conventional procedures: high yield (specific immuno-binding); reduced contamination (non-specific binding); and minimal damage to the bound materials.

The high specific binding is obtained by optimizing each step individually in the production of the immunoadsorbant (a solid support + a linker molecule + a specific antibody). The 3-μm monodisperse, magnetic beads described by Ugelstad et al. (1983) are used as the solid support. The linker molecule, affinity purified sheep antibody against the Fc fragment of either rabbit or mouse IgG, is hydrophobically adsorbed on the beads and retains its activity to immuno-bind the specific antibody. Use of antibody against the Fc regions as the linker provides orientation of the specific antibody, so that all of the antigen-binding sites are available. The remaining hydrophobic sites are quenched in 5 mg/ml bovine serum albumin before immuno-binding of the specific antibody, which was either affinity purified rabbit polyclonal or mouse monoclonal against the viral surface protein, G.

Reduced non-specific binding is achieved by using a 'free flow' technique, where the beads are maintained in a dilute suspension throughout the isolation and subsequent washings. After the binding step the glass chamber (magnetic bottle) containing the suspension of immunoadsorbant is placed at 4°C in the magnetic field generated by a solenoid ($B = 0.1$ T). This allows the washing solutions to flow freely through the magnetic bottle, while the immunoadsorbant plus bound materials is contained. In addition, this procedure prevents damage to the bound vesicles when subcellular compartments are being isolated, since the need to pellet and resuspend the immunoadsorbant is eliminated. Such a process causes the organelles to break and reseal into small vesicles, significantly reducing the recovery.

Under the best conditions, 1 mg of immunoadsorbant with 4 μg of specific antibody bound, resulted in the isolation of 50 μg of VSV from 100 μg input fraction. The experiment was done in the presence of high concentrations of various subcellular fractions used to assess the non-specific binding, which remained less than 1%. Morphological evaluation at the electron microscopic level showed a uniform single layer binding of the VSV to the surface of the beads with approximately 50% of the bead surface occupied.

Reference

Ugelstad, J., Söderberg, L., Berge, A. and Bergström, J. (1983) Nature 303, 95–96.

Subject index

Note, The original terms used by the authors to describe (variously) microparticles, microspheres, nanoparticles and particles, have been used in compiling this index.